STP 1403

Environmental Toxicology and Risk Assessment: Science, Policy, and Standardization—Implications for Environmental Decisions: Tenth Volume

B. M. Greenberg, R. N. Hull, M. H. Roberts, Jr., and R. W. Gensemer, editors

ASTM Stock Number: STP1403

ASTM
100 Barr Harbor Drive
PO Box C700
West Conshohocken, PA 19428-2959

Printed in the U.S.A.

ISBN: 0-8031-2886-X
ISSN: 1071-720X

Peer Review Policy

Each paper published in this volume was evaluated by two peer reviewers and at least one editor. The authors addressed all of the reviewers' comments to the satisfaction of both the technical editor(s) and the ASTM Committee on Publications.

To make technical information available as quickly as possible, the peer-reviewed papers in this publication were prepared "camera-ready" as submitted by the authors.

The quality of the papers in this publication reflects not only the obvious efforts of the authors and the technical editor(s), but also the work of the peer reviewers. In keeping with long-standing publication practices, ASTM maintains the anonymity of the peer reviewers. The ASTM Committee on Publications acknowledges with appreciation their dedication and contribution of time and effort on behalf of ASTM.

Printed in Chelsea, MI
April 2001

Foreword

This publication, *Environmental Toxicology and Risk Assessment: Science, Policy, and Standardization—Implications for Environmental Decisions: Tenth Volume,* contains papers presented at the symposium of the same name held in Toronto, Ontario, Canada, on 10-12 April 2000. The symposium was sponsored by ASTM Committee E47 on Biological Effects and Environmental Fate. The symposium co-chairpersons were Dr. Bruce M. Greenberg, University of Waterloo, Ruth N. Hull, Cantox Environmental, Inc., Morris H. Roberts, Jr., Virginia Institute of Marine Science College of William and Mary, and Robert W. Gensemer, ENSR Corporation.

Contents

ASTM STANDARDS AND THEIR APPLICATIONS

BIOMONITORING OF SEDIMENTS AND AQUATIC SYSTEMS

CURRENT ISSUES IN SOIL TOXICITY AND REMEDIATION

Overview

The Tenth Symposium on Environmental Toxicology and Risk Assessment was held April 10-12, 2000 in Toronto, Ontario, Canada. This conference was the 27th symposium addressing the area of environmental toxicology that has been sponsored by ASTM Committee E47 on Biological Effects and Environmental Fate. Because of the advances in the field of environmental toxicology over the past decade, we felt it was an appropriate time to look beyond science, and thus chose the theme "Science, Policy, and Standardization—Implications for Environmental Decisions" for the symposium. This Special Technical Publication (STP) contains 26 peer-reviewed papers from the symposium. There are papers from each of the seven platform sessions and the two poster sessions. They cover the major topics of environmental toxicology (e.g., aquatic, sediment, terrestrial, and biomonitoring) and they cover the specialty topics of the symposium (environmental science, policy, and standards). The authors also represent a cross-section of the community of environmental toxicology and risk assessment, including scientists from academia, government, and the private sector.

The symposium theme, "Science, Policy, and Standardization—Implications for Environmental Decisions," was chosen to focus on a key aspect of the mission of committee E47 of ASTM. That mission is to develop standards that can be used by the environmental science community to collect coherent data and apply that data to make scientifically sound decisions. The background for this theme was elegantly established in the Plenary Session by presentations on risk evaluation, human health, generation of policy for large multi-jurisdictional environments, and the impacts of environmental policy on Native communities. This led to lively discussions throughout the symposium on problems of carrying scientific findings forward to sound policy decisions.

The firsr two platform sessions were "Aquatic Toxicology" and "Interface Between Policy, Science and Risk Assessment." Aquatic toxicology is one of the most active areas of environmental science, and is central to committee E47. It brings together many topics, and these were represented by the contributions to that session. There are three chapters from that session reflecting that diversity. The paper by Welsh et al. addresses the ionic composition of water used in toxicity tests and how that impacts on metal toxicity. The chapter by Schirmer et al. examines how modified PAHs impact on EROD levels, extending this important test to a novel class of compounds. The paper by Marwood et al. examines how UV radiation in natural aquatic settings impacts on photosynthesis in phytoplankton. In addition, there was one chapter from the poster session related to the aquatic toxicology session; Heyer et al. on the toxicity of chlorinated compounds to crawfish.

The session on the interface between science and policy dealt with the theme of the symposium. From that session, there were three chapters contributed to this STP. Sigal et al. address the question of using appropriate data in environmental modeling, which must be understood if risk assessment is to have real meaning. This topic is continued with statistical procedures to find real risk drivers (Tchounwou et al.), and a chapter from the poster session on statistical evaluation of terrestrial non-target organisms (Habig et al.). The subject then shifts to a comparison of fish and human toxicity by Tchounwou et al.

The next platform session was "ASTM Standards and Their Applications." This was central to the symposium, as it dealt with how ASTM standards can be used in science and policy. There were three chapters contributed to this volume from that session. The first, by Smrchek and Zeeman, deals with interagency harmonization of test methods. The other two chapters are on proper selection of plant toxicity test methods (Petrie, and Stephenson et al.).

The next two platform sessions were "Biomonitoring of Sediments and Aquatic Systems" and "Current Issues in Soil Toxicity and Remediation." Biomonitoring is central to the standardization process, as most standards in E47 begin as biomonitor assays that ultimately become well enough established such that a standard method can be generated. Two chapters were contributed from this session. The paper by El-Alawi et al. describes an extension of the Microtox assay, allowing photobacteria to be used in long term assays. The paper by Neff et al. deals with assessing PAH bioavailability at off-shore oil wells. In addition, two chapters from the poster session on biomonitoring are included. The paper by Diener et al. presents a new, powerful molecular bioindicator (differential display polymerase chain reaction) that is coming into use by environmental biologists. The paper by Lee et al. is a comparison of EROD and fibronectin levels.

The soil toxicity and remediation session recognizes on the one hand how important the evaluation of soil toxicity is becoming, and on the other hand how such contaminated sites can be cleaned for reuse. Chapters were contributed in both areas. Soil toxicity is examined by Boyd and Williams, and by Stephenson et al. Contributions by Wells and Lanno, and Huang et al. are on bioavailability of contaminants in soil and their remediation, respectively.

The last two platform sessions were "Hazards of Sediments and Sediment Derived Materials" and "New Directions in Environmental Assessment and Recovery." Sediment toxicology is an important theme for committee E47 of ASTM. There was one chapter from this session. In it Lampi et al. show how contaminant hazards in sediments can be elevated by structural modification after chemical deposition into the environment.

The goal of the session on new directions in environmental assessment and recovery was to bring many of the concepts of the symposium together. The idea was to consider how one uses environmental assessment data to make decisions on risk and restoration. The paper from the session chair (Landis and McLaughlin) sets the stage by discussing if recovery is even a appropriate concept for environmental science. The paper by Sunahara looks at an emerging problem for reuse of military bases: the toxic hazards of residue explosive substances. Babu et al. presents material on the toxicity of co-contaminants, showing a mechanism for synergistic toxicity of metals and PAHs. Lee et al. assess the success of a remediation project using three biological endpoints. Lastly, Dudal and Deschénes examine how bioavailability of contaminants changes in dynamic systems.

The papers of this volume give an excellent cross section of the topics presented at the symposium. They show the diversity of the field of environmental toxicology and risk assessment, and indicate many of the new directions being taken in the environmental sciences. Many of the chapters presented are likely to become the foci of future ASTM standards. This shows how ASTM symposia and STPs are critical steps in spearheading standards for ecotoxicology.

We gratefully acknowledge the efforts of the session chairs for developing the stimulating and comprehensive platform and poster sessions, and for encouraging the preparation of manuscripts provided in this volume. We are deeply indebted to ASTM staff, who worked tirelessly to bring the symposium and this volume to fruition. They are Dorothy Fitzpatrick and Hannah Sparks in symposium operations, Eileen Gambetta in publications, and the committee E47 staff manager Len Morrissey. We also thank the executive committee of E47 for their strong support and input on the symposium.

Bruce M. Greenberg
Department of Biology
University of Waterloo
Waterloo, Ontario, Canada.

Ruth N. Hull
Cantox Environmental Inc.
Mississauga, Ontario, Canada.

Morris H. Roberts, Jr.
Virginia Institute of Marine Sciences
College of William and Mary
Glaucester Point, VA.

Robert W. Gensemer
ENSR Corporation
Fort Collins, CO.

AQUATIC TOXICOLOGY

Paul G. Welsh,[1] Gary A. Chapman,[2] James A. Hansen,[1] and Joshua Lipton[1]

Importance of Ionic Composition of Reconstituted Laboratory Test Water in Interpreting Metal Toxicity Test Results

---

Reference: Welsh, P. G., Chapman, G. A., Hansen, J. A., and Lipton, J., "**Importance of Ionic Composition of Reconstituted Laboratory Test Water in Interpreting Metal Toxicity Test Results**," *Environmental Toxicology and Risk Assessment: Science, Policy, and Standardization — Implications for Environmental Decisions: Tenth Volume, ASTM STP 1403*, B. M. Greenberg, R. N. Hull, M. H. Roberts, Jr., and R. W. Gensemer, Eds., American Society for Testing and Materials, West Conshohocken, PA, 2001.

Abstract: We compare the ionic composition of ASTM reconstituted water with surface waters of the United States. The relative concentrations of major cations in surface waters are variable: Ca:Mg molar ratios range from 0.3 to 12.9, and Na:K molar ratios range from 1.4 to 600. However, the relative concentrations of these cations in ASTM reconstituted water are constant: the Ca:Mg molar ratio is 0.7 and the Na:K molar ratio is 21.3. Recent research has demonstrated that Ca is more important than Mg in modifying metal toxicity to salmonids. Hence, differences in the relative concentrations of these cations between surface waters and ASTM reconstituted waters may bias metal toxicity results. We also evaluate the potential for Na to modify Cu toxicity in salmonids. Sodium concentrations as high as 32.5 mg/L did not influence Cu toxicity. These results indicate that ASTM reconstituted water may not be appropriate for metal toxicity tests.

Keywords: reconstituted water, calcium, magnesium, sodium, copper toxicity, metals.

Introduction

A specific freshwater reconstituted laboratory water, first recommended by Marking and Dawson (1973), has been adopted by the U.S. Environmental Protection Agency (U.S. EPA 1993) and the American Society for Testing and Materials (Standard Guide for Conducting Acute Toxicity Tests with Fishes, Macroinvertebrates, and Amphibians ASTM E729-88a$^{\epsilon 1}$) for conducting acute toxicity tests in freshwater. This reconstituted water is often used for both research and compliance testing (e.g., whole effluent toxicity testing and EPA's water-effect ratio testing).

Marking and Dawson (1973) first used this reconstituted water to study the toxicity of quinaldine sulfate to several fish species. The test solution was prepared by adding specific quantities of sodium bicarbonate, calcium sulfate, magnesium sulfate, and

---

[1]Stratus Consulting Inc., P.O. Box 4059, Boulder, CO 80306.
[2]Paladin Water Quality Consulting, 3725 NW Polk Avenue, Corvallis, OR 97330.

potassium chloride to deionized water. If required, the pH of the water could be adjusted and maintained by adding chemical buffers. While any alkalinity/hardness water can be prepared, ASTM E729-88a$^{\epsilon 1}$, provides guidance on preparing four types of reconstituted water based on hardness: very soft, soft, hard, and very hard (Table 1).

Table 1 — *Water quality of ASTM reconstituted water based on relative hardness.*

Hardness Classification	Hardness, mg/L as $CaCO_3$	Alkalinity, mg/L as $CaCO_3$	pH[1]
Very Soft	10-13	10-13	6.7-6.8
Soft	40-48	30-35	7.3-7.5
Hard	160-180	110-120	7.8-8.0
Very Hard	280-320	225-245	8.0-8.2

[1] Approximate equilibrium pH after aeration but before adding fish to test water.

Water hardness is often treated as a defined chemical parameter. However, hardness is a qualitative, descriptive term that was originally used to quantify the ability of water to prevent soap from foaming (Carroll et al. 1979). Chemically, total hardness is defined as the total amount of dissolved calcium (Ca) and magnesium (Mg) in the water (APHA 1992). However, the relative amounts of Ca and Mg as constituents of total water hardness are often ignored, even though Ca has a much greater effect than Mg in modifying the toxicity of copper (Cu), cadmium (Cd), and zinc (Zn) (Carroll et al. 1979, Davies et al. 1993, Erickson et al. 1996, Alsop and Wood 1999, Welsh et al. 2000).

Sodium (Na) and potassium (K) concentrations can also influence copper toxicity. Acute copper toxicity in fish primarily involves net Na plasma loss as a result of disruption of osmoregulation (Lauren and McDonald 1996). In acute toxicity tests conducted with fathead minnows (*Pimephales promelas*), elevated external Na was found to assist, and elevated external K to oppose, the net K/Na exchange at the gill surface (Erickson et al. 1996). Hence, elevated Na decreases, and elevated K increases, acute Cu toxicity (Erickson et al. 1996). Sodium concentrations greater than 23 mg/L were necessary to modify Cu toxicity in fathead minnows (Erickson et al. 1987, as cited in Erickson et al. 1996). Limited data are available on the effect of Na and K on metal toxicity in salmonids. However, research conducted with salmonids indicated that elevated Na as high as 69 mg/L did not influence Cd toxicity in brook trout (*Salvelinus fontinalis;* Carroll et al. 1979).

Varying Na concentrations was a potential confounding factor in tests that evaluated the relative importance of Ca and Mg (expressed as Ca:Mg molar ratios) on Cu toxicity in salmonids (Welsh et al. 2000). In three of the four toxicity tests, conducted at a constant total hardness but varying Ca:Mg molar ratios, Na concentrations were positively correlated with Ca concentrations (Welsh et al. 2000). However, in one test, Na concentrations were held constant and Ca concentrations varied. Welsh et al. (2000)

concluded that Na did not adversely influence their test results because the same generalized relationship between Ca:Mg molar ratios and Cu toxicity was observed in all four paired toxicity tests regardless of the Na concentration. However, the role of Na was never directly tested in that study.

In this study, we compare the ionic composition of ASTM reconstituted water and natural surface waters in the United States and critically evaluate the relative importance of Ca, Mg, and Na to hardness-based modification of metal toxicity. The role of Ca and Mg in modifying acute Cd, Cu, and Zn toxicity is evaluated based on previously published information. The potential role of Na in modifying acute Cu toxicity in salmonids is evaluated by examining Cu sensitivity in rainbow trout at constant Ca and Mg concentration but varying Na concentrations. Finally, we discuss the implications of using existing ASTM reconstituted water for conducting and interpreting metal toxicity tests.

Methods

Natural Surface Waters

Water quality data representative of natural surface waters in the United States (including Alaska, Hawaii, and territories) were obtained from the United States Geological Survey (USGS) water quality network (WQN). The WQN includes water chemistry information collected between 1962 and 1995 from the National Stream Quality Accounting Network (NASQAN) and the Hydrological Benchmark Network (HBN). NASQAN consists of 618 stations located on major U.S. rivers and streams; WQN consists of 63 stations located in small, minimally disturbed watersheds (Alexander et al. 2000).

Data on selected water chemistry parameters were collected from the WQN database for all 681 stations for all sampling times available. In total, water chemistry data were collected for Ca, Mg, K, Na, alkalinity (measured from an unfiltered sample in the field by the fixed endpoint method), and hardness. Mean concentrations and other summary statistics (e.g., standard deviation, sample size) were determined for each of these water chemistry parameters for each sampling station. Variation associated with each mean estimate was primarily a result of temporal (i.e., seasonal) variability in the concentration or level of the parameter of interest. For example, the coefficient of variation for hardness ranged from 0% to 283% (median 24%). Only mean values are used in subsequent analysis in this study; these values are assumed to provide a suitable measure of central tendency of the relative ionic composition of natural surface waters for comparative purposes to ASTM reconstituted water.

Na Toxicity Tests

Fish Source and Acclimation Conditions — Eagle Lake rainbow trout were obtained as eggs from Dubois State Fish Hatchery, Dubois, WY, and hatched in hatching jars in well water (hardness, 220 mg/L). All fish were cultured in rectangular troughs receiving a continuous supply of well water at 7°-8°C. Following resorption of the yolk sac, fry were fed a vitamin-fortified commercial trout starter diet (BioDiet Starter Crumbles, Bio-Oregon, Inc., Warrenton, OR) at the manufacturer's recommended rate (at 8°C) of 3.5% total biomass per day. Fish were acclimated to appropriate test water conditions (e.g., hardness, alkalinity, pH, and temperature) for a minimum of 14 days prior to testing (see Table 2 for test water quality conditions). Fish were not acclimated to elevated Na or chloride (Cl) levels as present in the high Na test (see below). Mean Cu concentrations in the acclimation water ranged from 0.17 μg/L (SD, 0.06; n, 7) to 0.21 μg/L (SD, 0.02; n, 5); mean Cd and Zn concentrations in the acclimation water were less than detection limits (detection limits provided below). Feeding was discontinued 48 h before test initiation. All culture and acclimation water was monitored daily for hardness, alkalinity, pH, temperature, and dissolved oxygen.

Table 2 — *Test water quality [Mean (SD, n)].*

Water Quality Parameter	Low Na Test	High Na Test
Alkalinity (mg/L as $CaCO_3$)	87.9 (1.2, 10)	91.2 (3.2, 10)
Hardness (mg/L as $CaCO_3$)	98.2 (2.2, 10)	97.7 (1.3, 10)
Dissolved Oxygen (mg/L)	9.21 (0.22, 5)	9.39 (0.23, 5)
Temperature (°C)	8.49 (0.24, 30)	8.49 (0.26, 30)
pH	7.89 (0.05, 30)	7.91 (0.04, 30)
Calcium (mg/L)	22.3 (0.21, 5)	21.3 (0.22, 5)
Potassium (mg/L)	0.90 (0.00, 5)	3.86 (3.80, 5)
Magnesium (mg/L)	11.2 (0.15, 5)	10.7 (0.11,5)
Sodium (mg/L)	3.58 (0.04, 5)	32.2 (0.40, 5)
Chloride (mg/L)	2.85 (0.03, 5)	54.1 (1.44, 4)
Sulfate (mg/L)	11.5 (0.11, 5)	11.7 (0.37, 4)
Cadmium (μg/L)[1]	< dl (-, 6)	< dl (-, 6)
Zinc (μg/L)[1]	< dl (-, 6)	< dl (-, 6)

[1] Detection limits for metals were 0.013 μg Cd/L and 6 μg Zn/L.

Toxicity Test Methods — Toxicity tests were conducted at Red Buttes Environmental Biology Laboratory, University of Wyoming, Laramie, WY. Well water was continuously mixed with deionized water in a 190-L head tank to produce a target hardness concentration of 100 mg/L. Test water pH was controlled to pH 7.9 in each head tank with a Signet pH controller (Signet Scientific, Tustin, CA) that controlled the addition of sulfuric acid or potassium hydroxide using metering pumps. Target temperatures were achieved by chilling or heating deionized water before delivery to the head tank. All fish were maintained and tested under a 16-h light/8-h dark illumination cycle.

Each test used a continuous-flow proportional diluter designed to provide six replicates of six treatment concentrations (five Cu treatments and a control). Fresh copper chloride stock solutions ($CuCl_2 \cdot 2H_2O$) were metered into the diluter using a Fluid Metering Inc. (Syosset, NY) QG20 laboratory metering pump at 3 mL/min. Within a diluter, each treatment was split into six replicate exposure tanks. The placement of treatments within the bank was by randomized block design. Each side of the bank contained three complete replicate blocks. Each exposure tank contained 7.6 L of exposure water with 150 mL/min exposure water replacement. This flow rate provided 216 L/day, or over 28 volume replacements per day, and a 99% molecular replacement time of approximately 4 h. For the low Na test, only three replicate blocks were used (all from one side of the test bank); six replicate blocks were used in the high Na test.

Twenty fish were loaded, two at a time, into each exposure tank to provide a random distribution of fish in the tanks. Fish loading into each exposure tank did not exceed 4.0 g/L of tank volume or 0.15 g/L/24-h of total flow through the tank. Mean wet weights ranged from 430 mg (SD, 91; n, 20) in the low Na test to 602 mg (SD, 73; n, 20) in the high Na test. Copper exposures were conducted for 120 h, a time period sufficient to approximate the incipient lethal level (i.e., the time independent acute LC50). During exposures, mortality (i.e., cessation of opercular movement) was monitored at 0, 3, 6, 9 h, and then at each 12-h interval to the end of the test. Dead fish were removed and discarded at each observation.

Water Chemistry — Routine water quality parameters (hardness, alkalinity, pH, temperature, and dissolved oxygen), cations (Ca, Mg, Na, K), anions [Cl, sulfate (SO_4)], and metals (Cd, Cu, Zn) were analyzed throughout fish culture, acclimation, and test exposures using standard techniques. Samples for cation, anion, and metal analysis were collected in precleaned, certified Level 1 polyethylene sample bottles (Eagle-Picher); cation and total metals samples were acidified with 0.1% addition of Ultrex II nitric acid. Dissolved metal samples were collected, filtered through a Gelman ACRO 50 (0.45 μm pore) in-line filter before acidification. Copper and Cd were analyzed by graphite furnace atomic absorption spectrophotometry. Zinc and all other cations were analyzed by flame atomic absorption spectrophotometry. Anions were analyzed by ion chromatography. Detection limits for metals were 0.16 μg Cu/L, 0.013 μg Cd/L, and 6 μg Zn/L.

Data Analysis and Statistics — Mortality data were analyzed using the 10% trimmed Spearman-Karber procedure using Toxstat v.3.5 (WEST 1996). Dosages were log transformed to provide more equal spacing between treatments. Control data were included. LC50 values were calculated using mean analyzed dissolved Cu concentrations, and 95% confidence intervals were compared to determine significantly different responses between tests. LT50 values (e.g., median time to death) for each treatment were calculated using the Kaplan-Meier method for estimating a survival function (Kalbfleisch and Prentice 1980). Mortality records from replicate exposure tanks were pooled before curve estimation. In this procedure, the LT50 was defined as the least elapsed time at which the estimated survival function fell below 50%, and 95% confidence limits on these values were defined as fiducial limits. LT50 calculations were performed using S-PLUS v4.5 (Mathsoft Inc, Seattle, WA).

Results

ASTM Reconstituted Water and Natural Surface Waters

In ASTM reconstituted water, hardness and alkalinity levels are positively correlated: as hardness levels increase, alkalinity levels also increase but to a lesser degree (Table 1).[3] In general, the relationship between hardness and alkalinity in natural surface waters is similar to that of ASTM reconstituted water (Figure 1). However, the relative amounts of Ca, Mg, K, and Na in ASTM reconstituted water are fixed; Ca:Mg molar ratios are 0.7 and Na:K molar ratios are 21.3. These molar ratios in ASTM reconstituted water are different from those observed in natural surface waters (Figures 2 and 3). The Ca:Mg molar ratio of natural surface waters in the WQN database ranged from 0.3 to 12.9, with a median value of 2.0. These Ca:Mg molar ratios are much higher than those in ASTM reconstituted water (Figure 2). Similarly, the Na:K molar ratios in natural surface waters ranged from 1.4 to 600, with a median value of 10.7. These Na:K molar ratios are generally lower than those in ASTM reconstituted water at hardness values less than approximately 300 mg/L; at higher hardness levels, Na:K ratios increase above those in ASTM reconstituted water (Figure 3).

Na Toxicity Tests

Water Chemistry — With the exception of Na, Cl, and K, water chemistry results were similar between the two Na toxicity tests (Table 2). Changes in Na and Cl concentrations were anticipated and were the result of the experimental design of the test (Na concentrations were adjusted by adding NaCl). Changes in K concentrations, however, were unexpected and resulted from the saturation of the cation and anion exchange resins in the dual bed deionizing water system and subsequent addition of large amounts of potassium hydroxide to maintain the test pH. Potassium concentrations ranged from 7.5 to 8.5 mg/L on the first two days of the test and then dropped to typical values of 1.1 mg/L on the remaining test days after the deionized water system was recharged.

Acute Cu Toxicity Results — Acute toxicity was similar between the two Na tests; dissolved Cu 120-h LC50s ranged from 34.9 μg Cu/L (95% CI, 31.7-38.6) at 3.6 mg/L Na to 39.1 μg Cu/L (95% CI, 35.6-42.9) at 32.2 mg/L Na. The time to death was delayed in the high Na test; LT50 values were higher in the high Na test at all concentrations tested (Figure 4).

---

[3]The pH of ASTM reconstituted water is also positively correlated with both alkalinity and hardness. However, since pH can be adjusted in ASTM reconstituted water by adding chemical buffers, and the role of pH in modifying metal toxicity is well studied (e.g., Campbell and Stokes 1985, Cusimano et al. 1986, Welsh et al. 1993), we do not evaluate the relationship between pH and other cations/anions in this study.

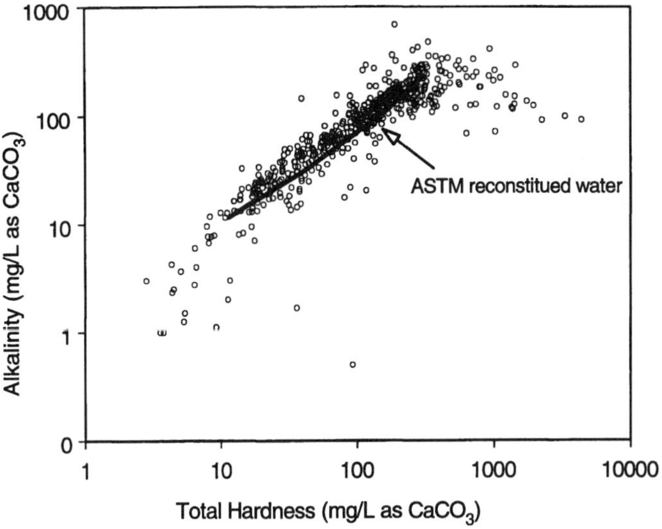

Figure 1 — *Relationship between Hardness and Alkalinity*

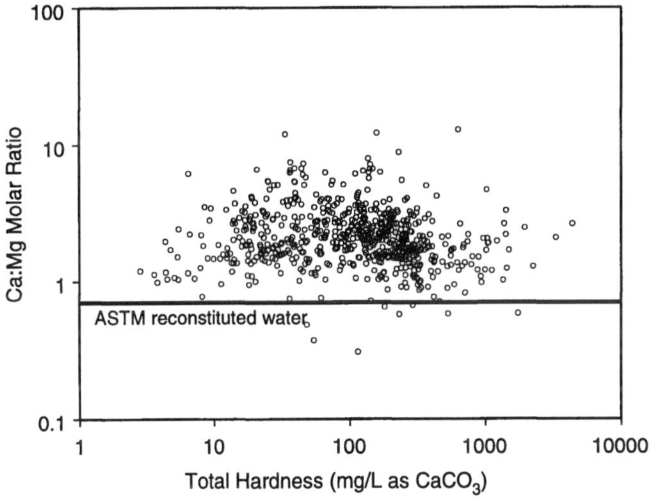

Figure 2 — *Relationship between Ca:Mg Molar Ratios and Hardness.* Reprinted with permission from *Environmental Toxicology and Chemistry*, 2000. Relative importance of calcium and magnesium in hardness-based modification of copper toxicity, by P.G. Welsh, J. Lipton, G.A. Chapman, and T.L. Podrabsky. Volume 19 (6). Copyright Society of Environmental Toxicology and Chemistry (SETAC), Pensacola, FL. 2000.

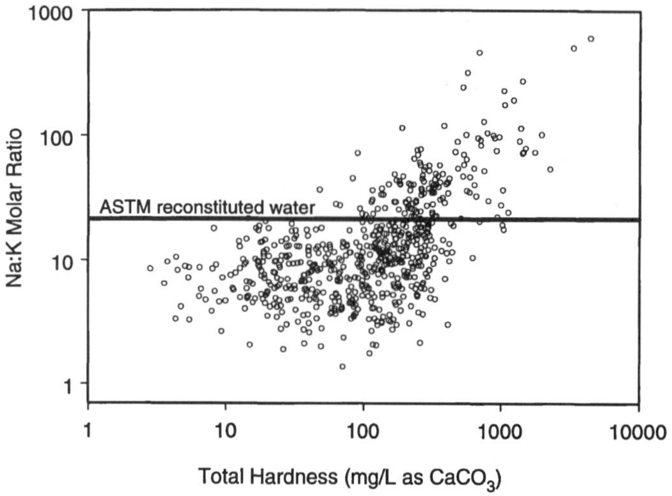

Figure 3 — *Relationship between Na:K Molar ratios and hardness.*

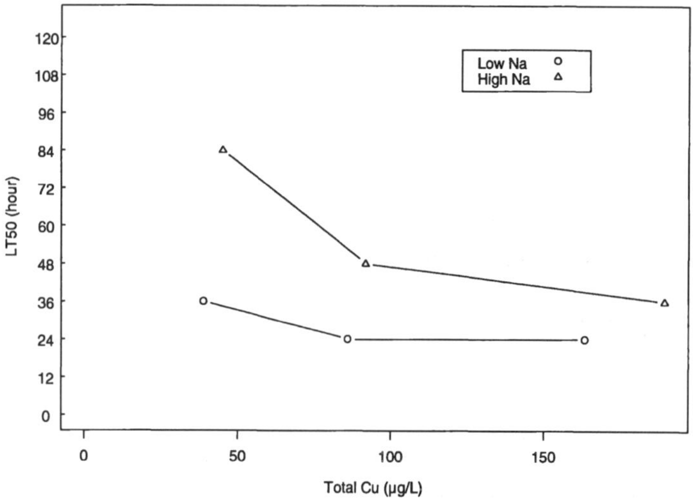

Figure 4 — *Median lethal time (LT50) for rainbow trout exposed to copper at low Na or elevated Na concentrations in water at a hardness of 100 mg/L.*

Discussion

With respect to alkalinity and hardness, ASTM reconstituted water and natural surface waters appear to be well matched; the relationship between alkalinity and hardness is similar between the two types of water (Figure 1). Closer examination of the ionic composition of these waters indicates that there are differences between the relative amounts of Ca, Mg, Na, and K in these waters. In natural surface waters, the relative amounts of Ca and Mg (and Ca:Mg molar ratios) vary; Ca:Mg molar ratios range from 0.3 to 12.9 (Figure 2). However, the relative amounts of Ca and Mg in ASTM reconstituted water are constant at a Ca:Mg molar ratio of 0.7. Similarly, the relative amounts of Na and K (and Na:K molar ratios) also vary; Na:K molar ratios range from 1.4 to 600 (Figure 3). As with Ca and Mg, the relative amounts of Na and K in ASTM reconstituted water are constant at a Na:K molar ratio of 21.3.

Calcium is an important ion in modifying metal toxicity (Carroll et al. 1979, Davies et al. 1993, Erickson et al. 1996, Alsop and Wood 1999, Welsh et al. 2000). Calcium can modify metal exposure by three mechanisms: (1) competition with metal ions for biological binding sites (Playle et al. 1992), (2) alteration in the permeability of the gill membrane to ions (McDonald et al. 1989), and (3) physiological changes at the gill as a result of acclimation to ambient Ca conditions (Laurén and McDonald 1986). For example, soft water acclimated fish demonstrate a physiological adaptation to low Ca water through proliferation of chloride cells on the gill apical membrane, production of a thicker mucous coat on secondary lamellae, and higher concentrations of the Ca-binding protein calmodulin (Laurén and McDonald 1985, 1986).

The effect of hardness on toxicity is primarily a function of Ca rather than Mg. For example, Erickson et al. (1996) showed that adding calcium chloride increased the 96-h LC50 of Cu to fathead minnows by a factor of 3.26, whereas adding an equivalent amount of magnesium chloride increased the LC50 by a factor of only 1.09. A recent study by Welsh et al. (2000) evaluated the role of Ca and Mg on copper toxicity to rainbow trout and chinook salmon (*O. tshawytscha*) by modifying the relative concentration of Ca and Mg while maintaining constant hardness. In four paired toxicity tests in which Ca:Mg molar ratios were varied, Ca, but not Mg, was identified as being primarily responsible for observed changes in Cu toxicity (Welsh et al. 2000). A similar role of Ca has also been observed with salmonids exposed to Cd and Zn. In toxicity tests with trout exposed to Cd, Carroll et al. (1979) observed that Ca, but not Mg, was protective against Cd toxicity in brook trout. Similarly, in a study with rainbow trout where hardness was manipulated by adding magnesium sulfate, Davies et al. (1993) observed only a modest decrease in acute and chronic Cd toxicity over a hardness range of 50 to 400 mg/L. The lack of stronger antagonistic effects of hardness in their study was attributed to the use of Mg over Ca to adjust hardness levels. In a study evaluating Zn toxicity to rainbow trout, Alsop and Wood (1999) concluded that Ca was more important than Mg in modifying Zn toxicity. These studies clearly demonstrate that Ca is more important than Mg in modifying hardness-dependent metal toxicity.

In three of the four paired Cu toxicity tests conducted by Welsh et al. (2000), Na concentrations were positively correlated to Ca concentrations, potentially confounding their test results (in one paired toxicity test, Na concentrations was held constant).

Overall, Na concentrations in the four paired toxicity tests ranged from 4.8 mg/L to 32.5 mg/L (Welsh et al. 2000). Sodium has been associated with decreased Cu toxicity in fathead minnows at concentrations greater than 23 mg/L (Erickson et al. 1987, as cited in Erickson et al. 1996); toxicity tests conducted with Na concentrations of 46 mg/L were associated with a twofold decrease in Cu toxicity, whereas no change in toxicity was observed at Na concentrations of 23 mg/L. However, the concentration of Na sufficient to modify copper toxicity to salmonids is not known.

The Na toxicity tests presented here specifically address whether elevated Na concentrations as measured in Welsh et al. (2000) influence Cu toxicity to salmonids. As previously described, Cu toxicity was examined at two Na concentrations (3.6 mg/L and 32.2 mg/L), with hardness, Ca, and Mg held constant. Copper toxicity estimates to rainbow trout were similar at both Na concentrations tested; 120-h LC50s ranged from 34.9 μg Cu/L (95% CI, 31.7-38.6) at 3.6 mg/L Na to 39.1 μg Cu/L (95% CI, 35.6-42.9) at 32.2 mg/L Na. Since there is substantial overlap between the 95% confidence intervals of these toxicity estimates, the estimates are not considered significantly different. Overall, the test results indicate that Na concentrations up to 32.2 mg/L do not influence acute Cu toxicity in rainbow trout and that the results presented in Welsh et al. (2000) are representative of the effects of elevated Ca concentrations on Cu toxicity, not elevated Na concentrations.

Interestingly, the high Na test was associated with a delay in Cu toxicity, as illustrated by an increase in the LT50 values in the high Na test at constant Cu exposure concentrations (Figure 4). Since no change in time to death was observed in the Cu toxicity tests conducted by Welsh et al. (2000; unpublished data) where Na concentrations ranged up to 32.5 mg/L, we do not attribute the increase in LT50 values to the elevated Na concentrations. Instead, we attribute the delay in toxicity to the elevated K concentrations that occurred during the first 2 days of the test. Hence, the delay in toxicity in the high Na test was most likely caused by the elevated K concentration and not by the elevated Na concentration.

Conclusions and Recommendations

Overall, ASTM reconstituted water is a poor surrogate for natural surface waters. While hardness and alkalinity relationships are similar between ASTM reconstituted water and natural surface waters, differences in the ionic composition of major cations (Ca, Mg, Na, K) exist. These differences in ionic composition may have implications for conducting and interpreting metal toxicity tests that use ASTM reconstituted water (e.g., water effect ratio tests or whole effluent toxicity tests). Calcium is a very important ion in modifying metal toxicity. While elevated concentrations of Na and K may modify Cu toxicity, Mg appears to have very little effect on the toxicity of Cu, Cd, and Zn, three important metals whose water quality criteria are hardness dependent. Hence, differences in Ca concentrations between ASTM reconstituted water and natural surface waters may inappropriately influence metal toxicity test interpretation and subsequent environmental management decisions. Future metal criteria development should examine the advantages of Ca-dependent criteria rather than hardness-dependent criteria. This approach is currently being addressed with development of the Biotic Ligand Model, in which the role of individual ions is expressly considered when predicting the acute toxicity of metals.

Future guidance for using ASTM reconstituted water in metal toxicity tests should explicitly state the role of Ca in "hardness-based" modification of metal toxicity. In addition, an alternative ASTM reconstituted water should be developed that is more appropriately matched with the ionic composition of natural surface waters. This new reconstituted water could be an alternative to or could supplement the existing ASTM reconstituted water. The importance of ionic composition for other toxicants could then be evaluated by performing comparison toxicity tests in both reconstituted waters. The ultimate use of toxicity test results should be carefully considered by the researcher before using any reconstituted water as a surrogate for a site water. If ionic composition is important (i.e., may influence test results), then a site-specific reconstituted water should be considered.

Acknowledgments

Laboratory testing was conducted at the University of Wyoming's Red Buttes Environmental Laboratory in Laramie, WY, and at the California Department of Fish and Game's Aquatic Toxicology Laboratory in Elk Grove, CA. We are grateful to the entire project staff from both facilities. The research was funded in part by the State of California and the State of Montana.

References

Alexander, R. B., Slack, J. R., Ludtke, A. S., Fitzgerald, K. K., and Schertz, T. L., 2000, Data from selected U.S. Geological Survey national stream water-quality monitoring networks (WQN). United States Geological Survey Digital Data Series DDS-37. Downloaded from <http://wwwrvares.er.usgs.gov/wqn96cd> February 7, 2000.

Alsop, D. H. and Wood, C. M., 1999, "Influence of Waterborne Cations on Zinc Uptake and Toxicity in Rainbow Trout, *Oncorhynchus mykiss,*" *Canadian Journal of Fisheries and Aquatic Sciences,* Vol. 56, pp. 2112-2119.

APHA, AWWA, and WEF, 1992, *Standard Methods for the Examination of Water and Wastewater*, 18th Edition, M. A. H. Franson (ed.), American Public Health Association, American Water Works Association, and Water Environment Federation, Washington, DC.

Campbell, P. G. C. and Stokes, P. M., 1985, "Acidification and Toxicity of Metals to Aquatic Biota," *Canadian Journal of Fisheries and Aquatic Sciences,* Vol. 42, pp. 2034-2049.

Carroll, J. J., Ellis, S. J., and Oliver, W. S., 1979, "Influences of Total Hardness Constituents on the Acute Toxicity of Cadmium to Brook Trout (*Salvelinus fontinalis*)," *Bulletin of Environmental Contamination and Toxicology,* Vol. 22, pp. 575-581.

Cusimano, R .F., Brakke, D. F., and Chapman, G. A., 1986, "Effects of pH on the Toxicities of Cadmium, Copper, and Zinc to Steelhead Trout," *Canadian Journal of Fisheries and Aquatic Sciences,* Vol. 43, pp. 1497-1503.

Davies, P. H., Gorman, W. C., Carlson, C. A., and Brinkman, S. F., 1993, "Effect of Hardness on Bioavailability and Toxicity of Cadmium to Rainbow Trout," *Chemical Speciation and Bioavailability,* Vol. 5, pp. 67-77.

Erickson, R. J., Benoit, D. A., Mattson, V. R., Nelson, H. P., Jr., and Leonard, E. N, 1996, "The Effects of Water Chemistry on the Toxicity of Copper to Fathead Minnows," *Environmental Toxicology and Chemistry,* Vol. 15, pp. 181-193.

Kalbfleisch, J. D. and Prentice, R. L., 1980, *The Statistical Analysis of Failure Time Data*, John Wiley and Sons, New York.

Laurén, D. J. and McDonald, D. G., 1985, "Effects of Copper on Branchial Ionoregulation in the Rainbow Trout, *Salmo gairdneri*: Richardson," *Journal of Comparative Physiology,* Vol. 155, pp. 635-644.

Laurén, D.J. and McDonald, D.G., 1986, "Influence of Water Hardness, pH, and Alkalinity on the Mechanisms of Copper Toxicity in Juvenile Rainbow Trout, *Salmo gairdneri,"* *Canadian Journal of Fisheries and Aquatic Science,* Vol. 43, pp. 1488-1496.

Marking, L.L. and Dawson, V.K., 1973, "Toxicity of Quinaldine Sulfate to Fish," in *Investigations in Fish Control*, No. 48 Final Report, U. S. Department of the Interior, Fish and Wildlife Service, Washington, DC, pp. 3-8.

McDonald, D.G., Reader, J.P., and Dalziel, T.R.K., 1989, "The Combined Effects of pH and Trace Metals on Fish Ionoregulation," in *Acid Toxicity and Aquatic Animals*, R. Morris, E.W. Taylor, D.J.A. Brown, and J.A. Brown (eds.), Cambridge University Press, New York.

Playle, R. C., Gensemer, R. W., and Dixon, D. G., 1992, "Copper Accumulation on Gills of Fathead Minnows: Influence of Water Hardness, Complexation and pH of the Gill Micro-environment," *Environmental Toxicology and Chemistry*, Vol. 11, pp. 381-391.

U.S. EPA. 1993, "Methods for Measuring the Acute Toxicity of Effluents and Receiving Waters to Freshwater and Marine Organisms," Fourth edition, EPA/600/4-90/027F, Final Report, U.S. Environmental Protection Agency, Office of Research and Development, Washington, DC.

Welsh, P. G., Skidmore, J. F., Spry, D. J., Dixon, D. G., Hodson, P. V., Hutchinson, N. J., and Hickie, B. E., 1993, "Effect of pH and Dissolved Organic Carbon on the Toxicity of Copper to Larval Fathead Minnow (*Pimephales promelas*) in Natural Lake Waters of

Low Alkalinity," *Canadian Journal of Fisheries and Aquatic Sciences*, Vol. 50, pp. 1356-1362.

Welsh, P. G., Lipton, J., Chapman, G. A., and Podrabsky, T. L., 2000, "Relative Importance of Calcium and Magnesium in Hardness-based Modification of Copper Toxicity," *Environmental Toxicology and Chemistry*, Vol. 19, pp. 1624-1631.

WEST, 1996, *Toxstat v3.5 Documentation,* Western EcoSystems Technology, Cheyenne, WY.

Kristin Schirmer,[1] Elizabeth M. Joyce,[2] D. George Dixon,[2] Bruce M. Greenberg,[2] and Niels C. Bols[2]

Ability of the Quinones Arising from the UV Irradiation of Anthracene to Induce 7-Ethoxyresorufin-O-Deethylase Activity in a Trout Liver Cell Line

---

Reference: Schirmer, K., Joyce, E. M., Dixon, D. G., Greenberg, B. M., and Bols, N. C., "**Ability of the Quinones Arising from the UV Irradiation of Anthracene to Induce 7-Ethoxyresorufin-O-Deethylase Activity in a Trout Liver Cell Line,**" *Environmental Toxicology and Risk Assessment: Science, Policy, and Standardization – Implications for Environmental Decisions: Tenth Volume, ASTM STP 1403*, B. M. Greenberg, R. N. Hull, M. H. Roberts, Jr., and R. W. Gensemer, Eds., American Society for Testing and Materials, West Conshohocken, PA, 2001.

Abstract: Quinone derivatives of the polycyclic aromatic hydrocarbon, anthracene, were investigated for their ability to induce 7-ethoxyresorufin-*O*-deethylase (EROD) activity in a cell line from rainbow trout liver, RTL-W1. Of the 11 anthracene quinones tested, five were capable of inducing EROD activity. From most to the least potent, the order of induction potency, based on EC50 values, was 2,6-dihydroxyanthraquinone = 1,2,4-trihydroxyanthraquinone < 1,2-dihydroxyanthraquinone = 1,3-dihydroxyanthraquinone = 2-hydroxyanthraquinone. The 1,2,10-trihydroxylated anthracene also induced EROD activity whereas anthraquinone did not, indicating that the quinone structure alone was not adequate for EROD induction to occur. The current results show that UV irradiation of an AhR-inactive PAH, such as anthracene, can yield derivatives that are AhR active and induce EROD activity in fish cells and presumably in fish. Thus, responses mediated by the AhR and/or P4501A should be considered in the environmental risk assessment of UV/PAH interactions.

Keywords: anthracene quinones, UV irradiation, EROD induction, fish cells

---

[1]Postdoctoral research associate, UFZ Centre for Environmental Research Leipzig-Halle, Department of Chemical Ecotoxicology, Permoserstr. 15, 04318 Leipzig, Germany.

[2]Research technician and professors, respectively, Department of Biology, University of Waterloo, Waterloo, ON, N2L 3G1, Canada.

Introduction

Polycyclic aromatic hydrocarbons (PAHs) are common environmental contaminants for which a number of adverse biological effects has been discovered. One is carcinogenicity which, at least in mammals, has been associated with the induction of cytochrome P4501A (Ioannides and Parke 1993). Although in fish information about a relationship between carcinogenicity and P4501A induction is rather limited, knowledge of whether a PAH induces P4501A is useful in environmental risk analysis for a number of reasons. Firstly, due to the involvement of the aryl-hydrocarbon receptor (AhR) (Sadar et al. 1996), induction of P4501A in fish indicates a pathway through which PAHs act on the cellular level in a manner similar to dioxins, and a possible route to the expression of toxicity. Secondly, inasmuch as there are many different PAHs or PAH derivatives, knowledge about the spectrum of PAHs that induce P4501A in fish can strengthen the usefulness of P4501A as a biomarker. Thirdly, the induction of P4501A can be used as a common response to derive toxic equivalency factors (Bols et al. 1999, 1997; Delistraty 1997), which are central to the toxic equivalency approach for evaluating the toxicity of complex mixtures (Eadon et al. 1986).

It was the goal of the current paper to investigate the ability of 12 derivatives of anthracene to induce P4501A activity in the rainbow trout liver cell line RTL-W1. The response of this cell line to PAHs appears to be similar to the in vivo response of rainbow trout (Bols et al. 1999). In a previous study with this cell line, anthracene (Figure 1) was found to be a non-inducer of cytochrome P4501A, which was measured by monitoring its catalytic activity as 7-ethoxyresorufin-*O*-deethylase (EROD) activity (Bols et al. 1999). The 11 anthraquinones and one hydroxylated anthracene were selected based on their potential occurrence following exposure of the PAH to natural or simulated solar ultraviolet (UV) radiation (Mallakin et al. 1999, 2000). Thus, this is the first study to investigate systematically whether UV treatment of a parent PAH that is unable to induce EROD activity can yield products capable of inducing EROD- and thus P4501A-activity. Elaborating this question is the more important as none of these photo-oxidized products are currently accounted for in environmental surveillance and risk assessment.

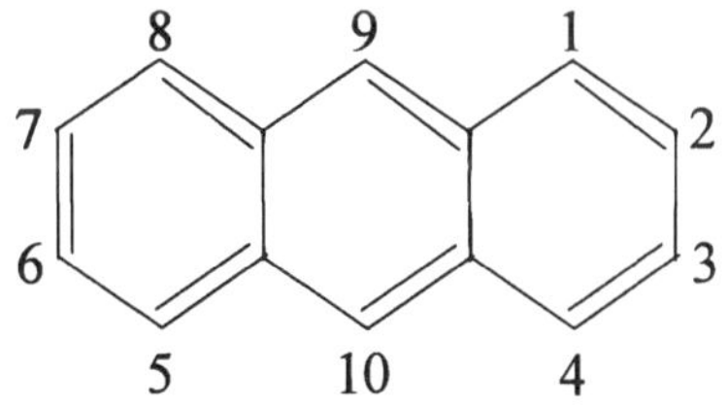

Figure 1 – *Structure of the PAH anthracene.*

Materials and Methods

Anthracene Derivatives

With the exception of 1-hydroxy-, 2-hydroxy- and 1,3-dihydroxyanthraquinone, which were synthesized at the University of Waterloo as described by Wang and Sniekus (1990), all quinones and the 1,2,10-trihydroxyanthracene were purchased in high purity from Sigma (St. Louis, MO) or Aldrich (Milwaukee, WI). High performance liquid chromatography was used to confirm the purity of the chemicals (Mallakin et al. 1999). Stock solutions of all compounds were prepared in dimethyl sulfoxide (DMSO, BDH, Toronto, ON) and serially diluted in DMSO to give 200 times the final concentration required by each design treatment. The concentration of the anthracene derivatives in these working solutions was also confirmed by HPLC (Mallakin et al. 1999).

RTL-W1 Cell Culture and Exposure to Anthracene Derivatives

The rainbow trout (*Oncorhynchus mykiss*) liver cell line, RTL-W1, was grown in Leibovitz's L-15 culture medium with 5% fetal bovine serum (FBS), as detailed in the original description of this cell line (Lee et al. 1993). Routine maintenance was done in 75-cm^2 flasks and subcultivations were made from confluent flasks with 0.1% trypsin. Prior to exposure of RTL-W1 to anthracene and the oxygenated derivatives, confluent cell monolayers were obtained in 48-well tissue culture plates by adding 30 000 cells per well in 500 µL L-15 with 5% FBS and allowing the cells to grow at 22°C for three days. Exposures began by the addition to each well of 2.5 µL of the appropriate working solution or the DMSO control. Exposures were terminated 24 h later and cells assayed directly for EROD activity (Bols et al. 1999). The amount of protein in each microwell was determined with fluorescamine as described by Lorenzen and Kennedy (1993) in order to express EROD activity as specific activity (pmol resorufin/mg protein/min).

As judged from their absorption spectra (Mallakin et al. 1999), several of the anthracene derivatives tested were expected to absorb radiation at 530±30 nm, the wavelength used to excite resorufin in the EROD assay. Inasmuch as absorption at this wavelength may also lead to a fluorescent signal by the anthracene derivatives at the emission wavelength used for resorufin, 595±35 nm, plates were checked periodically for autofluorescence of the anthracene-derived compounds at excitation/emission of 530±30 nm/595±35 nm at the end of the exposure period immediately prior to the EROD assay.

Analysis of EROD Data and Dose-Response Curves for EROD Induction

Data from each experiment over an exposure range were analyzed by a one-way analysis of variance (ANOVA). The exposure range usually consisted of 8 to 14 concentrations, with the upper limit of the range being determined by one of three factors. The first factor was the derivation of a complete sigmoidal dose-response curve that included a maximal level of EROD activity. The second factor influencing the upper limit of the concentration range was the formation of crystals in the culture wells, which indicated that the solubility limit of the compound had been surpassed. Examination of cultures with either the naked eye or by phase-contrast microscopy revealed the presence of crystals. Finally, the third factor restricting the upper limit of the concentration range was the observation of fluorescence at excitation/emission of 530±30 nm/595±35 nm in the absence of resorufin. With the concentration range being determined in this way, a compound was concluded not to be an EROD inducer if the P-value of the ANOVA was greater than 0.05. If the P-value was less than 0.05, the compound was concluded to be an EROD inducer provided that a multiple comparison test (Student-Newman-Keuls) confirmed that the EROD activities for two or more consecutive concentrations were significantly higher than the EROD activities for the two lowest concentrations being tested (Bols et al. 1999).

For those test compounds that significantly induced EROD activity, dose-response curves were used to calculate maximum levels of EROD activity (ERODmax), and the effective concentration that caused 50% of the maximal EROD response (EC50). This was done by fitting the dose-response data to a four parameter logistic equation, using the SigmaPlot nonlinear regression curve-fitting module (Jandel Scientific, San Rafael, CA). The logistic equation was:

$$y(d) = Ymin + (Ymax - Ymin)\{1 + exp[-g(ln(d) - ln(EC50))]\}^{-1} \quad (1)$$

where y(d) is the response at a given concentration d, Ymin is the minimum response, Ymax is the maximum response, and g is a slope parameter.

The EC50s and the EROD maxima for the different anthracene derivatives were compared by ANOVA. As the P values for the ANOVA tests were less than 0.05, the data were further examined by the Student-Newman-Keuls multiple comparison test.

Calculation of Toxic Equivalency Factors (TEFs)

The relative ability of the anthracene derivatives to induce EROD activity was expressed in two ways. The TCDD TEF was the mean EC50 for TCDD divided by the mean EC50 for the compound being evaluated. The BaP TEF was the mean EC50 for BaP divided by the mean EC50 for the compound being evaluated. Both the mean EC50 for TCDD and the mean EC50 for BaP were obtained from a previous study by Bols et al. (1999) that used RTL-W1 cells and similar experimental procedures.

Results

Eleven anthracene quinones that potentially arise from the UV irradiation of the parent compound, anthracene, and one hydroxylated anthracene were tested for their ability to induce EROD activity in the fish liver cell line, RTL-W1. Five of the eleven anthracene quinones as well as the hydroxylated anthracene, 1,2,10-trihydroxyanthracene, were capable of inducing EROD activity (Table 1). When the EC50 for EROD induction was used to judge potency, these six compounds fell into two groups. The most potent group consisted of 2,6-dihydroxyanthraquinone (anthraflavic acid), 1,2,4-trihydroxyanthraquinone (purpurin), and 1,2,10 trihydroxyanthracene (anthrarobin). The second group, which had about half the potency of the first group, was made up of 1,2-dihydroxyanthraquinone (alizarin), 1,3-dihydroxyanthraquinone, and 2-hydroxyanthraquinone. When the maximum induced EROD activity was used to judge potency, six compounds induced to a similar low level, but the seventh, 1,2-dihydroxyanthraquinone, stood out as a strong inducer.

Table 1 – *Anthracene derivatives that induced EROD activity in RTL-W1.*

Compound being tested	Structure	No. of EROD experiments	EC50, nM (±S.D.)	ERODmax, pmol/mgP/min (±S.D.)
Quinones				
2,6-dihydroxy anthraquinone (anthraflavic acid)	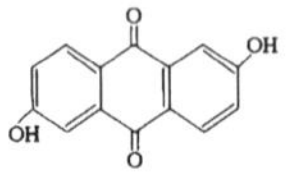	5	1,363.61 (±540.44)	8.79 (±2.74)
1,2,4-trihydroxy anthraquinone (purpurin)	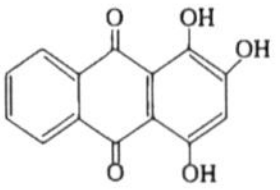	2	2,455.62 (±230.07)	10.84 (±0.82)
1,2-dihydroxy anthraquinone (alizarin)	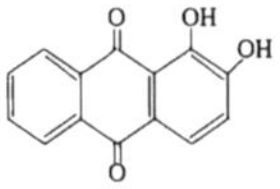	6	4,276.51 (±1,029.55)	29.69 (±8.13)
1,3-dihydroxy anthraquinone	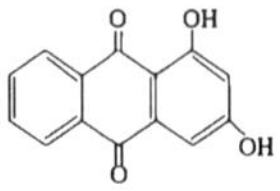	2	4,875.26 (±358.79)	13.38 (±3.16)
2-hydroxy anthraquinone	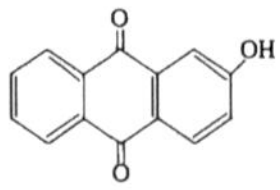	2	5,171.79 (±995.90)	11.68 (±1.59)
Non-quinone				
1,2,10-trihydroxy anthracene (anthrarobin)	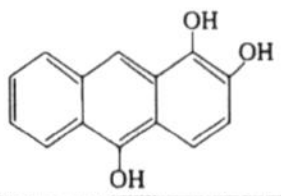	2	2,484.49 (±610.31)	13.71 (±5.19)

The TEF values for the six anthracene derivatives capable of inducing EROD activity in RTL-W1 are listed in Table 2 from most to the least potent. For each compound, TEFs were calculated relative to the EC50 derived previously in RTL-W1 for both TCDD and BaP (Bols et al. 1999). The range from the most potent anthracene derivative, 2,6-dihydroxyanthraquinone, to the least potent, 2-hydroxyanthraquinone, was approximately four-fold.

For six anthracene quinones, no evidence of EROD induction was observed. These quinones are listed in Table 3 along with the range of concentrations tested without EROD activity being induced. As judged from phase-contrast microscopy, signs of cytotoxicity in the cultures were not seen in these experiments. In most cases, the upper limit of the concentration range was dictated by the formation of crystals in the culture wells and/or the potential interference of the compounds with the EROD assay through the emission of fluorescence light.

Table 2 – *TEFs for anthracene derivatives derived from EROD induction in RTL-W1 cells.*

Compound being tested	TCDD TEF[1]	BaP TEF[2]
2,6-dihydroxyanthraquinone	0.000 004 261	0.034
1,2,4-trihydroxyanthraquinone	0.000 002 366	0.019
1,2,10-trihydroxyanthracene	0.000 002 338	0.019
1,2-dihydroxyanthraquinone	0.000 001 358	0.011
1,3-dihydroxyanthraquinone	0.000 001 192	0.010
2-hydroxyanthraquinone	0.000 001 123	0.009

[1]TCDD TEFs were derived by dividing the EC50 for TCDD (5.81 pM, see Bols et al. 1999) by the EC50 for each of the anthracene derivatives.
[2]BaP TEFs were derived by dividing the EC50 for BaP (46.74 nM, see Bols et al. 1999) by the EC50 for each of the anthracene derivatives.

Discussion

Five of the anthracene quionones tested were capable of inducing EROD activity in the cell line from rainbow trout liver, RTL-W1. Their ability to induce EROD activity was in contrast to the inability of the parent compound, anthracene, to act as an EROD inducer in the fish cell line (Bols et al. 1999). The five EROD-inducing quinones, 2,6-dihydroxyanthraquinone, 1,2,4-trihdydroxyanthraquinone, 1,2-dihydroxyanthraquinone, 1,3-dihydroxyanthraquinone and 2-hydroxyanthraquinone, have recently been confirmed as products of the anthracene photodegradation pathway (Mallakin et al. 2000). Upon exposure of an anthracene solution to simulated solar radiation for 9 h, all five quinones were present in the mixture of anthracene and photooxidized anthracene products although their contribution varied, with the 2,6- and the 2-hydroxyanthraquinone being much more prevalent than the 1,2-, 1,3-, and 1,2,4-hydroxyanthraquinones (Mallakin et al. 2000). None of the quinones appear to have previously been studied for their ability to induce EROD activity in fish and only 2,6-dihydroxyanthraquinone was identified as an EROD inducer in rat hepatic microsomal preparations upon intraperitoneal injection

(Ayrton et al. 1988). For the study on rats, 2,6-dihydroxyanthraquinone was selected as a plant-derived anthraquinone with potential anticarcinogenic activities. In the current study, 2,6-dihydroxyanthraquinone and the other anthraquinones were selected as anthracene-derived products that may form upon UV irradiation of anthracene in the environment. In that respect, the current research illustrates an important point for environmental risk assessment: UV treatment of a parent PAH that is not an EROD inducer can yield at least some photomodified products that are EROD inducers.

Table 3 – *Anthracene derivatives that did not induce EROD activity in RTL-W1.*

Compound being tested (all quinones)	Structure	No. of EROD experiments	Concentration range tested, nM	Specific observations
anthraquinone	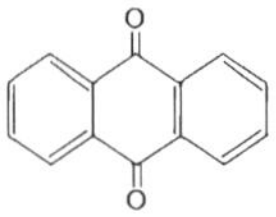	3	0.012-12,481	-
1-hydroxy anthraquinone	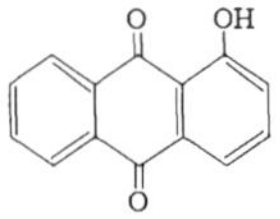	2	0.39-51,066	- crystal formation above 6,383 nM
1,4-dihydroxy anthraquinone (quinizarin)	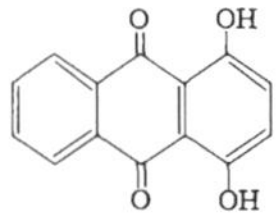	2	2.5-20,815	- crystal formation above 2,602 nM - fluorescence[1] above 650 nM
1,5-dihydroxy anthraquinone (anthrarufin)	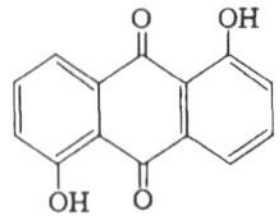	2	0.96-7,904	- crystal formation above 3,952 nM
1,8-dihydroxy anthraquinone (danthron)	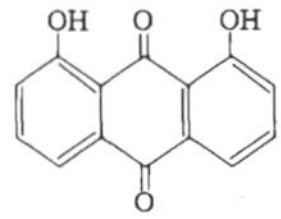	2	8.4-136,880	- crystal formation above 17,110 nM
1,2,5,8-tetrahydroxy anthraquinone (quinalizarin)	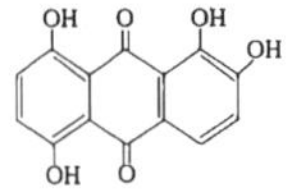	2	4.3-70,350	- crystal formation above 8,794 nM - fluorescence above 275 nM

[1] Fluorescence by the compound was determined for the excitation/emission wavelengths used for resorufin (530±30 nm/595±35 nm) at the end of the exposure period immediately prior to the EROD assay.

Among the five quinones capable of inducing EROD activity in RTL-W1, 2,6-dihydroxyanthraquinone and 2-hydroxyanthraquinone appear to be the most important to consider for their impact in the environment. This is because, in addition to being EROD inducers, these two compounds are photostable and thus are among the end-products of anthracene photomodification (Mallakin et al. 2000, 1999). As such they may persist and potentially accumulate in the environment. Based on the combination of chemical stability and high toxicity to *Lemna gibba*, 2-hydroxyanthraquinone has been suggested previously to be included in the assessment of PAH contaminated environments as an indicator of potentially harmful PAH photooxidation products (Mallakin et al. 1999). The data presented here are in support of this suggestion. However, due to its greater potency, 2,6-dihydroxyanthraquinone may be a more appropriate indicator specifically for PAH photooxidation products that are EROD inducers.

Although not the focus of this study, a few generalizations about the structural requirements for the anthracene derivatives to be EROD inducers in RTL-W1 can be made. The fact that the only non-quinone tested, 1,2,10-trihydroxyanthracene, was an EROD inducer but anthraquinone was not indicates that the quinone structure alone was not adequate for EROD induction to occur but that the hydroxylation pattern was of importance. Hydroxylation in the C1 position appeared not to be a requirement for EROD induction because, except for anthraquinone, all of the non-inducers were C1-hydroxylated. As well, hydroxylations in the 1,4 or 5,8 para-positions did not seem to be of importance. However, one characteristic common to all inducers was the hydroxylation in either the C2 or the C3 position whereas none of the non-inducers were hydroxylated in these position with one exception: 1,2,5,8-tetrahydroxyanthraquinone. However, this quinone could be interfering with the EROD assay due to its autofluorescence at relatively low concentrations. Therefore it cannot entirely be ruled out that, due to high background fluorescence, a small induction of EROD activity by 1,2,5,8-tetrahydroxyanthraquinone might have gone unnoticed in the current study.

As judged from their TCDD- and BaP-TEFs, the potency of the anthracene-derived photooxidation products to act as EROD inducers was low relative to some other classes of environmental contaminants. Previously, TEFs have been derived in RTL-W1 for four dioxins, four furans, seven polychlorinated biphenyls (PCBs) and thirteen PAHs (Bols et al. 1999, 1997; Clemons et al. 1997). The TCDD TEFs for the anthracene derivatives were in the range of the TCDD TEF derived for the least potent PAH, triphenylene, whose TEF again was in the range of TEFs derived for mono-ortho PCBs. For the BaP TEFs, the most potent anthraquinone, 2,6-dihydroxyanthraquinone, was about as potent as triphenylene but was 100-fold less potent than benzo[*k*]fluoranthene. Despite their relatively low potency to induce EROD activity, however, anthracene- and potentially other PAH-photooxidation products should still be investigated for their importance from an environmental risk assessment point of view. This is because the oxidation and hydroxylation reactions of photomodification generally increase the aqueous solubility of the photo-oxidized products, thereby increasing their mobility and potential to interfere with biota (Duxbury et al. 1997). Thus, when toxic equivalency concentrations are being calculated for an environmental sample, the lower potency of the photooxidation products to induce EROD activity might be compensated by their greater presence in the water column.

The ability of some of the anthracene photooxidation products to induce EROD activity, which is a measure of their ability to activate the aryl-hydrocarbon receptor (AhR) signal transduction pathway, should be studied in the future in the light of other modulating processes that have been ascribed to anthraquinones. Most previous reports on anthraquinones have focussed on their biological activities as plant- or fungi-derived, naturally occurring derivatives. For example, 2,6-dihydroxyanthraquinone, the most potent EROD inducer in the current study, has also been shown to be a potent inhibitor of cytochrome P450 activity, thereby inhibiting the mutagenicity of several bay-region diol-epoxides of PAHs (Ayrton et al. 1987; Das et al. 1987). The 1,2-diyhroxyanthraquinone exerted an uncoupling and inhibitory effect on isolated rat liver mitochondria (Kawai et al. 1986). Among the anthraquinones that were unable to induce EROD activity in the current study, 1- and 1,8-hydroxyanthraquinone were genotoxic in the hepatocyte/DNA repair test (Kawai et al. 1986), and induced various tumors in rats (Mori et al. 1990, 1985). These latter two hydroxyanthraquinones were also among those stable under continued UV-irradiation (Mallakin et al. 1999) and thus, they too may be persistent organic chemicals. Only future research that includes a surveillance of photooxidized PAHs in the environment can elucidate the real risk that these chemicals may pose.

Acknowledgment

This research was supported by an NSERC Strategic Grant and by the Canadian Network of Toxicology Centres.

References

Ayrton, A. D., Ioannides, C., and Walker, R., 1988, "Induction of Rat Hepatic Cytochrome P-450 Proteins by the Antimutagen Anthraflavic Acid," *Food Chemistry and Toxicology*, Vol. 26, No. 11/12, pp. 909-915.

Ayrton, A. D., Lewis, D. F. V., Ioannides, C., and Walker, R., 1987, "Anthraflavic Acid is a Potent and Specific Inhibitor of Cytochrome P-448 Activity," *Biochimica et Biophysica Acta*, Vol. 916, pp. 328-331.

Bols, N. C., Schirmer, K., Joyce, E. M., Dixon, D. G., Greenberg, B. M., and Whyte, J. J., 1999, "Ability of Polycyclic Aromatic Hydrocarbons to Induce 7-Ethoxyresorufin-*o*-Deethylase Activity in a Trout Liver Cell Line," *Ecotoxicology and Environmental Safety*, Vol. 44, pp. 118-128.

Bols, N. C., Whyte, J. J., Clemons, J. H., Tom, D. J., van den Heuvel, M., and Dixon, D. G., 1997, "Use of Liver Cell Lines to Develop Toxic Equivalency Factors and to Derive Toxic Equivalent Concentrations in Environmental Samples," *Ecotoxicology: Responses, Biomarkers and Risk Assessment* (J. T. Zelikoff, Ed.), pp. 329-350, SOS Publications, Fair Haven, NJ.

Clemons, J. H., Dixon, D. G., and Bols, N. C., 1997, "Derivation of 2,3,7,8-TCDD Toxic Equivalency Factors (TEFs) for Selected Dioxins, Furans and PCBs with Rainbow Trout and Rat Liver Cell Lines and the Influence of Exposure Time," *Chemosphere*, Vol. 34, pp. 1105-1119.

Das, M., Mukhtar, H., Bik, D. P., and Bickers, D. R., 1987, "Inhibition of Epidermal Xenobiotic Metabolism in SENCAR Mice by Naturally Occurring Plant Phenols," *Cancer Research*, Vol. 47, pp. 760-766.

Delistraty, D., 1997, "Toxic Equivalency Factor Approach for Risk Assessment of Polycyclic Aromatic Hydrocarbons," *Toxicology and Environmental Chemistry*, Vol. 64, pp. 81-108.

Duxbury, C. I., Dixon, D. G., and Greenberg, B. M., 1997, "The Effects of Simulated Solar Radiation on the Bioaccumulation of Polycyclic Aromatic Hydrocarbons by the Duckweed *Lemna gibba*," *Environmental Toxicology and Chemistry*, Vol. 16, 1739-1748.

Eadon, G., Kaminsky, L., Silkworth, J., Aldous, K., Hilker, D., O'Keefe, P., Smith, R., Gierthy, J., Hawley, J., Kim, N., and DeCaprio, A., 1986, "Calculation of 2,3,7,8-TCDD Equivalent Concentrations of Complex Environmental Contaminant Mixtures," *Environmental Health Perspectives*, Vol. 70, pp. 221-227.

Ioannides, C., and Parke, D. V., 1993, "Induction of Cytochrome P4501A as an Indicator of Potential Chemical Carcinogenesis," *Drug Metabolism Reviews*, Vol. 254, pp. 485-501.

Kawai, K., Mori, H., Sugie, S., Yoshimi, N., Inoue, T., Nakamaru, T., Nozawa, Y., and Matsushima, T., 1986, "Genotoxicity in the Hepatocyte/DNA Repair Test and Toxicity to Liver Mitochondria of 1-Hydroxyanthraquinone and Several Dihydroxyanthraquinones," *Cell Biology and Toxicology*, Vol. 2, No. 4, pp. 457-467.

Lee, L. E. J., Clemons, J. H., Bechtel, D. G., Caldwell, S. J., Han, K.-B., Pasitschniak-Arts, M., Mosser, D. D., and Bols, N. C., 1993, "Development and Characterization of a Rainbow Trout Liver Cell Line Expressing Cytochrome P450-Dependent Mono-Oxygenase Activity," *Cell Biology and Toxicology*, Vol. 9, pp. 279-294.

Lorenzen, A., and Kennedy, S. W., 1993, "A Fluorescence-Based Protein Assay for Use with a Microplate Reader," *Analytical Biochemistry*, Vol. 214, pp. 346-348.

Mallakin, A., Dixon, D. G., and Greenberg, B. M., 2000, "Pathway of Anthracene Modification Under Simulated Solar Radiation," *Chemosphere*, Vol. 40, No. 12, pp. 131-137.

Mallakin, A., McConkey, B. J., Miao, G., McKibben, B., Sniekus, V., Dixon, D. G., and Greenberg, B. M., 1999, "Impacts of Structural Photomodification on the Toxicity of Environmental Contaminants: Anthracene Photooxidation Products," *Ecotoxicology and Environmental Safety*, Vol. 43, No. 2, pp. 204-212.

Mori, H., Yoshimi, N., Iwata, H., Mori, Y., Hara, A., Tanaka, T., and Kawai, K., 1990, "Carcinogenicity of Naturally Occurring 1-Hydroxyanthraquinone in Rats: Induction of Large Bowel, Liver and Stomach Neoplasms," *Carcinogenesis*, Vol. 11, pp. 799-802.

Mori, H., Sugie, S., and Takahashi, K., 1985, "Induction of Intestinal Tumors in Rat by Chrysazin," *British Journal of Cancer*, Vol. 52, pp. 781-783.

Sadar, M. D., Ash, R., Sundqvist, J., Olsson, P-E., and Andersson, T. B., 1996, "Phenobarbital Induction of CYP1A1 Gene Expression in a Primary Culture of Rainbow Trout Hepatocytes," *Journal of Biological Chemistry*, Vol. 271, No. 30, pp. 17635-17643.

Wang, X., and Sniekus, V., 1990, "Regioselective Synthesis of Substituted Anthraquinones by Tandem Directed *Ortho* Metalation-Metal Halogen Exchange," *Synlett*, Vol. 6, pp. 313-316.

Christopher A. Marwood,[1] Evan Dobson,[2] Ralph E. H. Smith,[1] Keith R. Solomon,[2] and Bruce M. Greenberg[1]

Chlorophyll Fluorescence as a Bioindicator of Photosynthesis Inhibition from Solar Ultraviolet Radiation in Plants and Algae

---

Reference: Marwood, C. A., Dobson, E., Smith, R. E. H., Solomon, K. R., and Greenberg, B. M., **"Chlorophyll Fluorescence as a Bioindicator of Photosynthesis Inhibition from Solar Ultraviolet Radiation in Plants and Algae,"** *Environmental Toxicology and Risk Assessment: Science, Policy and Standardization – Implications for Environmental Decisions: Tenth Volume, ASTM STP 1403*, B. M. Greenberg, R. N. Hull, M. H. Roberts, Jr., and R. W. Gensemer, Eds., American Society for Testing and Materials, West Conshohocken, PA, 2001.

Abstract: Chlorophyll fluorescence is a simple, rapid technique for measuring photosynthetic efficiency in plants and algae. Pulse-amplitude modulated chlorophyll fluorescence was examined in aquatic plants and natural assemblages of Lake Erie phytoplankton exposed to solar ultraviolet (UV) radiation. UV-exclusion studies were performed in which plastic films were used to screen sunlight to remove ultraviolet-B radiation (295-320 nm), or UVB plus ultraviolet-A radiation (320-400 nm) in outdoor aquatic microcosms and ship exposure chambers. UV had negligible impacts on photosynthesis and growth in the aquatic macrophyte *Myriophyllum spicatum* in microcosms. However, photosynthetic electron transport in natural assemblages of Lake Erie phytoplankton was substantially diminished by short exposures to full sunlight. Phytoplankton exposed to full sunlight for 30 min lost 90 % of maximum photosystem II efficiency (F_v/F_m) and 75 % of the effective yield of photosystem II photochemistry ($\Delta F/F_m'$). Diminished photosynthetic electron transport was primarily due to UVB wavelengths in sunlight. UVA and visible wavelengths also diminished photosynthetic electron transport to a lesser extent. Thus, this assay represents a general bioindicator of effects from environmental stress in freshwater plants and algae that is able to detect impacts due to current and increasing levels of UVB.

Keywords: Plants, ultraviolet radiation, microcosms, phytoplankton, chlorophyll fluorescence, photosynthesis, bioindicator

[1]Post-doctoral fellow, professor, and professor, respectively, Department of Biology, University of Waterloo, Waterloo, Ontario, N2L 3G1, Canada.
[2]Research technician and professor, respectively, Centre for Toxicology, University of Guelph, Guelph, Ontario, N1G 2W1, Canada.

Introduction

Although there are abundant biological assays for assessing exposure to contaminants and environmental stresses, laboratory studies alone are insufficient to predict effects in the environment. There is a need in ecotoxicology for bioindicators that have been validated in the field. Bioindicators are biochemical or physiological endpoints of exposure to, or effects of, environmental stress which can be measured rapidly. Chlorophyll-*a* (Chl_a) fluorescence induction is a well understood approach for measuring photosynthesis in plants and algae. This assay is a potential bioindicator of effects, as impacts on photosynthesis generally result in deleterious effects on plant growth or development. Chl_a fluorescence possesses several advantages over conventional techniques for measuring photosynthesis. Measurements can be taken rapidly from plant leaves in situ, with little or no preparation, and without extensive experience in the technique. Several useful parameters, each describing the efficiency of a specific photosynthetic process, can be calculated within minutes from Chl_a fluorescence measurements using a pulse-amplitude modulated (PAM) fluorometer. F_v/F_m, measured from plants in the dark, describes the maximum efficiency of PSII electron transport. The corresponding PSII efficiency in light-adapted plants, $\Delta F/F_m'$, is equivalent to the quantum yield of PSII photosynthesis, and is closely correlated with carbon assimilation (Genty et al. 1989). The extent of fluorescence quenching due to photochemical (i.e., electron transport) and nonphotochemical processes (dissipation of excess energy) are described by the parameters qP and qN, respectively.

Chl_a fluorescence has been found to be remarkably consistent in many different higher plants and algal groups, reflecting the strict conservation of photosynthetic mechanisms throughout the plant kingdom (Bolhàr-Nordenkampf et al. 1989). At the same time, Chl_a fluorescence parameters have been found to be sensitive to various environmental stresses such as strong light, drought, low temperature, pathogen infection and acid rain, as well as exposure to various herbicides (Lichtenthaler and Rinderle 1988, Huner et al. 1998). Despite the widespread use of Chl_a fluorescence in plant physiology and agricultural research, this technique has not been used extensively in environmental risk assessment because effects of many environmental stresses on Chl_a fluorescence have not been assessed in natural systems, and links between effects at the suborganismal level and effects at higher levels of biological organization (e.g., organism, population, community) have not been demonstrated.

Ultraviolet-B radiation (UVB, 290-320 nm) is one environmental stress that has received much attention recently. Depletion of stratospheric ozone has resulted in increased solar UVB radiation in the environment (Kerr and McElroy 1993). Although UVB is attenuated in freshwater systems, effects on organisms near the surface can be substantial (Kirk 1994). Detrimental effects of UVB have been demonstrated in a variety of freshwater and marine macrophytes and algae. In almost all species examined, primary productivity and growth is diminished by exposure to UV (Strid et al. 1990, Herrmann et al. 1997, Nilawati et al. 1997). Photosynthesis appears to be a primary target of UV radiation. Elevated UV levels result in increased turnover of the photosystem II (PSII) D1 protein (Greenberg et al. 1987), reduced pigment content (Marwood and Greenberg 1996), and diminished rates of photosynthetic electron transport (Herrmann et al. 1997, Marwood et al. 2000).

Artificial lighting supplemented with UV lamps has often been used in laboratory studies of UVB impacts (Chalker-Scott 1995, Gerber and Häder 1995). However, laboratory studies can not reproduce the high photon fluence rates of ultraviolet-A (UVA, 320-400 nm) and photosynthetically active radiation (PAR, 400-700 nm) found in natural sunlight. These wavebands have been shown to ameliorate UVB damage in higher plants by photoactivation repair of DNA lesions (Britt 1995). Moreover, effects on individual species cannot predict complex ecosystem responses to UV radiation. In natural systems, allocation of photosynthetic products in phytoplankton is affected by UV (Furgal et al. 1998), which can affect the grazing rates of zooplankton (Hessen et al. 1997). UV can also directly affect species composition and interactions between trophic levels of natural communities (Bothwell et al. 1994).

Freshwater microcosms, experimental ponds and limnocorrals are the most useful approach for studying effects of environmental stresses such as UVB radiation and chemical contaminants on freshwater communities (Solomon et al. 1986, Shaw and Manning 1996). Microcosms are semi-natural systems designed to represent natural ecosystems, while still retaining a sufficiently small size that parameters of interest can be controlled practically. Two experimental approaches may be used in field studies with UV radiation: natural light can be supplemented with UV radiation from lamps, or UV can be selectively excluded from natural sunlight. Enhancing UV may be more predictive of future trends as ozone depletion continues; however, that experimental strategy is technically complex because it requires uniform illumination of the system and simulation of daily UV irradiance cycles. Also, interpretation of results is difficult because the quantity and quality of the supplemental UV radiation produced by lamps is always different than natural UV radiation (Greenberg et al. 1995). Alternatively, UV exclusion experiments are useful in mechanistic studies of UV effects. These types of studies have none of the problems associated with interpreting differences between natural and artificial sources of UV. However, studies using exclusion designs are limited by the UV radiation levels currently found in sunlight, and subtle effects may be difficult to discern.

This paper describes UV-exclusion studies in which Chl_a fluorescence was used to examine the relative effects of PAR, UVA and UVB radiation on photosynthesis and growth of freshwater plants. Filters consisting of plastic films with specific transmission properties were used to exclude solar UV radiation from large outdoor freshwater microcosms. A similar system of filters was used to examine the effects of UV exposure in natural assemblages of phytoplankton from Lake Erie.

Materials and Methods

Freshwater Microcosms

UV exclusion experiments were performed using rooted Eurasian Milfoil (*Myriophyllum spicatum* L.) growing in freshwater microcosms approximately 3.9 m in diameter and 1 m deep. Polymer films were suspended over six microcosms using wooden frames onto which sheets of plastic film were affixed (Fig. 1). Ten frames were constructed of untreated spruce to cover each microcosm. Frequent sampling and other requirements such as water evaporation necessitated elevating the screens above the microcosms and offsetting the rows of screens. The frames were suspended 0.5 m over the microcosms on stainless steel cables supported by posts driven into the ground (Fig. 1). Four sets of cables were suspended over each pond, at 0.5 m and 0.66 m above the water, allowing the polymer films to be positioned at an angle of 8° to the south horizon when the northern edge of the frame was placed on the higher cable and the southern edge on the lower cable. The frames supporting the polymer films were suspended over each microcosm in an overlapping pattern which provided complete overhead coverage while minimizing the shade cast on the microcosm. The three rows of frames overlapped by approximately 20 cm, ensuring complete coverage of the microcosm during most of the day.

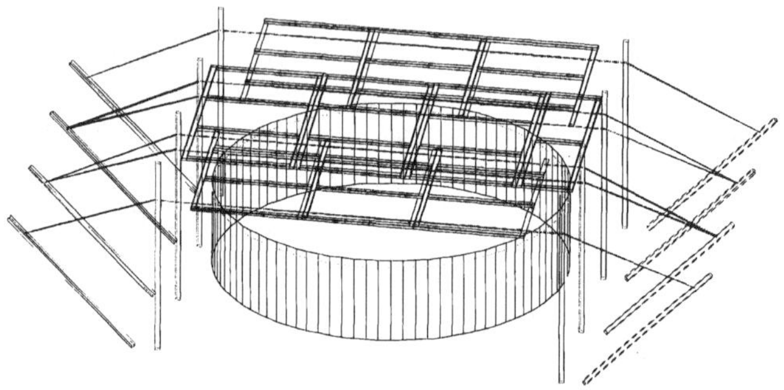

Figure 1 – *System for suspending polymer films over outdoor microcosms.*

Three light regimes were established by using three different polymer films which attenuated specific wavelengths in the UV region (Greenberg et al. 1995). One pair of microcosms was screened with a layer of polyethylene (PE) film (0.08 mm, Johnston Plastics, Mississauga, ON) which was transparent in both UVB (290-320 nm) and UVA (320-400 nm) regions. A second pair of microcosms was screened with a layer of polyester film (Mylar-D; 0.08 mm, Johnston Plastics) which removed UVB radiation. A third pair of microcosms was covered with a polycarbonate (PC) sheet (1.6 mm, Johnston Plastics) which removed both UVA and UVB wavelengths. The transmission of all three films to PAR (400-700 nm), as measured with a scanning spectrophotometer was 90 to 95 %. In outdoor UV exclusion studies, frequent replacement of polymer films is desirable to compensate for deterioration of transmission properties in prolonged sunlight exposure (Greenberg et al. 1995). However, the expense of the film material prohibits frequent replacement. Therefore, films were replaced once during the study, after six weeks.

The effectiveness of the UV-screening system was tested by measuring solar spectra beneath the polymer films on a clear, cloudless day in August between 12:00 h and 14:00 h. A calibrated diode array spectroradiometer with an integrating sphere (Oriel Inc., Stratford, CT) was used to record spectra from 280-780 nm. Measurements were taken 20 cm above the water surface. For each microcosm, four spectra 30 cm from the sides of the microcosm, plus one spectrum at the center of the microcosm were measured. The irradiance of UVB, UVA and PAR wavebands were converted to photon fluence rates. For each microcosm, five spectra measurements were averaged. A generalized plant damage spectrum (Caldwell et al. 1980) was used to calculate biologically effective UVB (UVB_{BE}) values based on an eight-hour exposure to sunlight.

Short (3 cm) lengths from terminal shoot tips of *M. spicatum* were sampled for Chl_a fluorescence at midday after one, two and four weeks in the microcosms. Chl_a fluorescence was measured from whole plant tips immersed in pond water in petri dishes. Measurements were taken from three plants in each microcosm. The means of the two replicate microcosms were calculated for each treatment. A one-way ANOVA was used to test for significant differences between light treatments.

Seasonal plant growth was determined by harvesting all *M. spicatum* biomass above the sediment at the end of the experiment. Excess water was removed using a salad spinner, and plant material was weighed. A one-way ANOVA was used to test for significant differences between treatments.

Lake Erie Phytoplankton

Experiments were performed aboard C.C.G.S. *Limnos* (Canada Center for Inland Waters, Burlington, Ontario, Canada) between July 6-10, 1998. Whole water was sampled from the central basin (Fig. 2) from a depth of 5 m at 06:00 h and stored in carboys in the dark. Aliquots of 200 mL of water were transferred into clear polyethylene bags (First Brands Corporation, Scarborough, Ontario), which were floated in shipboard exposure chambers consisting of shallow boxes fastened to the ship's deck, with continuous lake water circulation to maintain samples at the surface water temperature. Samples were exposed for 30, 60 and 120 minutes at solar noon to direct sunlight screened through cellulose acetate film, which transmitted all wavelengths, or through Mylar-D or PC. Following exposure, samples were transferred to exposure chambers screened with black plastic to allow recovery for one, two, or four hours in low (5 %) light. Phytoplankton from 200 mL of exposed water samples and dark control samples were concentrated on 25 mm glass fiber filters (GF/C; Whatman, Springfield Mill, UK) under low vacuum. Chl_a fluorescence was measured directly from phytoplankton on moist filters floating on filtered lake filter.

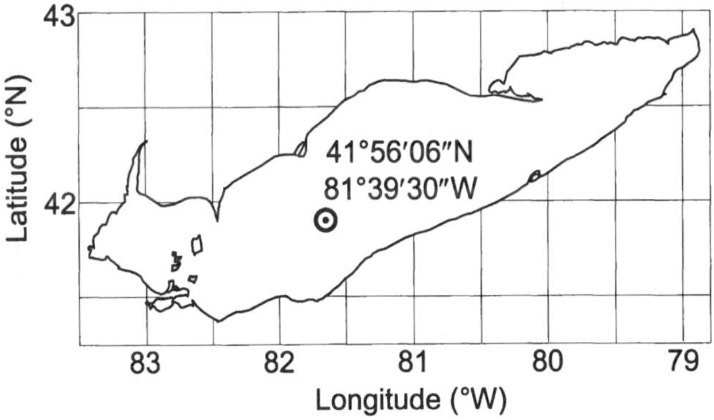

Figure 2 – *Lake Erie sampling site for UV-exclusion experiments.*

Solar spectra from 280-780 nm were recorded midway through the exposure using a calibrated diode array spectroradiometer (Oriel Inc.). Photon fluence rates for each exposure were calculated for each waveband (PAR, UVA and UVB). Biologically effective UVB (UVB_{BE}) was calculated using a weighting function for the inhibition of phytoplankton photosynthesis (Cullen et al. 1992) normalized at 300 nm.

*Chlorophyll-*a *Fluorescence*

A pulse-amplitude modulated fluorometer (PAM-2000, Walz, Effeltrich, Germany) was used to measure Chl_a fluorescence from plants or algae which had been dark-adapted for 15 min prior to measurement. Initial fluorescence (F_o) was measured with a weak red light (< 1 μmol m^{-2} s^{-1}). Dark-adapted maximum fluorescence (F_m) was produced by a single 0.6 s saturating pulse of white light (3400 μmol m^{-2} s^{-1}). Red light (655 nm, 22 μmol m^{-2} s^{-1}) was used to induce photosynthesis. Steady-state fluorescence (F_s) and light-adapted maximum fluorescence (F_m') were measured after 10 min. $\Delta F/F_m'$ (the effective yield of photosystem II photochemistry) was calculated according to Genty et al. (1989). The Chl_a fluorescence parameters F_v/F_m (the maximum efficiency of electron transport in photosystem II), qP (photochemical quenching) and qN (nonphotochemical quenching) were calculated according to standard equations (van Kooten and Snel 1990). Because nonphotochemical quenching is elevated in stressed plants, the normalized parameter 1–qN was compared with other parameters. It was not possible to accurately measure qP and qN parameters from Lake Erie phytoplankton samples with a low fluorescence signal.

Results

Freshwater Microcosms

Ultraviolet radiation was attenuated to varying degrees in all three light treatments. PE did not substantially alter the spectral quality of sunlight (Table 1). Mylar-D films attenuated negligible amounts of UVA radiation, but reduced UVB radiation to less than 25 % of the PE-covered microcosms. PC filters removed about 75 % of the UVA radiation compared to PE, and reduced fluence rates of UVB to about 10 % of the level in PE-screened microcosms. PAR fluence rates in all three light regimes were comparable. Shading from the suspension system used to support the films over the microcosms resulted in 15 to 25 % attenuation of PAR (Table 1).

The biologically effective UVB fluence rate (UVB_{BE}) was calculated for each microcosm using an action spectrum for generalized plant damage (Caldwell et al. 1980). UVB_{BE} in Mylar- and PC-screened microcosms was negligible, but UVB_{BE} in unscreened sunlight was about 1.5 times greater than the PE-screened microcosms (Table 1). Thus, although PE filtered a small amount of the solar UVB waveband, it altered the spectral quality by selectively removing lower wavelength photons.

Table 1 – *Surface solar photon fluence rates and biologically effective UVB (UVB_{BE}) in screened microcosms. The means of five measurements (± standard error) are shown.*

Light Treatment	Screen[1]	Photon Fluence Rate, μmol m^{-2} s^{-1} PAR[2]	UVA	UVB	UVB_{BE}, μmol m^{-2} s^{-1}
Full Sunlight	None	1965.1	144.5	5.64	0.501
PAR+UVA+UVB	PE	1519.6	99.5	4.34	0.304
		(117.0)	(5.4)	(0.49)	(0.083)
PAR+UVA	M	1701.5	103.5	1.05	0.0497
		(59.8)	(6.7)	(0.06)	(0.0144)
PAR	PC	1652.1	26.1	0.50	0.0999
		(80.1)	(0.03)	(0.05)	(0.0594)

[1]PE = Polyethylene; M = Mylar-D polyester; PC = polycarbonate.
[2]PAR = photosynthetically active radiation (400-700 nm); UVA = ultraviolet-A (320-400 nm); UVB = ultraviolet-B (290-320 nm).

All four Chl_a fluorescence parameters measured from *M. spicatum* in the different light treatments were similar, with the exception of 1–qN, which was significantly ($\alpha = 0.05$) lower in unscreened microcosms compared to all other treatments (Table 2). All parameters were consistently higher in plants from PE-screened microcosms compared to the other treatments, but the differences were small and not statistically significant ($\alpha = 0.05$).

Table 2 – *Effect of light quality on Chl_a fluorescence parameters in* M. spicatum. *The means from three plants in each microcosm are shown (± standard errors).*

Light Treatment[1]	Screen[2]	F_v/F_m	$\Delta F/F_m'$	qP	1–qN
Full Sunlight	None	0.759	0.673	0.947	0.687
		(0.013)	(0.021)	(0.017)	(0.043)
PAR+UVA+UVB	PE	0.740	0.676	0.949	0.810
		(0.011)	(0.014)	(0.006)	(0.031)
PAR+UVA	M	0.691	0.620	0.935	0.802
		(0.021)	(0.026)	(0.010)	(0.033)
PAR	PC	0.695	0.614	0.923	0.792
		(0.016)	(0.026)	(0.010)	(0.046)

[1]PAR = photosynthetically active radiation, 400-700 nm; UVA = ultraviolet-A, 320-400 nm; UVB = ultraviolet-B, 295-320 nm.
[2]PE = Polyethylene; M = Mylar-D polyester; PC = polycarbonate.

M. spicatum biomass in unscreened microcosms was lower than any of the screened microcosms (Table 3). The greatest plant biomass was found in microcosms receiving PAR plus UVA. The mean biomass accumulation for this treatment was 63 % greater than microcosms receiving PAR only, and 32 % greater than those receiving PAR+UVA+UVB. However, there was moderate variability in replicate samples, and no statistically significant differences ($\alpha = 0.05$) between light treatments was found.

Table 3 – *Biomass accumulation (± standard error) of* M. spicatum *plants in freshwater microcosms.*

Treatment[1]	Screen	Biomass, g
Full Sunlight	None	64.2 (6.8)
PAR+UVA+UVB	Polyethylene	103.1 (21.1)
PAR+UVA	Mylar-D	137.0 (18.4)
PAR	Polycarbonate	84.3 (10.2)

[1]PAR = photosynthetically active radiation, 400-700 nm; UVA = ultraviolet-A, 320-400 nm; UVB = ultraviolet-B, 295-320 nm.

Lake Erie Phytoplankton

The UV-screened shipboard exposure chambers used for the exposure of Lake Erie phytoplankton had the same transmission properties as the filters covering the freshwater microcosms, but Lake Erie samples received greater sunlight fluence rates because no frame system was required to hold the filters. Sunlight measured during the exposure period contained 2002, 136 and 5.5 μmol m^{-2} s^{-1} of PAR, UVA and UVB, respectively. The UVB_{BE} using Cullen's phytoplankton weighting factor was 1.33 μmol m^{-2} s^{-1}.

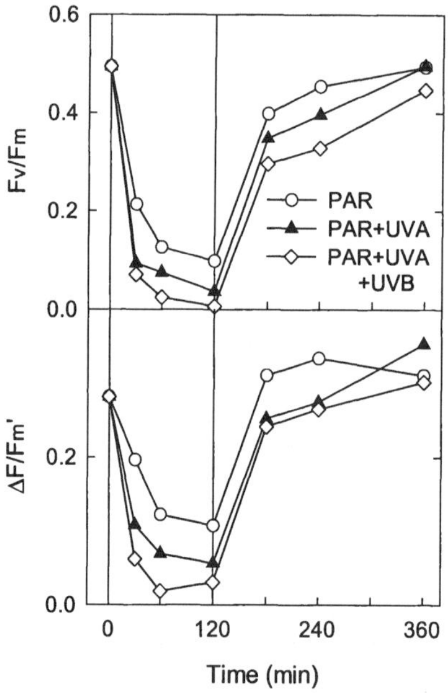

Figure 3 – *Photoinhibition and recovery of photosynthesis in natural assemblages of Lake Erie phytoplankton exposed to solar radiation. Efficiency of PS II electron transport (F_v/F_m) and effective quantum yield of PSII photochemistry ($\Delta F/F_m'$) were measured from phytoplankton exposed to direct sunlight for various times up to 120 min and allowed to recover in low light for up to 4 h.*

Exposure to sunlight caused rapid and strong inhibition of photosynthesis (Fig. 3). Phytoplankton exposed to UVB consistently exhibited greater inhibition of photosynthetic efficiency than samples exposed to UVA, which were inhibited more than those exposed to PAR only. After 120 min in sunlight, phytoplankton exposed to PAR had F_v/F_m values that were only 20 % of those measured in unexposed controls, while cells exposed to PAR plus UVA were inhibited to 7 % of control values. Phytoplankton exposed for the same length of time to the entire solar spectrum including UVB were diminished to only 1 % of unexposed F_v/F_m values, indicating extensive photoinhibition. $\Delta F/F_m'$ measured in the same samples followed a similar trend as F_v/F_m, although $\Delta F/F_m'$ was diminished less than unexposed samples. For both parameters, most of the inhibition occurred within the first 30 min exposure.

Recovery of photosynthetic efficiency was somewhat slower than the kinetics of exposure, with full recovery of F_v/F_m requiring 4 h in low light conditions (Fig. 3). Recovery from photoinhibition proceeded at the same rate in each of the three light treatments: the magnitude of recovery during each time period was the same for each treatment. Thus, phytoplankton exposed to UVB had consistently lower F_v/F_m and $\Delta F/F_m'$ compared to the PAR and PAR plus UVA treatments, up to 4 h recovery, at which point Chl_a fluorescence had returned to control levels in all treatments. After 4 h recovery, samples exposed to PAR plus UVA had the highest values of $\Delta F/F_m'$.

Discussion

One difficulty in the assessment of plant responses to UV in the field is the construction of screening systems on a large scale. The system of polymer films described here was effective at excluding UVA and UVB radiation from outdoor microcosms. This design could easily be modified to allow the incorporation of lamps to supplement UV radiation in freshwater microcosms. The overall transmission of the screening system to PAR wavelengths was similar for the three materials used, and the small area of the frames in relation to the area of the microcosms produced minimal shading. However, shade effects, or possibly the removal of low-wavelength UVB from screened ponds, may have influenced photosynthesis in *M. spicatum*, as the most substantial difference in Chl_a fluorescence parameters was observed between plants in unscreened microcosms *vs.* other treatments. Additionally, plant biomass accumulation was greater in screened microcosms, suggesting the minor quantity of UVB photons screened by the polyethylene were the most effective at inhibiting photosynthesis, and thus, plant growth. Plant growth in all microcosms demonstrated high variability, which is often observed in microcosm studies. Although the filters effectively removed UVB and UVA, differences in Chl_a fluorescence parameters or growth were insignificant compared to natural variability, and no significant differences between any of the light treatments were seen. There was a trend toward higher values in plants exposed to more of the solar spectrum (i.e., PAR+UVA+UVB) for all parameters, but it may have been due to the differences in PAR transmitted by each filter, rather than due to the presence or absence of any particular waveband. These results underscore the difficulty of minimizing confounding effects in outdoor UV studies.

In Lake Erie phytoplankton, effects of UV wavelengths in sunlight were substantial and distinct from PAR effects. Although PAR also diminished F_v/F_m and $\Delta F/F_m'$, the greatest inhibition was in algae exposed to the full solar spectrum. On a quantum basis, UVB effects were much stronger than PAR or UVA, as there was much less UVB in sunlight. The distinct effects of PAR and UVB are consistent with different targets for inhibition of photosynthesis by PAR and UV. Reduced photosynthetic efficiency from exposure to high PAR fluence is due to short-term down-regulation of electron transport in PSII and increased dissipation of energy to xanthophyll pigments which do not contribute to photosynthesis (Long et al. 1994). If the photon fluence rate exceeds the capacity of the xanthophyll cycle to successfully dissipate excess energy as heat, increased degradation of the D1 protein occurs (Long et al. 1994). Like PAR photoinhibition, increased degradation of D1 is a major effect of UV photodamage, but UVB has many other targets, including DNA (Gieskes and Buma 1997), proteins such as Rubisco (Wilson et al. 1995), membrane components (Hessen et al. 1997), and the D2 protein of PSII (Jansen et al. 1996). In the marine diatom *Phaeodactylum tricornutum*, excess PAR and UVB have been shown to have different effects on Chl_a fluorescence parameters, suggesting a different mechanism for photodamage from UVB (Wilhelm et al. 1997).

Although previous studies have demonstrated photoinhibition in phytoplankton exposed to sunlight for up to one photoperiod (Gala and Giesy 1991, Furgal and Smith 1997), in this study substantial inhibition of Chl_a fluorescence was detected within just 30 min. Rapid detection of photoinhibition is one advantage of PAM fluorescence over traditional methods of measuring photosynthesis. ^{14}C-incorporation experiments in particular require several hours to perform, and therefore do not have the time resolution required to detect rapid effects of light exposure on photosynthesis.

Photoinhibition in Lake Erie phytoplankton occurred with faster kinetics than recovery. Cells exposed to the full solar spectra were completely inhibited after only 30 min exposure, but recovery back to the level found in unexposed samples required 2 h under low light conditions for $\Delta F/F_m'$, and 4 h for F_v/F_m. The length of exposure seemed to have little effect on recovery, in that shorter exposures required the same recovery time as longer exposures. This effect has been noted previously in green algae exposed to sunlight for short time periods similar to this study (Herrmann et al. 1997).

Greater inhibition of Chl_a fluorescence parameters in samples exposed to PAR plus UVA than PAR alone indicate UVA was responsible for a portion of photoinhibition in Lake Erie phytoplankton. In some environments, UVA has been reported to be responsible for a major fraction of photoinhibition (Hessen et al. 1997, Smith et al. 1998), but UVA may also be beneficial for attenuating UVB effects (Quesada et al. 1995). UVA is not attenuated in the water column as much as UVB, and thus UVA penetrates to greater depths (Kirk 1994). In freshwater systems where vertical mixing rates are lower, UVA may be a more important factor than UVB in the inhibition of primary production.

The short exposure times used here were likely a realistic exposure scenario for phytoplankton in a shallow mixed water column which can cycle in less than an hour (Long et al. 1994, Smith et al. 1998). Vertical mixing, combined with the shading effects of clouds, creates a variable light environment for phytoplankton in the water column, and photoinhibition is likely to occur frequently during each photoperiod. However, mixing of the water column can mitigate the effects of light on phytoplankton assemblages by reducing the exposure time at the surface to full sunlight and allowing exposed cells to recover at a lower light fluence. Thus, the overall effect of mixing on primary production in the water column will depend on mixing rates and the kinetics of photoinhibition and recovery. However, short periods of photosynthetic inhibition would be expected to have deleterious effects on overall water column primary production, due in part to the short life span of phytoplankton.

Because PSII is the first step in photosynthetic electron transport, inhibition of electron transport at any point after PSII will exert excitation pressure on PSII, and can be detected as diminished $\Delta F/F_m'$ (Huang et al. 1997, Huner et al. 1998). $\Delta F/F_m'$ estimates PSII photosynthetic yield (ϕ_{PSII}) and is strongly correlated with carbon assimilation by electron transport downstream from PSII (Genty et al. 1989). This parameter is a function of both electron transport through PSII and non-photochemical quenching (qN) which attenuates PSII efficiency (Genty et al. 1989). Thus, this parameter integrates effects on many processes which contribute to inhibition of electron transport, either by decreasing the quantum yield of photochemistry or by increasing the yield of non-photochemical, thermal decay processes. The ability of Chl_a fluorescence to detect diminished electron transport resulting from UV radiation suggests this assay may be a general bioindicator of effects from a variety of environmental stressors with non-specific modes of action.

Acknowledgments

This work was supported by grants from the Canadian Network of Toxicology Centres (K.R.S. and B.M.G.) and the Natural Sciences and Engineering Research Council (B.M.G.), as well as ship time, equipment and a Science Horizons grant from Environment Canada.

References

Bolhàr-Nordenkampf, H. R., Long, S. P., Baker, N. R., Öquist, G., Schreiber, U., and Lechner, E. G., 1989, "Chlorophyll Fluorescence as a Probe of the Photosynthetic Competence of Leaves in the Field: A Review of Current Instrumentation," *Functional Ecology,* Vol. 3, pp. 497-514.

Bothwell, M. L., Sherbot, D. M. J., and Pollock, C. M., 1994, "Ecosystem Response to Solar Ultraviolet-B Radiation: Influence of Trophic-Level Interactions," *Science,* Vol. 265, pp. 97-100.

Britt, A. B., 1995, "Repair of DNA Damage Induced by Ultraviolet Radiation," *Plant Physiology,* Vol. 108, pp. 891-896.

Caldwell, M. M., Robberecht, R., and Billings, W. D., 1980, "A Steep Latitudinal Gradient of Solar Ultraviolet-B Radiation in the Arctic-Alpine Life Zone," *Ecology,* Vol. 61, pp. 601-611.

Chalker-Scott, L., 1995, "Survival and Sex Ratios of the Intertidal Copepod, *Tigriopus californicus*, Following Ultraviolet-B (290-320 nm) Radiation Exposure," *Marine Biology,* Vol. 123, pp. 799-804.

Cullen, J. J., Neale, P. J., and Lesser, M. P., 1992, "Biological Weighting Function for the Inhibition of Phytoplankton Photosynthesis by Ultraviolet Radiation," *Science,* Vol. 258, pp. 646-650.

Furgal, J. A. and Smith, R. E. H., 1997, "Ultraviolet Radiation and Photosynthesis by Georgian Bay Phytoplankton of Varying Nutrient and Photoadaptive Status," *Canadian Journal of Fisheries and Aquatic Sciences,* Vol. 54, pp. 1659-1667.

Furgal, J. A., Taylor, W. D., and Smith, R. E. H., 1998, "Environmental Control of Photosynthate Allocation in the Phytoplankton of Georgian Bay (Lake Huron)," *Canadian Journal of Fisheries and Aquatic Sciences,* Vol. 55, pp. 726-736.

Gala, W. R. and Giesy, J. P., 1991, "Effects of Ultraviolet Radiation on the Primary Production of Natural Phytoplankton Assemblages in Lake Michigan," *Ecotoxicology and Environmental Safety,* Vol. 22, pp. 345-361.

Genty, B., Briantais, J.-M., and Baker, N. R., 1989, "The Relationship Between the Quantum Yield of Photosynthetic Electron Transport and Quenching of Chlorophyll Fluorescence," *Biochimica et Biophysica Acta,* Vol. 990, pp. 87-92.

Gerber, S. and Häder, D. P., 1995, "Effects of Artificial UV-B and Simulated Solar Radiation on the Flagellate *Euglena gracilis*: Physiological, Spectroscopical and Biochemical Investigations," *Acta Protozoologica,* Vol. 34, pp. 13-20.

Gieskes, W. W. C. and Buma, A. G. J., 1997, "UV Damage to Plant Life in a Photobiologically Dynamic Environment: The Case of Marine Phytoplankton," *Plant Ecology,* Vol. 128, pp. 16-25.

Greenberg, B. M., Dixon, D. G., Wilson, M. I., Huang, X.-D., McConkey, B. J., Duxbury, C. L., Gerhardt, K., and Gensemer, R. W., 1995. "Use of Artificial Lighting in Environmental Assessment Studies," *Environmental Toxicology and Risk Assessment: 4th Volume, ASTM STP 1262*, LaPoint, T. M., Price, F. T. and Little, E. E., Eds., American Society for Testing and Materials, West Conshohocken, PA, U.S.A., pp. 55-70.

Greenberg, B. M., Gaba, V., Mattoo, A. K., and Edelman, M., 1987, "Identification of a Primary *In Vivo* Degradation Product of the Rapidly-Turning-Over 32 kDa Protein of Photosystem II," *EMBO Journal,* Vol. 6, pp. 2865-2869.

Herrmann, H., Häder, D.-P., and Ghetti, F., 1997, "Inhibition of Photosynthesis by Solar Radiation in *Dunaliella salina*: Relative Efficiencies of UV-B, UV-A and PAR," *Plant, Cell and Environment,* Vol. 20, pp. 359-365.

Hessen, D. O., De Lange, H. J., and Van Donk, E., 1997, "UV-Induced Changes in Phytoplankton Cells and its Effects on Grazers," *Freshwater Biology,* Vol. 38, pp. 513-524.

Huang, X.-D., McConkey, B. J., Babu, T. S., and Greenberg, B. M., 1997, "Mechanisms of Photoinduced Toxicity of Photomodified Anthracene to Plants: Inhibition of Photosynthesis in the Aquatic Higher Plant *Lemna gibba* (Duckweed)," *Environmental Toxicology and Chemistry,* Vol. 16, pp. 1707-1715.

Huner, N. P. A., Öquist, G., and Sarhan, F., 1998, "Energy Balance and Acclimation to Light and Cold," *Trends in Plant Science,* Vol. 3, pp. 224-230.

Jansen, M .A. K., Greenberg, B. M., Edelman, M., Mattoo, A. K., and Gaba, V., 1996, "Accelerated Degradation of the D2 Protein of Photosystem II Under Ultraviolet Radiation," *Photochemistry and Photobiology,* Vol. 63, pp. 814-817.

Kerr, J. B. and McElroy, C. T., 1993, "Evidence for Large Upward Trends of Ultraviolet-B Radiation Linked to Ozone Depletion," *Science,* Vol. 262, pp. 1032-1034.

Kirk, J. T. O., 1994, *Light and Photosynthesis in Aquatic Ecosystems*, Cambridge University Press, Cambridge, UK.

Lichtenthaler, H. K. and Rinderle, U., 1988. "The Role of Chlorophyll Fluorescence in the Detection of Stress Conditions in Plants," *CRC Critical Reviews in Analytical Chemistry*, Vol. 19, Supplement 1, CRC Press, Boca Raton, Florida, U.S.A., pp. 29-85.

Long, S. P., Humphries, S., and Falkowski, P. G., 1994, "Photoinhibition of Photosynthesis in Nature," *Annual Review of Plant Physiology and Plant Molecular Biology,* Vol. 45, pp. 633-662.

Marwood, C. A. and Greenberg, B. M., 1996, "Effect of Supplementary UVB Radiation on Chlorophyll Synthesis and Accumulation of Photosystems During Chloroplast Development in *Spirodela oligorrhiza*," *Photochemistry and Photobiology,* Vol. 64, pp. 664-670.

Marwood, C. A., Smith, R. E. H., Furgal, J. A., Charlton, M. N., Solomon, K. R., and Greenberg, B. M., 2000, "Photoinhibition of Natural Phytoplankton Assemblages in Lake Erie Exposed to Solar Ultraviolet Radiation," *Canadian Journal of Fisheries and Aquatic Sciences,* Vol. 57, pp. 371-379.

Nilawati, J., Greenberg, B. M., and Smith, R. E. H., 1997, "Influence of Ultraviolet Radiation on Growth and Photosynthesis of Two Cold Ocean Diatoms," *Journal of Phycology*, Vol. 33, pp. 215-224.

Quesada, A., Mouget, J.-L., and Vincent, W. F., 1995, "Growth of Antarctic Cyanobacteria Under Ultraviolet Radiation: UVA Counteracts UVB Inhibition," *Journal of Phycology,* Vol. 31, pp. 242-248.

Shaw, J. and Manning, J. P., 1996, "Evaluating Macroinvertebrate Population and Community Level Effects in Outdoor Microcosms: Use of In Situ Bioassays and Multivariate Analysis," *Environmental Toxicology and Chemistry,* Vol. 15, pp. 608-615.

Smith, R. E. H., Furgal, J. A. and Lean, D. R. S., 1998, "The Short-Term Effects of Solar Ultraviolet Radiation on Phytoplankton Photosynthesis and Photosynthate Allocation Under Contrasting Mixing Regimes in Lake Ontario," *Journal of Great Lakes Research,* Vol. 24, pp. 427-441.

Solomon, K. R., Yoo, J. Y., Lean, D., Kaushik, N. K., Day, K. E., and Stephenson, G. L., 1986, "Methoxychlor Distribution, Dissipation, and Effects in Freshwater Limnocorrals," *Environmental Toxicology and Chemistry,* Vol. 5, pp. 577-586.

Strid, Å., Chow, W. S., and Anderson, J. M., 1990, "Effects of Supplementary Ultraviolet-B Radiation on Photosynthesis in *Pisum sativum*," *Biochimica et Biophysica Acta*, Vol. 1020, pp. 260-268.

van Kooten, O. and Snel, J. F. H., 1990, "The Use of Chlorophyll Fluorescence Nomenclature in Plant Stress Physiology," *Photosynthesis Research,* Vol. 25, pp. 147-150.

Wilhelm, C., Bida, J., Domin, A., Hilse, C., Kaiser, B., Kesselmeier, J., Lohr, M., and Müller, A. M., 1997, "Interaction Between Global Climate Change and the Physiological Responses of Algae," *Photosynthetica,* Vol. 33, pp. 491-503.

Wilson, M. I., Ghosh, S., Gerhardt, K. E., Holland, N., Babu, T. S., Edelman, M., Dumbroff, E. B., and Greenberg, B. M., 1995, "*In Vivo* Photomodification of Ribulose-1,5-bisphosphate Carboxylase/Oxygenase Holoenzyme by Ultraviolet-B Radiation. Formation of a 66-kilodalton Variant of the Large Subunit," *Plant Physiology,* Vol. 109, pp. 221-229.

Martin E. Arhelger,[1] Faust R. Parker, Jr.,[2] Paul A. Jensen,[1] Claude E. Boyd[3]

Estero Salado / Guayaquil Ship Channel Contaminant Assessment

---

Reference: Arhelger, M. E., Parker, F. R., Jr., Jensen, P. A., and Boyd, C. E., **"Estero Salado / Guayaquil Ship Channel Contaminant Assessment,"** *Environmental Toxicology and Risk Assessment: Science, Policy, and Standardization - Implications for Environmental Decisions: Tenth Volume, ASTM STP 1403*, B. M. Greenberg, R. N. Hull, M. H. Roberts, Jr., and R. W. Gensemer, Eds., American Society for Testing and Materials, West Conshohocken, PA, 2001.

Abstract: Testing of maintenance material from the Estero Salado and some side bays off the Bay of Guayaquil was conducted, including chemical and bacteriological analyses of sediment and suspended particulate phase (SPP) bioassays, using both the Pacific white shrimp, *Penaeus vannamei*, in Guayaquil, Ecuador and the "opossum shrimp", *Mysidopsis bahia* in Houston, Texas. The SPP was prepared from channel or bay sediments and shrimp farm intake water. The work was designed to determine the potential environmental short-term (acute) impact of the proposed open-bay disposal of maintenance material to be dredged from the Estero Salado.

The chemical analyses demonstrated no cause for concern relative to usual estuary sediments but demonstrated metals concentrations well above those normally found in sediments from shrimp ponds near Guayaquil. The bioassays with *P. vannamei* showed almost no acute toxicity but, did show some sublethal effects, including counts of *Vibrio* bacteria, a bacteria of concern to shrimp farmers worldwide. The mysid bioassays demonstrated both lethal and sublethal effects from the 100% SPP of several channel stations.

An analysis of the material to be dredged suggests that the plume from the proposed discharge can generate a significant and easily detectable increase over background turbidity near the discharge. The area affected by the increase in suspended sediment could encompass many of the shrimp farm intakes, which could provide an environmental stress to shrimp in the farms. All of this leads to the conclusion that the open bay discharge of material from the Estero Salado may cause problems to the shrimp farms that fringe Guayaquil Bay. Measures to reduce the amount of additional turbidity that would be generated during disposal were suggested.

Keywords: bioassays, dredging, Ecuador, Estero Salado, Guayaquil, *Mysidopsis bahia*, *Penaeus vannamei*, shrimp farms, suspended particulate phase, toxicity, *Vibrio* bacteria.

---

[1] Vice President, PBS&J, Austin, TX 78746

[2] Director, PBS&J E-TOX Laboratory, Houston, TX 77042

[3] Professor, Dept. of Fisheries/Allied Aquacultures, Auburn Univ., Auburn, AL 36849.

Introduction

In April, 1999, PBS&J was retained by the Cámara Nacional de Acuacultura (Cámara) to conduct bioassays on the suspended particulate phase (SPP) prepared with sediments from portions of the Estero Salado where dredging is planned. The Scope of Work required specific testing of maintenance material from the Estero Salado and some side bays off the Bay of Guayaquil, an analysis of the movement of the turbidity plume, and recommendations to reduce impacts. The purpose of the work performed for this item was to determine the potential environmental short-term (acute) impact of the proposed open-bay disposal of maintenance material to be dredged from the Estero Salado.

The laboratory work performed consisted of chemical and bacteriological analyses of sediment and SPP bioassays, using both *Penaeus vannamei* in Guayaquil, Ecuador and *Mysidopsis bahia* in Houston, Texas. The SPP was prepared from channel or bay sediments and shrimp farm intake water to simulate worst-case conditions at a shrimp farm intake.

The emphasis was on bacteria that grew in the agar, TCBS, and on bacteria of the genus *Vibrio*. This is a bacteria of concern to shrimp farmers worldwide, since this genus of bacteria has been implicated in bacteriosis, or Vibriosis if caused by *Vibrio* spp., in various life stages of several species of shrimp in various parts of the world (*P. vannamei* in Ecuador and Texas (Lightner 1992; Mohney et al. 1994); *P. monodon* and *P. merguiensis* in Indonesia (Sunaryanto and Mariam 1986), Thailand (Tansutapanit and Ruangpan 1987), and the Philippines (Lavilla-Pitogo et al. 1990); *P. monodon* in Malaysia (Anderson et al. 1988) and Taiwan (Bell 1991); and *P. joponicus* in Japan (Takahashi et al. 1985; Egusa et al. 1988).

Chemical analysis of the sediments provided data concerning background levels of specified potential toxins. All chemical analyses were performed by Anacon Inc., Houston, Texas. The bacteriological analyses, which provided information on the presence of *Vibrio* bacteria, were performed by Dr. Roberto Jimenez and his staff at Acvactecnos Asesores, Guayaquil, Ecuador. Both histopathological and bacteriological analyses were performed.

The bioassays are designed to determine the potential impact of the disposal of the dredged material on designated sensitive marine organisms living in the water column or on the bay bottom. Since both *P. vannamei* and *M. bahia* are detrital-feeding epibenthic organisms, they intimately interact with both the water column and the sediments. *P. vannamei* were chosen as test organisms since they are the shrimp raised in Ecuadorian shrimp farms surrounding the Bay of Guayaquil. *M. bahia* were selected because they have been used consistently in dredged material testing under U.S. Environmental Protection Agency (USEPA) and U.S. Army Corps of Engineers (USACE) protocols, have been included as a "sensitive marine organism" in all USEPA/USACE protocols since 1977, and have been used for toxicity testing of dredged material more than any other species. Since the transport of suspended material could contribute to contamination, the potential movement of the turbidity plume was also discussed and recommendations for reducing the turbidity were made.

Methods and Materials

Station Locations

There were nine test stations, resulting in ten samples for the bioassays and chemical analyses (see Figure 1):

Station	Location
Site 1	Estero Sabana Grande
Site 2	Buoy 66
Site 3	Buoy 62
Site 4	Buoy 59
Site 5	Buoy 58
Site 6	Buoy 54
Site 7	Buoy 48I/C (Collected at Buoy 48 by INOCAR personnel)
Site 8	Buoy 48P (Collected at Buoy 48 by PBS&J personnel)
Site 9	Buoy 44
Site 10	Estero Grande

Since duplication was not possible, the site designation for each sample location was kept confidential until data analysis was complete and the draft report was released in June, 1999 (PBS&J 1999a) to provide for the equivalent of blind sampling.

Sample Collection and Storage

Water Samples - Water (Temperature 27.1 - 30.0 °C, salinity 10 - 20 ‰, dissolved oxygen 3.4 - 7.0 mg/L) for preparing the SPP was collected with a non-contaminating pump and placed into new 5-gallon polyethylene containers. The water samples were chilled within minutes of collection and stored in the dark at 2-4°C until allowed to warm to test temperature immediately before SPP preparation. Water was collected adjacent to the intake structures of Quiñonez and Exporklore shrimp farms (Figure 1). Since the Cañizares and Salem shrimp farms receive their intake water from the same small estuary, water was collected in that estuary from just outside the side channel leading to the Cañizares intake structure.

Sediment Samples - Sediment from the test stations and reference stations was collected with a stainless steel Ponar Grab. This grab sampler collects eight to nine liters of sediment to a depth of 16 to 20 cm. Test sediment was collected within the channel to ensure that maintenance material was collected. Duplicate sediment samples were placed in one-gallon, air-tight linear polyethylene containers which were filled to overflowing, sealed to exclude air, chilled within minutes of collection, and stored at 2-4°C until used. Samples sent to Houston were maintained on ice in the dark until shipped on the evening of 5/17/99. These samples were received in the USA on the morning of 5/20/99, at Anacon, Inc. Subsamples were removed for chemical analysis and the remainder was sent to the PBS&J E-TOX Laboratory, where the SPP bioassays were initiated on 5/26/99, two weeks after sample

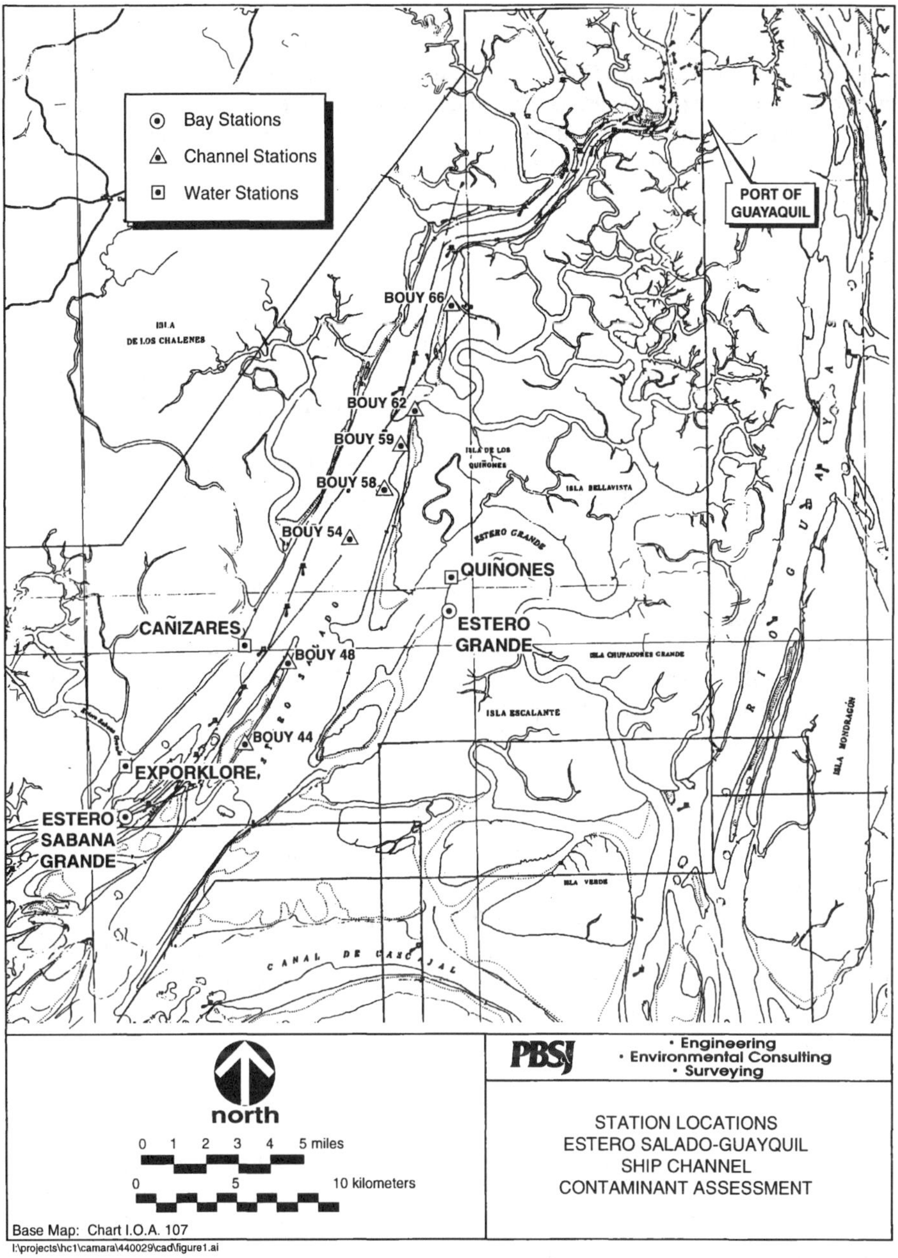

Figure 1 - *Station locations.*

collection.

In addition to the samples collected by PBS&J personnel, two additional samples were collected by INOCAR (Armada del Ecuador, Instituto Oceanográfico) personnel at Buoy 48 with a different type of sampler, for comparative purposes. A surficial sample was collected (48I) for chemical analysis and SPP bioassays, and a 30-cm core sample (48C), of smaller volume, was used only for chemical analyses. The sample collected by PBS&J personnel is identified as 48P throughout this report.

Laboratory Facilities

Guayaquil, Ecuador - The testing was conducted in a chemistry laboratory on the Prospina Campus of the Escuela Superior Polytécnica del Litoral (ESPOL), Guayaquil, Ecuador. The laboratory contained two rooms, one of which was used for temperature adjustment of water and sediment and for weighing of the shrimp food and the other, larger room was used for SPP preparation and the bioassays.

There was a window air conditioning unit which helped maintain a fairly constant temperature during the heat of the day. The unit and the lights were turned off at night. The temperature range for the bioassays was 22.8 - 26.6 °C.

Houston, Texas - The Laboratory has separate areas for water and sediment storage, culture of test organisms, and testing.

Upon receipt from Ecuador, sediments were stored in a darkened chamber maintained at 2-4°C. All testing was performed in a single 25°C test room (±1°C). Lighting was arranged so that light intensity was approximately 1200 $\mu w/cm^2$ using cool-white fluorescent bulbs with a 16-hour light and 8-hour dark cycle.

Organism Acquisition

Two species were tested in the SPP bioassays: the "opossum shrimp", *Mysidopsis bahia*, in the PBS&J E-TOX Laboratory and the Pacific white shrimp, *Penaeus vannamei*, in the ESPOL laboratory. *M. bahia* were cultured in the PBS&J E-TOX Laboratory and *P. vannamei* were cultured by El Rosario. *M. bahia*, 6-days of age, were acquired from the E-TOX culture facility immediately prior to test initiation and *P. vannamei*, 8-days of age, were transferred from the El Rosario culture facility on the morning the bioassays were initiated at ESPOL.

Test Media Preparation

The SPP was prepared by mixing site sediment and site water at a 1:4 ratio. The slurry was mixed vigorously, with aeration and occasional manual stirring for 30 minutes (USEPA/USACE 1991). After mixing, the suspension was allowed to settle overnight to allow the fine sediment to settle out. At the end of the settling period, the supernatant was siphoned off as the 100% SPP.

Chemical Analyses

Sediment samples were shipped directly from Ecuador to Anacon. The sediments from each channel and bay station were analyzed for the parameters listed in Table 1. The methods of analysis and the minimum detection limits are also found in Table 1.

Bioassessment Procedures

Randomization - Test and control vessel locations on the test benches were randomized using numbers from a PC random number generator.

7-Day Suspended Particulate Phase Bioassays - The SPP, after being prepared as described above was transferred to the test containers, and mixed with dilution water (intake water at ESPOL or laboratory-prepared seawater (Hawaiian Marine Mix®) in Houston) in appropriate amounts to give five replicates each of 10%, 50%, and 100% concentrations of SPP per channel site or Reference Control. The bay sites (Estero Sabana Grande and Estero Grande) were used as reference controls. Containers filled with 100% dilution water were used as True Control for the tests.

After the test containers were prepared and determined to be at 25 °C (Houston) or room temperature (Ecuador), ten *M. bahia* or *P. vannamei* were added randomly to each test vessel. The loading factor in all vessels was less than one-half gram per liter. Counts were made daily in the E-TOX Laboratory and on Days 4 and 7 at ESPOL to monitor the number of surviving organisms.

Temperature, dissolved oxygen, and salinity were recorded daily; pH was also recorded daily in the E-TOX Laboratory.

Statistical Analyses

Statistical analyses are described in detail in USEPA/USACE (1991) and are designed to determine whether the test results are significantly different from the results of the True Control (dilution water) or Reference Control (bay sediment SPP). All statistical comparisons are at the 95% confidence level.

Statistical calculations were performed for any bioassay where mortality in the 100% SPP was at least 10% greater than in the control.

The Shapiro-Wilkes test was used to determine if the data were normally distributed and Cochran's test was used to determine the homogeneity or heterogeneity of the variances. To determine if the difference among the mean survival of organisms in the tests and in either control was statistically significant the two-sample t-test (USEPA/USACE 1991) was used.

Histopathological and Bacterial Analyses of Sediment

Samples were removed with sterile tubes for placement in the proper agars to look for pathogens. For total bacterial counts, TSA agar was used, with incubation at 30 °C for 48 hours. For total Vibrio bacteria, TCBS agar was used. A luminescent agar (Peptona 5g, yeast extract 3 g., agar 18 g, glycerol 3 ml, seawater 750 ml, and distilled water 250 ml) was

TABLE 1
CHEMICAL PARAMETERS
ANALYTICAL METHODOLOGY AND MINIMUM DETECTION LIMITS

Parameter	Detection Limit	EPA Method
METALS		
Arsenic	0.10 mg/kg	7060A
Barium	0.10 mg/kg	6010B
Cadmium	0.10 mg/kg	7131A
Chromium	0.10 mg/kg	6010B
Copper	0.10 mg/kg	6010B
Lead	0.10 mg/kg	7421
Mercury	0.10 mg/kg	7471A
Nickel	0.10 mg/kg	6010B
Selenium	0.20 mg/kg	7740
Silver	0.10 mg/kg	7761
Zinc	0.10 mg/kg	6010B
PESTICIDES		
Aldrin	0.30 mg/kg	3550/8081A
Alpha-BHC	0.18 mg/kg	3550/8081A
Beta-BHC	0.18 mg/kg	3550/8081A
Gamma-BHC	0.19 mg/kg	3550/8081A
Delta-BHC	0.17 mg/kg	3550/8081A
Chlordane	0.17 mg/kg	3550/8081A
4,4'-DDD	0.29 mg/kg	3550/8081A
4,4'-DDE	0.21 mg/kg	3550/8081A
4,4'-DDT	0.41 mg/kg	3550/8081A
Dieldrin	0.27 mg/kg	3550/8081A
Endosulfan I	0.23 mg/kg	3550/8081A
Endosulfan II	0.69 mg/kg	3550/8081A
Endosulfan Sulfate	0.39 mg/kg	3550/8081A
Endrin	0.60 mg/kg	3550/8081A
Endrin Aldehyde	0.71 mg/kg	3550/8081A
Heptachlor	0.21 mg/kg	3550/8081A
Heptachlor Epoxide	0.18 mg/kg	3550/8081A
Toxaphene	10.5 mg/kg	3550/8081A
PCBs		
Arochlor 1016	1.50 mg/kg	3550/8081A
Arochlor 1221	3.45 mg/kg	3550/8081A
Arochlor 1232	3.45 mg/kg	3550/8081A
Arochlor 1242	1.50 mg/kg	3550/8081A
Arochlor 1248	3.90 mg/kg	3550/8081A
Arochlor 1254	3.45 mg/kg	3550/8081A
Arochlor 1260	1.35 mg/kg	3550/8081A

U.S. EPA, "Test Methods for the Evaluation of Solid Waste," SW-846, December, 1996.

also used. For identification of the bacteria, BIOLOG, API 20NE and API 20E were used for the identification of gram positive and gram negative bacteria. Confirming evidence was from biochemical responses and carbohydrate usage. Histopathological abnormalities found in the shrimp, after exposure to the SPP bioassays, included hemocyte enteritis, bacteremia, lesions, hyperplasia, and delamination of the hepatopancreas.

Results and Discussion

Chemical Analyses

Sediment concentrations (dry weight) of detected compounds are presented in Table 2. PCBs and pesticides were below detection limits in all sediment samples. An examination of the metals data indicates that there are no trends except that the metals concentrations in the Estero Sabana Grande sediment were consistently lower, numerically, that those at the other stations. However, the total range between the highest and lowest concentrations of all metals, except silver and cadmium, was less than a factor of three. Cadmium and silver both had one relatively high concentration versus the rest of the samples in which no cadmium or silver was detected. For silver, sample 48P contained 0.97 mg/kg while the two samples collected at Buoy 48 by INOCAR personnel contained no detectable silver. On the other hand, sample 48C contained 0.48 mg/kg cadmium while both samples 48I and 48P contained no detectable cadmium. This is not unusual given the patchy nature of estuarine sediments and the range of values found in this study is similar to those from Texas estuaries (TNRCC 1996). Boyd *et al.* (1994) measured the concentrations of numerous chemicals, including metals, from bottom sediments of 346 brackish water shrimp ponds. Of the metals measured by both Boyd *et al.* (1994) and this study, only lead was within the general range found by Boyd *et al.* (1994), while barium, chromium, copper, and zinc were higher than the upper limit of the "high" category (Table 2).

Bioassessment Studies

Lethality - Summary results of the SPP bioassays with *P. vannamei* are provided in Table 3, with indications of statistical significance provided by the footnotes.

There was no instance where survival in any concentration of SPP from any of the test stations was significantly less than survival in the Control for that station. Survival in the SPP for no channel station was significantly less than survival in the SPP prepared with Estero Sabana Grande Sediment.

Summary results of the SPP bioassays with *M. bahia* are also provided in Table 3. There were six instances where survival in the 100% SPP was (1) at least 10% less than control survival and (2) significantly less than control survival at the 95% confidence level (USEPA/USACE 1991): Buoy 66, Buoy 62, Buoy 59, Buoy 58, Buoy 48I, and Estero Grande. Survival in both the Estero Grande 50% and 100% SPP was zero. All of these sediments were stored on ice and in the dark from time of collection. However, two weeks had passed from time of collection until initiation of the SPP bioassays in Houston. While this meets the acceptability criterion found in USEPA/USACE (1991), the Estero Grande sediment contained excessive numbers of mussels (the only sample to contain any mussels),

TABLE 2
CONCENTRATIONS OF DETECTED COMPOUNDS (mg/kg, dry wt.)
SEDIMENT

Station\ Parameter	Buoy Number/ Bay Location	Arsenic	Barium	Cadmium	Chromium	Copper	Lead	Mercury	Nickel	Selenium	Silver	Zinc
Site 1	Estero Sabana Grande	2.49	16.5	<0.10	24.9	17.6	4.31	0.13	14.9	<0.20	<0.10	49.4
Site 2	Buoy 66	4.58	37.6	<0.10	49.6	40.7	13.0	<0.10	29.3	<0.20	<0.10	93.4
Site 3	Buoy 62	2.65	30.3	<0.10	31.2	28.7	5.36	<0.10	19.6	<0.20	<0.10	72.4
Site 4	Buoy 59	4.43	33.1	<0.10	45.0	40.0	7.47	<0.10	28.3	<0.20	<0.10	114
Site 5	Buoy 58	3.68	28.1	<0.10	26.3	36.7	7.81	0.13	31.4	<0.20	<0.10	76.9
Site 6	Buoy 54	3.97	31.6	<0.10	36.5	38.4	9.57	<0.10	26.2	<0.20	<0.10	91.9
Site 7	Buoy 48I*	4.13	34.9	<0.10	37.6	37.1	10.2	<0.10	26.9	<0.20	<0.10	87.0
Site 8	Buoy 48P*	3.78	27.9	<0.10	27.0	35.0	12.5	<0.10	27.0	<0.20	0.97	77.9
N/A	Buoy 48C*	5.51	29.1	0.48	30.9	35.0	9.17	0.13	25.3	0.31	<0.10	139
Site 9	Buoy 44	3.76	29.9	<0.10	30.4	41.2	7.56	<0.10	24.5	<0.20	0.65	80.2
Site 10	Estero Grande	2.94	25.7	<0.10	25.9	31.6	7.04	0.19	19.5	<0.20	<0.10	69.1
Boyd *et al.*, 1994	Low		0.5 - 1.0		1 - 2	1 - 2	2 - 4					2 - 5
	Medium		1.0 - 1.5		2 - 4	2 - 8	4 - 7					5 - 8
	High		1.5 - 3.5		4 - 7	8 - 11	7 - 9					8 - 14

which upon degradation, even on ice in the dark, may have been responsible for the extreme mortality in the Estero Grande 50% SPP (100% mortality at 24 hours) and 100% SPP (100% mortality at 24 hours in all but one replicate). By contrast, the sediment from Estero Sabana Grande did not contain high numbers of benthic organisms and survival in the 100% SPP after 7 days was 90%. This was significantly less than control survival (control survival was 100%), but the difference between test and control survival was not greater than 10% (USEPA/USACE 1991).

Excluding Estero Grande, the lowest survival in the 50% SPP was 96% and the lowest survival in the 10% SPP was 98%. Therefore, there was significant lethality to mysids only at 100% SPP. It is interesting that the surficial sediment sample collected by INOCAR personnel at Buoy 48 (48I) exhibited lethality in the 100% SPP while the surficial sediment sample collected by PBS&J personnel at Buoy 48 (48P) did not. The same samples for which the 100% SPP survival was significantly less than control survival also had survival in the 100% SPP that was significantly less than survival in the 100% Estero Sabana Grande SPP. In fact, an examination of the data demonstrates that, of the samples collected by PBS&J, samples from Buoy 54 and seaward did not have survival significantly less than that of Estero Sabana Grande, whereas all samples collected inshore from Buoy 54 did have survival significantly less than that of Estero Sabana Grande.

Sublethal Effects - For sublethal impacts to *P. vannamei*, both histopathological and bacteriological analyses were performed. All concentrations of SPP and the control from Sites 1 (Estero Sabana Grande), 2 (Buoy 66), and 3 (Buoy 62) were examined.

Only the Site 1 Control (Exporklore intake water) had no histopathological abnormalities. Site 2 and Site 3 Controls (Quiñonez intake water) exhibited hemocyte enteritis (from an abundance of gram negative bacteria in the intestine) and bacteremia (a bacterial infection with an immunological response), respectively. All SPP concentrations from all sites, including Estero Sabana Grande, exhibited pathological abnormalities, which appeared to be related to control versus SPP but did not appear to be related to SPP concentration. For example, the analysis of Site 1 indicated that the 10% SPP, 50% SPP, and 100% SPP exhibited 2, 3, and 3 types of the 5 types of abnormalities found. For Site 2, the 10% SPP, 50% SPP, and 100% SPP exhibited 2, 2, and 4 types of abnormalities, respectively, and for Site 3, the 10% SPP, 50% SPP, and 100% SPP exhibited 4, 5, and 3 types of abnormalities, respectively. Likewise, when a particular type of abnormality occurred, the percentage of samples analyzed which contained this type of abnormality did not appear to be related to SPP concentration; e.g., delamination of hepatopancreas canals for Site 2: 10% SPP - 24% occurrence, 50% SPP - 44% occurrence, and 100% SPP - 16% occurrence. Sites 2 and 3, made with channel sediment, generally exhibited a slight increase in the types of histopathological abnormalities than did Site 1, made with Estero Sabana Grande sediments, but it cannot be determined if the increase would be statistically significant.

The same 12 SPP samples were subjected to bacterial analysis. Both the 10% and 50% SPP had lower total bacteria counts than did the control or dilution water from which they were made for the Estero Sabana Grande sediment. For the Estero Salado channel sediments, the control had the lowest total bacteria count, although for the Buoy 66 sediment, the 50% SPP total bacteria count was intermediate between the control and the 10% SPP. For all three sites, the 100% SPP had noticeably larger total bacteria counts than either of the other concentrations or the controls. Total *Vibrio* bacteria counts were very mixed: the control had the highest count for the Estero Sabana Grande sample, the 100% SPP had the highest count for the Buoy 66 sample, and the 10% SPP had the highest count for the Buoy 62 sample.

The sublethal effect examined for *M. bahia* was growth, measured as average weight of organisms in the various concentrations of SPP versus average weight of control organisms. The average weight is calculated by taking the total weight of a replicate and dividing by the original number of organisms in the replicate. Thus a lethal effect is passed on to the sublethal effect, by protocol design. A summary of results can be found in Table 3.

The growth data generally parallel the survival data for *M. bahia*. Since there was no survival in the 50% and 100% SPP, there are no growth data for those concentrations of Estero Grande SPP, but the weight of the organisms exposed to the Estero Grande 10% SPP was not significantly different from the Estero Grande Control organisms. As would be expected, the same samples for which the 100% SPP survival was significantly different from control survival also had growth in the 100% SPP that was significantly less than Control growth and significantly less than growth of the Estero Sabana Grande 100% SPP organisms. Additionally, the 100% SPP for Buoy 48P was significantly less than Control growth and significantly less than growth of the Estero Sabana Grande 100% SPP organisms. By contrast, growth in most 10% and 50% SPP organisms was greater, often significantly so, than Control organism growth. This is not unusual and is normally attributed to added nutrition from preparation of the SPP from sterile laboratory-prepared sea water.

Discussion of the Turbidity Plume

Analysis of Dredging Turbidity Effects - There is no doubt that dredging of the navigation channel and disposal in the open bay adjacent to the channel will produce a short-term and localized increase in the concentration of suspended solids in the waters of the Estero Salado. While the impact of this increase in suspended solids is difficult to quantify with precision, it is more likely to have adverse biological effects than beneficial biological effects. This section briefly discusses these aspects as well as possible alternatives relative to dredged material disposal.

The proposed dredging procedure is to employ a hopper dredge in the navigation channel and dispose of the dredged material in deeper sections of the Estero Salado adjacent to the channel. INOCAR (1998) noted that there was no indication that the material disposed of during the previous dredging in 1989 remained in the disposal area. This suggests that the dredged material will be dispersed over a wide area by the strong tidal currents in Guayaquil Bay, which could provide an environmental stress to shrimp in the farms.

The Environmental Impact Statement (EIS: INOCAR 1998) prepared for the proposed dredging and disposal determined that, in general, currents are aligned with the axis of the Estero Salado and the navigation canal and have velocities in the range of 0.5 to 2 m/s.

The area to be dredged has a high silt content, but also substantial sand and clay. From INOCAR (1998), it was determined that the material to be dredged is 20% sand, 50% silt and 30% clay. It is assumed that the solids have a specific gravity of 2.7 and that the *in situ* sediment is about 50% solids with a solids concentration of 1,100 g/L.

The sand can be expected to settle within a few hundred meters of the discharge point.

TABLE 3
Survival of *P. vannamei* and Survival and Weight (mg) of *M. bahia* after Seven Days Exposure in SPP Bioassays

			Penneaus vannamei				*Mysidopsis bahia*			
Site	Sample	Dilution Water	Control	10%	50%	100%	Control	10%	50%	100%
1	Estero Sabana Grande	Exporklore	88%	96%	78%	92%	100%	100%	100%	90%*
							0.236	0.298	0.296	0.228
2	Buoy 66	Quiñonez	92%	98%	96%	96%	100%	100%	98%	54%*+
							0.236	0.280	0.268	0.106*+
3	Buoy 62	Quiñonez	94%	94%	96%	78%	100%	100%	96%	62%*+
							0.236	0.284	0.338	0.116*+
4	Buoy 59	Cañizares	90%	90%	80%	98%	100%	100%	100%	70*+
							0.236	0.256	0.300	0.138*+
5	Buoy 58	Cañizares	98%	98%	92%	98%	98%	100%	98%	46*+
							0.220	0.232	0.232	0.074*+
6	Buoy 54	Cañizares	84%	86%	82%	94%	98%	98%	98%	100%
							0.220	0.248	0.244	0.282
7	Buoy 48I	Cañizares	92%	86%	96%	92%	98%	100%	96%	50%*+
							0.254	0.298	0.278	0.090*+
8	Buoy 48P	Cañizares	96%	92%	94%	96%	98%	98%	98%	92%
							0.254	0.286	0.302	.0198*+
9	Buoy 44	Exporklore	94%	100%	100%	92%	100%	98%	100%	100%
							0.270	0.302	0.336	0.260
10	Estero Grande	Quiñonez	94%	92%	88%	96%	100%	96%	0%*	0%*+
							0.270	0.290	N/A	N/A

* Significantly less (α=0.05) than True Control.
\+ Significantly less (α=0.05) than Estero Sabano Grande sediments.

The other 80% of the dredged material will only settle where quiescent water conditions allow sufficiently low turbulence for the fine materials to drop out. This will happen for short periods at every tide reversal and when the water enters an inlet or other shallow water zone, but it will be a much slower process.

The dredge is noted to be able to remove about 600 m^3 per hour. This material is assumed to have a solids content of about 1,100 g/L in place and the poorly settleable fraction is estimated to be about 880 g/L, or kg/m^3. Moving 600 m^3/hr would produce 528,000 kg of poorly settleable material that would be placed in suspension in an hour. How this material would enter the water depends on the operation of the dredge. As the dredging begins, the hopper contains clean sea water and the overflow weir is above the water level in the hopper. As dredging proceeds, the hopper fills with water and suspended sediment, and turbid water begins to overflow the weir. It is normal to continue dredging, getting more solids to settle in the hopper while the concentration of fine material in the overflow increases. At some point a decision is made that an optimal load has been obtained. Dredging is then ceased and the vessel moves to the discharge point where the hopper doors are opened and the material dumped. Because of the varying nature of the sediment and the dredge operating procedures, it is not possible to specify the amount of turbidity that would be introduced to the dredging area and the disposal site. However, in general terms, a high proportion of the fine material that has accumulated in the channel would be placed in suspension, either in the channel area via the overflow weir or at the nearby disposal site.

The turbidity increase can be examined as if it were a continuous discharge. The poorly settleable fraction dredged in a second would be 147 kg. Assuming that, at the point of discharge, the Estero Salado is 2 km wide and 6 m deep, with a tidal current of 1 m/s, there will be a tidal flow of 12,000 m^3/s. Adding the continuous discharge to the tidal flow of 12,000 m^3/s gives a concentration increase when mixed over the entire cross-section of about 12 g/m^3 or mg/L. This would be at the limit of detectability if mixed over the entire cross-section, but would be quite visible as a turbidity plume in the immediate area of the discharge. In addition, the dredging supply of fine and poorly settleable material would be nearly continuous during times of operation. With little of the material settling, it would be added to in the next tidal oscillation. Within 10 tidal cycles the plume can be expected to be a significant and easily detectable increase over background in the area of the discharge. The area affected by the increase in suspended sediment would extend approximately 10 km up and downstream from the point of discharge and encompass many of the shrimp farm intake-water areas.

Actions to Reduce the Amount of Turbidity Increase from Dredging - From the standpoint of turbidity reduction, the preferable alternative would be confined upland disposal. With a confined disposal area most of the fine particles settle prior to discharge. In the United States, the discharge from confined disposal areas are typically limited to 300 mg/L of total suspended solids (TSS), which is not greatly different from background levels in the Estero Salado. For example, INOCAR (1998) notes that water column TSS is in the range of 100-500 mg/L. Pumping distances, availability of sites, and increased costs may make upland disposal impractical for the entire project in the short term. On the other hand, if an unused shrimp pond were available within reasonable distance, it would be desirable to use it as a confined disposal area to reduce turbidity.

If upland disposal is not used, utilizing suspension dredging, only during the ebb cycle could reduce potential problems. Another possibility would be to place material at key locations to redirect more of the flow down the navigation channel portion, increasing the velocity and reducing the amount of settling and the need for dredging. This could be evaluated with a numerical hydrodynamic model that would allow estimates to be made of the changes in current velocities that could be achieved with different amounts of changes in bathymetry. Another effort that should be considered is long-range planning to relocate new port infrastructure to a point closer to the ocean where maintenance dredging is not needed. This may well be necessary in any case to accommodate the increasingly larger vessels serving commercial traffic.

Another alternative to reduce overall impacts may be to increase the sediment load of the hopper by dredging for a longer period of time between dumps. This will increase the amount of fine material released via the overflow weir while dredging and the resulting turbidity in the channel, but it will reduce the amount released in the dump zone area. The overall effect should be to reduce the duration of the dredging by reducing the time spent in transit to and from the dump zones. The net reduction in dredging time would mean both a shorter period of elevated turbidity and a reduction in dredging costs.

Alternatives to Reduce Effects of Turbidity - Assuming no use of confined disposal or other methods that would actually reduce the amount of turbidity, there are some actions that could be taken to reduce effects of the turbidity that is produced. The increase in TSS levels in the Estero Salado from dredging and open bay disposal can be reduced to some degree by a coordinated effort between dredging and shrimp pond filling; *i.e.*, to coordinate and time operations to minimize effects. One component of this cooperative effort could be altering the times when shrimp water supply ponds are filled. If the pond operators are informed of the dredging location and dump cycles on a near real-time basis, and advised of the direction of the turbidity movement, it should be possible for individual pond operators to minimize the intake of high turbidity water. Another component could be timing most of the dredging to occur from near high tide through the ebb cycle, when most of the material would be moved initially towards the ocean. Such activities would have value in reducing to some extent the TSS concentrations of the water taken in to shrimp ponds.

Conclusions

The chemical analyses demonstrated no cause for concern relative to usual estuary sediments but demonstrate metals concentrations well above those normally found in shrimp pond sediments. The bioassays with *P. vannamei* showed no acute toxicity except that the histopathology and bacterial analyses demonstrated some sublethal effects, including highest total bacteria counts in the 100% SPP. The mysid bioassays demonstrated both lethal and sublethal effects from the 100% SPP of several channel stations.

An analysis of the material to be dredged suggests that the plume from the proposed discharge can be expected to generate a significant and easily detectable increase over background turbidity in the area of the discharge. Based on the calculations provided above, the area affected by the increase in suspended sediment would be expected to extend approximately 10 km up and downstream from the point of discharge and encompass many of the shrimp farm intake-water areas, which could provide an environmental stress to shrimp in the farms. Based on the area of open-bay disposal, 10 km up- and down-stream would range from Posorja to Buoy 58. Additionally, recent dredging in Thailand apparently caused mortality in shrimp farms (Tim Flegel, pers comm to C.E. Boyd 1999). All of this leads to the conclusion that the open bay discharge of material from the Estero Salado has the potential to cause problems to the shrimp farms that fringe Guayaquil Bay.

References

Anderson, I.G., M.N. Shamsudin, M. Shariff, and G. Nash. 1988. "Bacterial Septicemia in Juvenile Tiger Shrimp, *Penaeus monodon*, Cultured in Malaysian Brackish Water Ponds." *Asian Fisheries Science*, Vol. 2, pp. 93-108.

Bell, T.A. 1991. "Overview of Diseases and Drug Needs for Major Aquaculture Species: Shrimp." *Veterinary and Human Toxicology*, Vol. 33, Suppl. 1, pp. 19-23.

Boyd, C.E., M.E. Tanner, M. Madkour, and K. Masuda. 1994. "Chemical Characteristics of Bottom Soils from Freshwater and Brackishwater Aquaculture Ponds." *J. World Aquaculture Soc.*, Vol. 25, No. 4, pp 517-534.

Egusa, S., Y. Takahashi, T. Itami, and K. Momoyama. 1988. "Histopathology of Vibriosis in the Kuruma Prawn, *Penaeus japonicus* Bate." *Fish Pathology*, Vol. 23, pp. 59-65.

INOCAR (Instituto Oceanografico de la Armada). 1998. *Estudio de Impacto Ambiental previo al Dregado del Canal de Acceso al Puerto Maritimo de Guayaquil.* Octubre 1998.

Lavilla-Pitogo, C.R., M.C.I. Batacados, E.R. Cruz-Lacierda, and L.D. de la Pena. 1990. "Occurrence of Luminous Vacteial Dsease of *Penaeus monodon* Larvae in the Philippines." *Aquaculture* Vol. 91, pp. 1-13.

Lightner, D.V. 1993. "Shrimp Pathology: Major Diseases of Concern to the Farming Industry in the Americas." In: *Memorias I Americas Congreso Ecuatoriano de Acuicultura*, 177-195. Escuela Superior Politécnica del Litoral, 1993.

Mohney, L.L., D.V. Lightner, and T.A. Bell. 1994. "An Epizootic Vibriosis in Ecuadorian Pond-reared *Penaeus vannamei* Boone (Crustacea: Decapoda)." *Journal World Aquaculture Society*, Vol. 25, pp. 116-125.

PBS&J. 1999a. *Estero Salado - Guayaquil Ship Channel Contaminant Assessment, Draft Report.* Doc. No. 990921. PBS&J, Austin, Texas. June 1999.

PBS&J. 1999b. *Estero Salado - Guayaquil Ship Channel Contaminant Assessment, Final Report.* Doc. No. 990921. PBS&J, Austin, Texas. July 1999.

Sunaryanto, A. and A. Miriam. 1986. "Occurrence of a Pathogenic Bacteria Causing Luminescence in Penaeid Larvae in Indonesian Hatch Eries." *Bull. Brackishwater Aquaculture Development Center*, Vol. 8, pp. 64-70.

Takahashi, Y., Y. Shimoyama, and K. Momoyama. 1985. "Pathogenicity and Characteristics of *Vibrio* sp. Isolated from Diseased Postlarvae of Kuruma Prawns, *Penaeus japonicus* Bate." *Bulletin of the Japanese Society of Scientific Fisheries*, Vol. 51, pp. 1639-1643.

Tansutapanit, D.S.O.A. and L. Ruangpan. 1987. "*Vibrio harveyi*, a Causitive Agent of White Shrimp Nauplii, *Penaeus merguiensis*." Abstract. Technical paper No. 6/30. Third National Seminar on Marine Science, 6-8 August 1986, NSRC, Bangkok, Thailand.

TNRCC (Texas Natural Resource Conservation Commission). 1996. *State of Texas Water Quality Inventory* (SFR-50).

U.S. Environmental Protection Agency/ U.S. Army Corps of Engineers. 1991. *Evaluation of dredged Material Proposed for Ocean Disposal, Testing Manual*. EPA-503/8-91/001. 205 pp + Appendices.

NTERFACE BETWEEN POLICY, SCIENCE AND RISK ASSESSMENT

E. A. Sigal,[1] G. M. Ferguson,[1] C. M. Bacigalupo,[1] R. D. Willis,[2] and L. Marshall[2]

Potential Implications of Inappropriate Assumption Selection on Environmental Modelling Results: An RBCA Case Study.

Reference: Sigal, E. A., Ferguson, G. M., Bacigalupo, C. M., Willis, R. D., and Marshall, L., **"Potential Implications of Inappropriate Assumption Selection on Environmental Modelling Results: An RBCA Case Study,"** *Environmental Toxicology and Risk Assessment: Science, Policy, and Standardization - Implications for Environmental Decisions: Tenth Volume, ASTM STP 1403*, B. M. Greenberg, R. N. Hull, M. H. Roberts, Jr., and R. W. Gensemer, Eds., American Society for Testing and Materials, West Conshohocken, PA, 2001.

Abstract: In the past decade, the field of environmental risk assessment has seen vast improvements in the technologies and tools available to aid with quantification of human health and ecological risks. The development of publicly-available computational modelling tools, such as those based upon the risk based corrective action (RBCA) framework, have allowed those with a potentially less sophisticated understanding of the scientific rationale, equations and methodologies used to simulate environmental fate, toxicology and risk characterization processes to conduct and complete multimedia environmental risk assessments for regulatory approval. However, in many cases, this lack of understanding may result in the selection of inappropriate parameter data (*i.e.*, chemical-, receptor-, or scenario-specific data), unknowingly increasing the uncertainty inherent within the overall assessment of potential risk. Accordingly, the use of inappropriate assumptions and parameters can result in an increase or decrease in the estimated risk, with significant implications on remediation costs or, more importantly, human or environmental health. Three case studies will be presented to illustrate the importance surrounding the selection of appropriate data input parameters, and the potential implications of this selection process on the results of an environmental risk assessment.

Keywords: environmental risk assessment, environmental modelling, RBCA, risk based corrective action, assumption selection, risk estimation.

---

[1]Senior scientist and environmental scientists, respectively. Cantox Environmental Inc., 2233 Argentia Road, Suite 308, Mississauga, Ontario, Canada, L5N 2X7.

[2]Environmental risk analyst and environmental scientist, respectively. Cantox Environmental Inc., 5475 Spring Garden Road, Suite 503, Halifax, Nova Scotia,Canada, B3J 3T2.

Introduction

In the past decade, the field of environmental risk assessment has seen vast improvements in the technologies and tools available to aid with quantification of human health and ecological risks. For example, the ASTM has developed a standard to provide a consistent decision-making process for the risk-based assessment of contaminated sites. The ASTM Standard Guide for Risk-Based Corrective Action Applied at Petroleum Release Sites (E 1739-95), commonly referred to as RBCA, has formed the basis of several commercially-available software packages (models) intended to assist landowners and their consultants in the assessment of contaminated sites. The RBCA standard provides a framework that integrates risk and exposure assessment practices, as suggested by the U.S. Environmental Protection Agency (EPA), with site assessment activities to ensure that appropriate risk management measures are taken that are protective of human health and the environment. The framework outlines a detailed and complex approach for the evaluation of potential health risks at contaminated sites. The models developed based on the RBCA standard, as well as other commercially available risk assessment tools, incorporate the equations and methodologies used to simulate environmental fate processes to conduct and complete multimedia environmental risk assessment for regulatory approval purposes.

When using any type of model it is important to understand how the model input variables can influence model results. The results of a risk assessment conducted using these RBCA models are only as good as the assumptions and parameters used to conduct the assessment. Furthermore, a model utilized at a specific site, can provide questionable results if improper site-specific parameters are used in the assessment. This inappropriate use of input parameters is commonly expressed by the adage '*garbage in garbage out*' (*i.e.*, your assessment results are only as good as the assumptions or data on which they are based). This could result in the overestimation of potential risk, which may lead to high remedial cost implications. Conversely, an underestimation of the overall risk could result in the potential for adverse health effects.

In an attempt to provide for the protection of human health on a generic basis, these RBCA-based models are designed to select default parameters and assumptions when site-specific data are lacking. While it is generally preferable to collect and use site-specific data, this is often difficult due to both time or fiscal constraints on the data collection. As a result, where site-specific data are lacking, default assumptions and parameters are utilized, which are typically conservative in nature and err on the side of caution to ensure the protection of human and environmental health. Models using these conservative parameters and assumptions would overestimate, rather then underestimate, predicted health risks. This also results in an increased level of uncertainty in the assessment. In order to minimize the uncertainties inherent in risk assessment, it is imperative that a risk assessor be aware of the relationship(s) that exist between input data (*i.e.*, site-specific environmental, receptor and chemical parameters) and human and environmental health risk estimates (*i.e.*, the output upon which health-based criteria are based). Understanding how certain input parameters affect the output of these models provides the risk assessor with the ability to identify those key parameters which may have the greatest impact on health risks.

Risk assessment encompasses a diverse array of scientific tools and information drawing on knowledge from the fields of toxicology, environmental chemistry, ecology, hydrogeology, environmental fate and transport, epidemiology and community medicine, and statistics (OMOE 1997). As such, risk assessments have historically been conducted by teams of scientists with training and/or expertise in these disciplines. The development of commercially-available modelling tools for risk assessment, such as those based upon the RBCA framework, have allowed individuals with a potentially less sophisticated understanding of these concepts to conduct and complete multimedia environmental risk assessments. This lack of understanding may result in the selection of inappropriate parameter data (*i.e.*, chemical, receptor, or scenario), unknowingly increasing the uncertainty inherent within the overall assessment of risk and potentially leading to inappropriate risk management decisions.

Three case studies will be presented as examples of the potential implications of inappropriately selected assumptions on the results of risk assessments.

Case Studies

To illustrate the potential implications of selecting inappropriate parameters and assumptions, three separate hypothetical test scenarios were developed and modelled using a commercially available RBCA-based modelling system. Furthermore, all default conditions and scenarios used in these assessments were based upon the RBCA standard. The three case studies evaluate the relative impact of uncertainty on assessment results due to: a) exposure parameters, b) the toxicity data, and c) site-specific soil and building parameters, respectively. It is important to remember that these case studies are hypothetical and generic in nature, and were designed to illustrate qualitatively the potential implications of inappropriate assumption selection.

Case Study 1: Exposure Parameters

Most commercially-available risk assessment models are intended for the assessment of commercial or residential exposure scenarios. However, for other scenarios (*i.e.*, a high school) input parameters may need to be modified to reflect the actual scenario-specific situation. Default parameters, such as exposure duration, averaging time, receptor body weights and breathing rates, will need to be modified to reflect a school situation. As a result, a variety of receptors such as teachers, janitors, and students would need to be considered.

To illustrate the importance of selecting relevant site-specific assumptions and parameters in the evaluation of a particular scenario, the following case study provides the results of an assessment comparing three separate scenarios involving: 1) a default commercial building; 2) a default residential house, and 3) a modified school building.

For all assessed scenarios, the potential impacts of naphthalene exposure *via* surface and subsurface soil pathways were evaluated (*i.e.*, direct soil ingestion, dermal contact with soil, and indoor inhalation of vapours). Naphthalene concentrations were assumed to range from 900 to 3000 ppm and 540 to 1900 ppm for surface and subsurface soil, respectively. The soil type in each scenario was assumed to be sand and gravel.

The following is an outline of each model scenario completed, including specific information with respect to the receptor- and building-specific parameters used within each of the scenarios.

Default Scenario I (Commercial Building) - This exposure scenario assumed all default parameters associated with a commercial scenario (*i.e.*, building parameters, commercial worker, *etc.*).

Default Scenario II (Residential House) - This exposure scenario assumed all default parameters associated with a residential house scenario (*i.e.*, building parameters, child receptor, *etc.*).

Test Scenario (High School) - This exposure scenario was modified to reflect the characteristics of a high school scenario (*i.e.*, building parameters, student receptor, *etc.*).

The altered parameters were as follows:

- An adolescent female student was the receptor of concern;
- The building parameters were modified in terms of size, air exchanges, volume, *etc.*, to represent a school;
- Averaging time and exposure durations were set to 5 years to reflect years spent at school (the high school was assumed to be located in Ontario, Canada, which currently consists of grades 7 through 13);
- Receptor body weight was set at 38.6 kg to reflect a reasonable worst case female student;
- Exposure frequency was set to 210 days (*i.e.*, students typically have 10 weeks off per year), and;
- Receptor inhalation rate was set at 20.7 m^3/day to reflect a reasonable worst case female student.

The following, Table 1, provides the results of the default and test scenario assessments conducted for this case study.

Table 1 - *Results of the default and test scenarios in Case Study 1.*

Model run	Hazard Quotient (HQ) Produced		
	Indoor Air Pathway	Soil Pathway	Total HQ
Default Scenario I (Commercial Building)	1.2	0.10	1.3
Default Scenario II (Residential House)	5.6	0.58	6.18
Test Scenario (School Building)	2.6	0.15	2.75

Based on the results of this case study, it is clear that these types of parameters can have a potential impact on the results of an assessment. Using default assumptions, either commercial or residential, results in either an under-estimate (2.1 x) or an over-estimate (2.2 x) of risk compared to the results of an assessment using more site-specific parameters and assumptions.

Case Study 2: Toxicity Data

Typically, chemical-specific data are supplied within these commercially available risk assessment models. It is important that users of these models understand that toxicity data can become outdated as new scientific information becomes available. When using these models, it is essential that the user select the most up-to-date and appropriate data to characterize the toxicity of the chemicals of concern. For users without a toxicology background, it may be useful to consult someone in the toxicology field when revising/updating toxicity data. Furthermore, different regulators have different preferences as to the appropriate toxicity data or exposure limits to be used within their jurisdiction.

For this case study, the parameters and assumptions outlined in Case Study I for the default residential house were used, with the only difference being that the new inhalation RfD from IRIS (U.S. EPA 2000) (*i.e.*, an inhalation RfD of 9.9×10^{-4} mg/kg/day) was used rather than the default value provided with the version of the model used in this case study (*i.e.*, the Health Canada (1996) value of 1.6×10^{-2} mg/kg/day).

The following, Table 2, provides the results of the default and test scenario assessments conducted for this case study.

Table 2 - *Results of the default and test scenario in Case Study 2.*

Model run	Hazard Quotient (HQ) Produced		
	Indoor Air Pathway	Soil Pathway	Total HQ
Default Residential House Scenario (Health Canada RfD)	5.6	0.58	6.18
Test Residential House Scenario (U.S. EPA IRIS RfD)	91	0.58	91.6

Based on the results of this case study, it is clear that the selected chemical-specific exposure limit can have a significant impact on the results of an assessment. Using the Health Canada exposure limit for naphthalene results in a significantly lower estimation of risk (14.8 x) compared to the results of the same assessment using the newer exposure limit for naphthalene proposed by IRIS. However, it should be noted that the use of a particular exposure limit in a given regulatory jurisdiction may reflect a preferred hierarchy of exposure limits. For example, many Canadian regulatory jurisdictions prefer to use Health Canada limits first, when available, followed by any different value recommended by the U.S. EPA (*i.e.*, IRIS or HEAST). In any event, a failure to recognize the availability of new or revised toxicological data can have significant implications on the results of a risk assessment.

Case Study 3: Site-specific Soil and Building Parameters

Both site-specific soil and building structural parameters can markedly influence exposure and risk estimates. While conservative in nature, available default soil parameter values included within a RBCA-based model may not adequately represent many actual site situations. For example, the defaults for soil f_{oc} (fraction of organic carbon within the soil) typically are 0.01 and 0.001 for silt/clay and sand/gravel soils, respectively. However, soils may have f_{oc} values much higher than 0.001, depending on site-specific conditions. Therefore, it is important that model users understand how fluctuations in f_{oc} can influence model results, and incorporate this knowledge into the study's conclusions.

The following is an outline of each model scenario completed, including specific information with respect to the environmental parameters used within each of the scenarios. Five model scenarios were completed in total, two of which used all of the RBCA default parameters, while the other three included modified input parameter(s).

Default Scenario I - This residential exposure scenario included naphthalene impacted subsurface soil, at a concentration of 200 mg/kg. Only the indirect indoor vapour infiltration pathway was assessed. All default parameters, including default characteristics for sand/gravel soil type (*i.e.*, f_{oc}, porosity, moisture content, *etc.*) were used.

Default Scenario II - This residential exposure scenario included naphthalene impacted subsurface soil, at a concentration of 200 mg/kg. Only the indirect indoor vapour infiltration pathway was assessed. All default parameters, including default characteristics for silt/clay soil type (*i.e.*, f_{oc}, porosity, moisture content, *etc*) were used.

Test Scenario I - The parameters and assumptions selected for this test scenario were equivalent to those used in *Default Scenario I*, except the crack area fraction of the building foundation was changed from the default of 0.001 to a typical mean value of 0.00056.

Test Scenario II - The parameters and assumptions selected for this test scenario were equivalent to those used in *Test Scenario I*, except the fraction of organic carbon (f_{oc}) was changed from the default of 0.001 for sand/gravel soil to a site-specific value of 0.003.

Test Scenario III - The parameters and assumptions selected for this test scenario were equivalent to those used in *Default Scenario II*, except the crack area fraction of the building foundation was changed from the default of 0.001 to a site-specific value of 0.00056.

The following, Table 3, provides a list of detailed parameters used to characterize the sand/gravel and silt/clay type soils within the assessed scenarios.

Table 3 - *Parameters used to represent sand/gravel and silt/clay soil types within the assessed scenarios.*

Parameters	**Sand/Gravel Soil Type**	**Silt/Clay Soil Type**
Soil Bulk Density (g/cm^3)	1.7	1.4
Fraction of Organic Carbon in the vadose zone (unitless)	0.001	0.01
Total Soil Porosity (unitless)	0.38	0.46
Volumetric Water Content in the vadose zone (unitless)	0.09	0.13
Volumetric Air Content in the vadose zone (unitless)	0.29	0.33

The following, Table 4, provides the results of the default and test assessments of the indoor vapour infiltration of napthalene into a residential building.

Table 4 - *Results of the default and test residential scenarios in Case Study 3.*

Model Run	Parameters Replacing Defaults	Hazard Quotient Produced
Default Scenario I (sand/gravel)	none	1.0
Default Scenario II (clay/silt)	none	0.11
Test Scenario I (sand/gravel)	Crack area fraction of 0.00056	0.58
Test Scenario 2 (sand/gravel)	Crack area fraction of 0.00056 and a f_{oc} of 0.003	0.20
Test Scenario 3 (silt/clay)	Crack area fraction of 0.00056	0.061

Results of the assessment indicate that a three-fold increase in the soil f_{oc} between Test Scenarios 1 and 2 (*i.e.*, 0.001 to 0.003) resulted in a nearly three-fold decrease in predicted risk. Thus, a small change in an assumed soil parameter (*e.g.*, from better site-specific characterization) can result in a significant impact on the overall predicted health risk.

This can be also be seen in the evaluation of the risk variance related to changes in the assumed crack area fraction for the hypothetical building. The value of 0.001 selected as the crack area fraction for both of the default scenarios corresponds to the 95% upper confidence level of 218 residential houses sampled throughout North America by Grimsrud *et al.* (1982). The value of 0.00056 selected for the test scenarios, on the other hand, corresponds to the mean value found during the study of 218 houses. By changing the crack area fraction from the 95% (*i.e.,* 0.001) to the mean value of 0.00056, the estimated Hazard Quotient for naphthalene in our sample assessments decreased from 0.11 to 0.061 and from 1.0 to 0.58 for silt/clay and sand/gravel soil types, respectively.

Thus, an approximate two-fold adjustment in the crack area fraction, from a conservative upper 95% confidence level to that representing an average building, can result in a corresponding two-fold decrease in predicted health risks. This, in combination with varying f_{oc} values, could result in up to a five-fold variance in the predicted health risks.

Discussion and Conclusions

The purpose of this paper was to demonstrate some of the pitfalls that can occur when inexperienced risk assessors use models, such as those based upon the RBCA framework, without an adequate understanding of the assumptions and parameters involved. As demonstrated in the case studies, inappropriate selection of model parameters and assumptions can lead to significant impacts on the results of a risk assessment. This could occur through the naive use of a "canned" commercial RBCA model, without making sufficient adjustments to adequately address site- and scenario-specific conditions, or through the blind use of default parameters when they clearly do not apply in the situation under assessment.

While an underestimation of the overall risk could result in the potential for adverse health effects, it is more likely, due to the conservative nature of the default assumptions, that the results of incorrect use of these models are assessments that are overly protective. Such assessment would likely result in the establishment of site-specific remediation criteria which are too stringent, potentially leading to needless increases in overall site clean-up costs. As such, clients and regulators must be aware of the potential health and remedial-cost implications resulting from the improper selection of assumptions and parameters when using RBCA-type risk assessment models.

References

Grimsrud, D.T., Sherman, M.H., and Sonderegger, R.C., 1983, "Calculating Infiltration: Implications for a Construction Quality Standard," In: ASHRAE, 1983, "Transactions". American Society of Heating, Refrigeration, and Airconditioning Engineers Inc.

Health Canada, 1996, "TDI/ADI/(MRIL)/RD Summary for Organic Contaminants," Health Canada. July 5, 1996.

OMOE, 1997, "Guidance on Site Specific Risk Assessment for Use at Contaminated Sites In Ontario," Ontario Ministry of the Environment, Revised April 1997.

U.S. EPA, 2000, "Naphthalene," Integrated Risk Information System (IRIS), U.S. Environmental Protection Agency. Online database.

Robert K. Johnston,[1] Wayne R. Munns, Jr.,[2] and Diane E. Nacci[2]

A Probabilistic Analysis to Determine Ecological Risk Drivers

---

Reference: Johnston, R. K., Munns, W. R. Jr., and Nacci, D. E., "**A Probabilistic Analysis To Determine Ecological Risk Drivers**," *Environmental Toxicology and Risk Assessment: Science, Policy, and Standardization - Implications for Environmental Decisions: Tenth Volume, ASTM STP 1403*, B. M. Greenberg, R. N. Hull, M. H. Roberts, Jr., and R. W. Gensemer, Eds., American Society for Testing and Materials, West Conshohocken, PA, 2001.

Abstract: A probabilistic analysis of exposure and effect data was used to identify chemicals most likely responsible for ecological risk. The mean and standard deviation of the natural log-transformed chemical data were used to estimate the probability of exposure for an area of concern and a reference area. Benchmarks of chemical effects were selected from criteria, standards, and toxicological thresholds in the literature and dose-response models developed for Pb were used to estimate the probability of an effect from Pb. Ecological risk, defined as the probability of exceeding a benchmark or causing an effect given the probability of exposure was calculated for the area of concern and reference area. The probability of an effect from Pb and probability of exceeding any combination of benchmarks were determined by Monte Carlo simulations. Chemicals that caused an incremental increase of risk ≥ 0.05 above the reference area were identified as potential "risk drivers."

Keywords: ecological risk assessment, probabilistic, Monte Carlo, exposure, effect

Introduction

In conducting an ecological risk assessment for Portsmouth Naval Shipyard, the primary objective was to define the magnitude and nature of risk to ecological receptors within the system (Johnston et al. 1994, MESO 2000). Exposure and effects data collected from areas around the shipyard and reference locations in the lower estuary were used

[1] Research scientist, Marine Environmental Support Office, Space and Naval Warfare Systems Center, Code D3621, San Diego, CA 92152-6326.

[2] Branch chief and research biologist, respectively, U. S. Environmental Protection Agency, National Health and Environmental Effects Research Laboratory, Atlantic Ecology Division, 27 Tarzwell Drive, Narragansett, RI 02882.

to determine that there was low risk to ecological receptors in Clark Cove (Figure 1). Since preliminary remediation goals were required, the next step was to identify the chemical contaminants that were most likely responsible for the risk — the risk drivers. This paper presents the procedures used to identify ecological risk drivers in Clark Cove.

Methods

Exposure Distributions

Data collected for the ecological risk assessment included chemical concentrations measured in samples of shore seeps, estuarine surface water, sediment, sediment porewater, and mussel (*Mytilus edulis*) tissue collected around the shipyard and at reference locations in the lower estuary. Initial sampling was conducted in fall 1991 followed by monthly monitoring of water and mussels at a subset of stations during 1992, and resampling of some stations for sediment and mussels during 1993 (MESO 2000). The raw data were grouped by areas of concern and the reference stations were combined to represent ambient conditions in the lower Piscataqua River (Figure 1). The mean (μ) and standard deviation (σ) of the natural logarithm-transformed raw data were used to estimate the exposure distributions for each chemical and exposure media for the areas of concern and the reference area. Due to the small sample size, the tendency of pollutants to conform to lognormal distributions (Gilbert 1987), the predominance of better fits to lognormal than normal distributions in the data, and the conservative estimate of exposure associated with lognormal distributions, the exposure distributions were assumed to be lognormal.

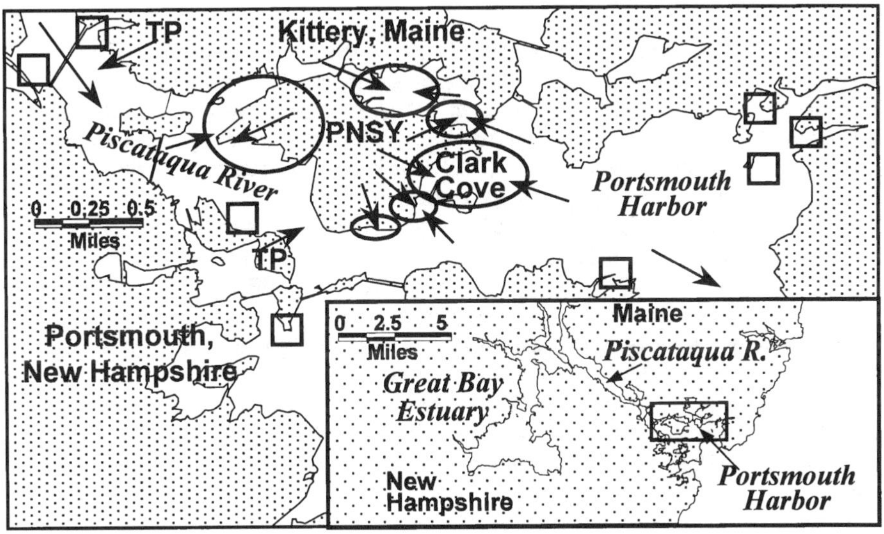

Figure 1 –*Conceptual model for the lower Piscataqua River showing the location of Portsmouth Naval Shipyard (PNSY), sewage treatment plants (TP), the areas of concern (circles), locations of reference stations (squares), and hypothesized transport pathways (arrows).*

Models of Exposure-Response for Pb

Because concentrations of Pb were high in the lower estuary, laboratory experiments were conducted to evaluate the effect of Pb on specific endpoints used in the risk assessment (Nacci et al. 2000) and develop exposure-response models for Pb (Bruce and Versteeg 1992)

$$R = R_0\ \Phi[(log(EC_x)\text{-}log(C))/\sigma+Z_x]\ for\ C > 0 \quad (1)$$

$$R = R_0\ for\ C = 0 \quad (2)$$

Where R is the predicted biological response at exposure concentration C, R_0 is the response measured in control treatments, Φ is a function that returns the cumulative area under the standard Gaussian distribution, Z_x is the normal deviate above which x percent of the Gaussian distribution lies, and EC_x and σ are the parameters that describe the position and slope of the cumulative Gaussian distribution. Fit to the EC_{20} effects levels (Figure 2), the models were developed for the effect of Pb exposure on sea urchin (*Arbacia punctulata*) larval fertilization, larval development, fecundity in adult females, and adult female survival (Nacci et al. 2000).

A sea urchin population model was also developed from the sea urchin toxicity data (Gleason et al. 2000). The population growth rate (λ) was used to relate Pb exposure to population level effects and it decreased as Pb tissue residues in adult urchins increased (Figure 2C, Gleason et al. 2000).

Benchmarks of Ecological Effect

Exposure-response data were not available for all the chemicals and biological effects that needed to be assessed. Therefore, toxicological thresholds (benchmarks) from the literature were used to estimate risk to selected biological receptors (Table 1). Benchmarks were selected to evaluate potential effects to a broad range of estuarine organisms. Unless otherwise noted, water benchmarks (W_B, Table 1) were set to national water quality criteria (WQC) for saltwater continuous (chronic) and maximum (acute) concentrations (U.S. EPA 1999). Water benchmarks for metals were based on total recoverable metal using the recommended dissolved to total metal conversion factor (U.S. EPA 1999). In accordance with the approach used to develop sediment quality criteria (U.S. EPA 1993), water quality criteria were used as benchmarks to evaluate porewater concentrations. The porewater concentrations of organic chemicals and metals were estimated by equilibrium partitioning (Di Toro et al. 1991) and by evaluating data on acid volatile sulfides (AVS) and simultaneously extracted metals (SEM, Di Toro et al. 1990), respectively. In the absence of water quality criteria values, the predicted interstitial water LC_{50} of polycyclic aromatic hydrocarbons (PAHs) determined for amphipods (Swartz et al. 1995) was used for pryene, flourene, benz(a)anthracence, and benzo(a)pryrene.

Sediment benchmarks (S_B, Table 1) consisted of the effects range-low (ERL) and effects range-median (ERM) sediment quality guidelines (Long et al. 1995) and the State of Washington sediment quality (WA-SQ) and cleanup (WA-CL) levels (Ginn and Pastorok 1992). Sediment benchmarks were developed for metals, individual PAHs, low (LPAH) and high (HPAH) molecular weight PAHs, the sum of the parent and alkyl homologs PAHs

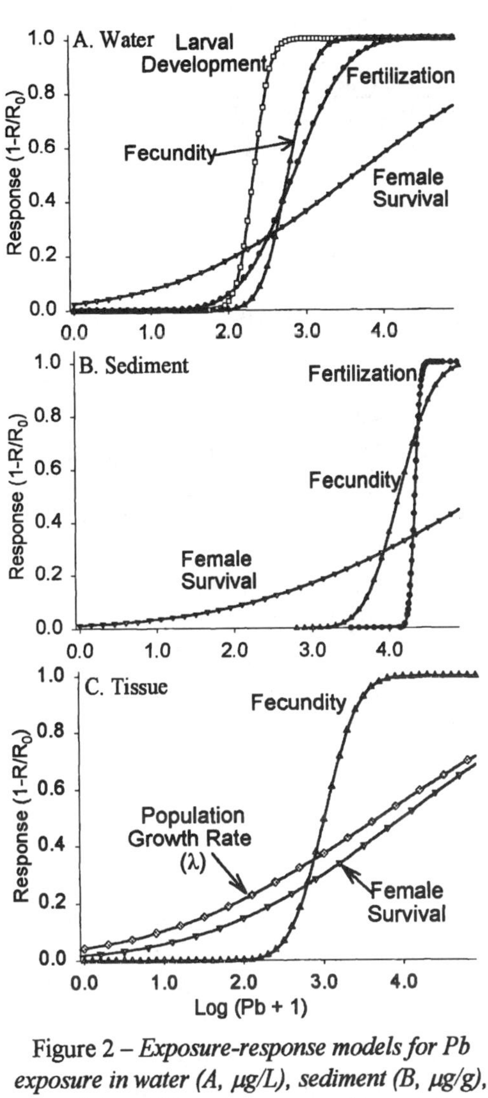

Figure 2 – *Exposure-response models for Pb exposure in water (A, µg/L), sediment (B, µg/g), and tissue (C, µg/g) to sea urchin toxicity endpoints. Model parameters from Nacci et al. (2000) and Gleason et al. (2000).*

(sumPAH), total PCB (tPCB), dichlorodiphenyl-trichloroethane (DDT), -dichloroethene (DDE), and -dichloroethane (DDD, Table 1). The sediment benchmarks were based on similar chemicals and ecological effects as those that were evaluated during the ecorisk assessment for the Portsmouth Naval Shipyard.

Water and sediment benchmarks were also used to develop benchmarks for mussel tissue residues (T_B, Table 1). The bioaccumulation critical value (B_{CV}) is the tissue concentration (µg/g dry weight) that would occur if water exposure levels exceeded the chronic or lowest available water benchmark

$$B_{CV} = W_B \cdot BCF/dw \qquad (3)$$

Where *BCF* is the bioconcentration factor (L/kg wet weight) and *dw* is the mass fraction of dry to wet tissue. The *BCF*s for Cd, Cu, Cr, Hg, Ni, and Zn were obtained from fitted values reported in Thomann et al. (1995) and the *BCF*s for PAHs were obtained from Pruell et al. (1986). A model of Pb uptake derived from mussels exposed to suspended sediments from Portsmouth Harbor (Nacci et al. 1994) was used to estimate the B_{CV} for Pb (Table 1).

For PCB exposure, 18 congeners were measured in sediment and mussel tissue samples. The PCB congener 153 (PCB153) was the most abundant congener, on average it accounted for 21% (range from 5 to 35%) of the sum of congeners (sumPCB) measured in mussels (MESO 2000). The B_{CV} for PCB was obtained using the BCF for PCB153 (Bergen et al. 1993) and assuming that PCB153 was proportional to sumPCB in mussels, and that the dissolved water concentration of tPCB could be approximated as 2×sumPCB (NOAA 1991).

Sediment bioaccumulation factors (BAF) measured in clams (*Macoma nasuta*, Boese et al. 1997) were used to develop the mussel tissue B_{CV} for DDT, DDE, and DDD. This

Table 1. *Benchmark concentrations for water, sediment, and mussel tissue (dry weight).*

	Water (W_B)		Sediment (S_B)				Tissue (T_B)	
	Chronic	Acute	ERL	ERM	WA-SQ[6]	WA-CL[6]	B_{CV}	D_{BD}
total metal	µg/L	µg/L	µg/g	µg/g	µg/g	µg/g	µg/g	µg/g
Ag		2.2	1.0	3.7	6.1	6.1		148.7[9]
As	36.0	69.0	8.2	70.0	57.0	93.0		460.6[10]
Cd	9.3	43.0	1.2	9.6	5.1	6.7	186.0	129.9[10]
Cr	50.0	1100.0	81.0	370.0	260.0	270.0	58.0	89.6[11]
Cu	3.7	5.8	34.0	270.0	390.0	390.0	20.0	4211.5[12]
Hg	1.1	2.1	0.2	0.7	0.4	0.6	0.6	40.3[13]
Ni	8.3	75.0	20.9	51.6			16.6	6935.5[10]
Pb	8.5	220.0	46.7	218.0	450.0	530.0	24.5[7]	101.3[13]
Zn	86.0	95.0	150.0	410.0	410.0	960.0	1720.0	1299.3[12]
fluorine		270.0[1]	0.019	0.540	23.0	79.0	801.8	90.5[14]
phenanthrene	3.8		0.240	1.500	100.0	480.0	20.4	5376.3[15]
anthracene		[3]	0.085	1.100	220.0	1200.0	952.6	
fluoranthrene	11.0		0.600	5.100	160.0	1200.0	106.2	
pyrene		14.0[1]	0.665	2.600	1000.0	1400.0	500.8	
chrysene		[3]	0.384	2.800	110.0	460.0	439.8	
benz(a)anthracene		6.6[1]	0.261	1.600	110.0	270.0	439.8	
benzo(a)pryene		1.9[1]	0.430	1.600	99.0	210.0	329.2	
dibenz(a,h)anthracene			0.036	0.260	12.0	33.0		
LPAH			0.552	3.160	370.0	780.0		
HPAH			1.700	9.600	960.0	5300.0		
sumPAH		300.0	4.022	44.792				4405.4[16]
PCB153							3.7	
tPCB		0.03	0.023	0.180	12.0	65.0		16.1[17]
DDT	0.001		0.002	0.046			0.005[8]	0.25[18]
DDE		3.6	0.002	0.020			0.05[8]	0.25[18]
DDD		14.0	0.002	0.027			0.03[8]	0.25[18]
tDDx[5]			0.003	0.350			0.3[8]	0.25[18]

[1] Amphipod LC_{50} (Swartz et al. 1995)
[2] (US EPA 1994)
[3] LC_{50} > solubility limit (Swartz et al. 1995)
[4] (US EPA 1993a)
[5] tDDx = DDT + DDE + DDD
[6] µg/g organic carbon for organics
[7] B_{CV}= antilog[1.495(Log W_B)] (Nacci et al. 1994)
[8] B_{CV}= BAF × Sediment ERM
[9] UF=0.2, duckling 4 wk NOEL (Van Fleet 1992)
[10] mallard duck NOEL (Sample et al. 1996)
[11] black duck NOEL (Sample et al. 1996)
[12] chicken NOEL (Sample et al. 1996)
[13] Japanese quail NOEL (Sample et al. 1996)
[14] UF=0.01, blackbird LD_{50} (Schafer et al. 1983)
[15] UF=0.1, mallard duck LOEL (Eisler 1987)
[16] UF=0.1, duck LOEL (Patton & Dieter 1980)
[17] ringneck pheasant NOEL (Sample et al. 1996)
[18] brown pelican NOEL (Sample et al. 1996)

assumed that the route of exposure between clams and mussels was similar, that bioaccumulation in clams was equal to bioaccumulation in mussels, and that the bivalve tissue concentrations were a result of exposure to sediment-bound DDT and its metabolites.

Toxicity reference values for black ducks (*Anas rubripes*) were used to develop benchmarks for dietary exposure from the consumption of mussel tissues (D_{BD}, Table 1). Dietary benchmarks were developed using the highest dose that caused no observed effect (NOEL) to the most sensitive bird species similar to black duck (Sample et al. 1996). Based on the similarity of toxicity values reported among avian species, the test species ($NOEL_T$) were assumed to be equivalent to the NOEL for black ducks (Sample et al. 1996, Table 1) and the benchmark was determined by

$$D_{BD} = (NOEL_T \cdot UF)/(F \cdot dw) \text{ ug/g (dry weight)} \quad (4)$$

$$F = aRdL = 0.09 \quad (5)$$

Where UF is an uncertainty factor and F is the dietary uptake factor (g/g body weight per day). The value for F was obtained by assuming assimilation efficiency ($a = 0.9$), fraction of diet ($d = 1.0$), fraction of life span ($L = 1.0$), and calculating the food ingestion rate (g/g body weight per day) as food consumption rate per day divided by body weight (125 g per day/1250 g = 0.1, Sample et al. 1996). For long term (> 7 wk) NOELs the UF was set to one. Short term NOELs, LOELs, and lethal doses were converted to NOELs by setting the UF to 0.2, 0.1, and 0.01, respectively (US EPA 1993b, Table 1).

Calculating Ecological Risk

The probability density function (Sokal and Rohlf 1995) was used to plot the exposure and effect distributions. The exposure distributions show the probability of exposure and the effect distributions show the probability that exposure will cause an effect. Ecological risk was defined as the probability of causing an effect *P(Effect)* given the probability of exposure *P(Exp)* or the probability $P(C_z)$ of exceeding a benchmark (B, Table 1)

$$P(Effect|Exp) = P(Effect \cap Exp)/P(Exp),\ P(Exp) \neq 0 \quad (6)$$

$$P(C_z) = \text{probability of exceeding } C_z \text{ of the Standard Normal Distribution} \quad (7)$$

$$C_z = (B - \mu)/\sigma \quad (8)$$

The exposure distributions of Pb for shore seeps, estuarine surface water, sediment, and mussel tissue concentrations were used to estimate the probability of an effect from Pb to sea urchins. Monte Carlo simulations (10 000 trials, CRYSTAL BALL,® Version 4.0, Decisioneering Inc., Denver, CO) were used to sample the exposure distributions and calculate the response to sea urchin fertilization, larval development, female fecundity, female survival, and population growth rate. A reduction greater than or equal to 1% in the control response was interpreted as an "effect."

Monte Carlo simulations were also used to simulate the probability of exceeding any combination of benchmarks for all chemicals in an exposure medium. The simulation also incorporated dependencies among the exposure distributions. Highly significant correlations ($p<0.0001$) between the chemicals that were detected in the data set were included as dependencies in the simulation. This caused the random numbers selected for the simulation to have the same correlations as was observed in the field data. If conflicts arose in obtaining the desired correlations during simulation, the program would make small adjustments to the correlation coefficients and continue the simulation (CRYSTAL BALL®).

Risk Drivers – The positive difference in the probability of exceeding a benchmark or an effect between Clark Cove and the reference area was defined as the incremental risk. Chemicals with an incremental risk greater than or equal to 0.05 were interpreted to signify a "meaningful" increase in risk and such chemicals were identified as "potential risk drivers." The conservative sediment benchmarks (ERL and WA-SQ) were not used to identify risk drivers.

Results

Exposure Distributions

Exposure distributions were calculated and tabulated for Clark Cove and Piscataqua River reference area. Generally, higher mean concentrations of chemicals were measured in Clark Cove, but for some of the chemicals the data from the reference area had more variation. The results obtained for Pb were typical (Table 2). There was about twice as much Pb in the mussel and sediment samples from Clark Cove than the samples from Piscataqua River, but there was more variation in the data from the reference area, resulting in a wider exposure distribution for Piscataqua River than for Clark Cove (Figure 3).

Risk Calculations

No risk from Pb exposure in the estuarine surface waters was calculated. However, Pb exposure in shore seeps resulted in notable increases in the probability of an effect on sea

Table 2 – *Exposure distributions of Pb for Clark Cove and Piscataqua River.*

	Clark Cove					Piscataqua River				
Pb	n	ln(μ)	ln(σ)	Gm[1]	max	n	ln(μ)	ln(σ)	Gm[1]	max
Shore Seeps[2] (μg/L)	28	0.63	1.82	1.88	39.46					
Surface Water (μg/L)	12	-2.39	0.16	0.09	0.12	39	-2.35	0.39	0.09	0.21
Bulk Sediment (μg/g)	28	4.09	0.53	60.03	123.00	18	3.37	1.53	29.16	116.10
Porewater[3] (μg/L)	6	0	0	0	0	9	0	0	0	0
Mussel Tissue (μg/g)	17	2.05	0.33	7.79	13.60	15	1.48	1.28	4.39	10.00

[1] Gm = geometeric mean $e^{\ln(\mu)}$ [2] No data for reference shore seeps
[3] AVS >> SEM no free metal present in porewater, risk not calculated.

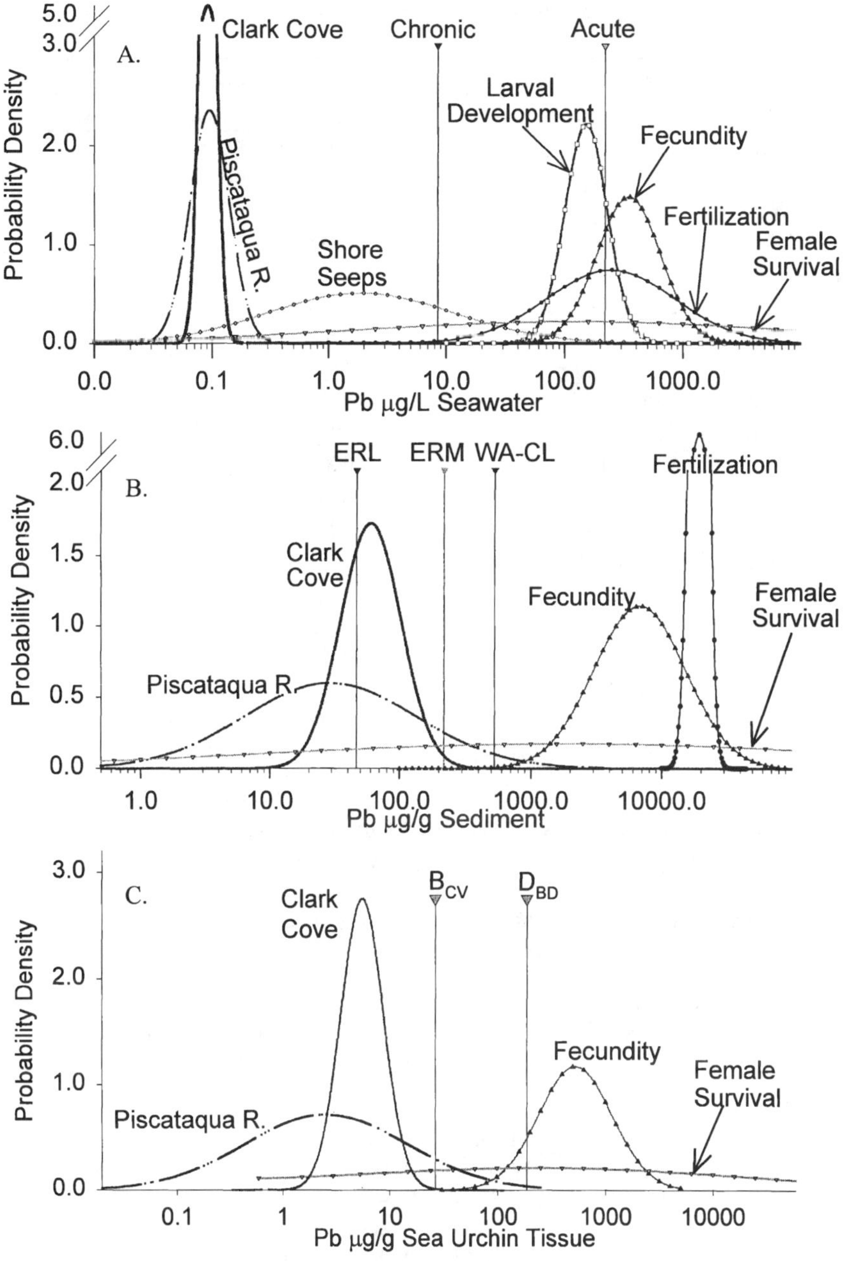

Figure 3 - *Probability density of Pb exposure and sea urchin EC20 effects levels and the corresponding benchmarks for exposure in seawater (A), sediment (B), and sea urchin tissue (C).*

Table 3 – *Risk of an effect or of exceeding a benchmark from Pb exposure.*

Media	Sea Urchin Endpoint or Benchmark	Clark Cove	Piscataqua River	Incremental Risk
Estuarine Water	Fertilization[1]	<0.0001	<0.0001	
Estuarine Water	Development[1]	<0.0001	<0.0001	
Estuarine Water	Fecundity[1]	<0.0001	<0.0001	
Estuarine Water	Female Survival[1]	0.0243	0.0558	
Shore Seep	Fertilization[1]	0.1101	[2]	
Shore Seep	Larval Development[1]	0.0395	[2]	
Shore Seep	Fecundity[1]	0.0286	[2]	
Shore Seep	Female Survival[1]	0.4158	[2]	
Bulk Sediment	ERL	0.6816	0.3792	0.3025
Bulk Sediment	ERM	0.0076	0.0944	
Bulk Sediment	WA-SQ	0.0001	0.0369	
Bulk Sediment	WA-CL	<0.0001	0.0291	
Bulk Sediment	Fertilization[1]	<0.0001	<0.0001	
Bulk Sediment	Fecundity[1]	0.0004	0.0186	
Bulk Sediment	Female Survival[1]	0.1689	0.3629	
Mussel Tissue	B_{CV}	0.0003	0.0900	
Mussel Tissue	D_{BD}	<0.0001	0.0072	
Mussel Tissue	Fecundity[1,3]	<0.0001	0.0096	
Mussel Tissue	Female Survival[1,3]	0.1171	0.3055	
Mussel Tissue	Population Growth Rate[1,3]	0.1288	0.3564	

[1] $R \leq 0.99R_0$ [2] No data from reference area for shore seeps.
[3] The Pb in mussel tissue was used to estimate bioaccumulation in sea urchin tissue $\log(Pb_{Urchin})=[\log(Pb_{Mussel}) - 0.34884]/0.7304$ (Nacci et al. 1994).

Table 4 – *Summary of potential risk drivers determined for Clark Cove. Probability of exceeding benchmarks in shore seeps, sediment, and mussel tissues.*

	Benchmark	Cu	Pb	Ni	Zn
Shore Seep	WQC - Chronic	0.484	0.204	0.213	0.530
Shore Seep	WQC - Acute	0.323	0.005	0.003	0.486

	Chemical	Benchmark	Clark Cove	Piscataqua River	Incremental Risk
Sediment	Cr	WA-CL	0.089	0.003	0.086
Sediment	Cu	ERM	0.046	0.002	0.044
Sediment	Ni	ERM	0.087	0.006	0.081
Sediment	DDD	ERM	0.082	0.004	0.077
Mussel Tissue	DDT	B_{CV}	0.951	0.873	0.078
Mussel Tissue	DDD	B_{CV}	0.129	0.000	0.129

urchin fertilization and female survival (Table 3, Figure 3). There was very low risk from Pb exposure in sediment to sea urchin fertilization, fecundity, and female survival. Using the relationship between Pb uptake in mussels and sea urchins reported by Nacci et al. (1994), the Pb concentration in mussel tissues were used to estimate the Pb concentration in sea urchin tissues and assess risk to sea urchin fecundity, survival, and population growth (Table 3). There were lower risks from Pb accumulation to sea urchin fecundity, survival, and population growth in Clark Cove than for the reference area (Figure 3, Table 3).

No risk was calculated from exposure to estuarine water but there was relatively high-risk ($P > 0.2$) of exceeding water quality criteria for Cu, Pb, Ni, and Zn in shore seeps (Table 4). For bulk sediment exposure in Clark Cove, all the metals, tPCB, DDD, DDE, DDT and tDDx had incremental risk ($P > 0.05$) of exceeding the ERL (MESO 2000), but only Ni, Cu and DDD had an incremental risk of exceeding the ERM and only Cr had an incremental risk of exceeding the WA-CL (Table 4). There was also an incremental risk ($P > 0.05$) of exceeding bioaccumulation critical values (B_{CV}) for DDT and DDD in mussel tissues (Table 4). No incremental risk was calculated for porewater exposure or for mussel tissue concentrations exceeding dietary (D_{BD}) benchmarks (MESO 2000).

There was about the same probability of exceeding one or more sediment benchmarks in Clark Cove as there was in the reference area, but the probability of exceeding multiple sediment benchmarks was higher for the reference area (PR) than for Clark Cove (CC). For mussel tissue residues, there was more risk of exceeding multiple benchmarks for Clark Cove than the reference area (Figure 4).

The consequence of assuming lognormal distributions for the data can be evaluated by examining the probability density functions for Cu in sediment displayed as both normal and lognormal distributions (Figure 5). The lognormal distribution obtained for Clark Cove had a much greater probability of exceeding the ERM benchmark ($P = 0.046$) than the normal distribution for Clark Cove ($P < 0.00001$). This is a function of the shape of the lognormal distribution, which tends to have a longer tail (Gilbert 1987, Sokal and Rohlf 1995) and will provide a more conservative estimate of exceeding benchmarks, especially nonconservative benchmarks, than the normal distribution.

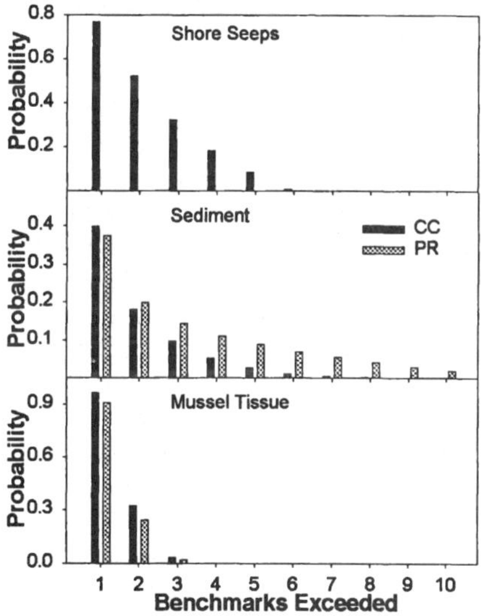

Figure 4. The probability of exceeding one or more benchmarks from shore seep, sediment, and tissue exposure.

Discussion

Risk from Exposure

Shore Seeps – The shore seeps were small streams that drained water from intertidal exchange areas, upland ground-water sources, or sources of surface water on the island into intertidal areas around the island. The seeps were a possible link

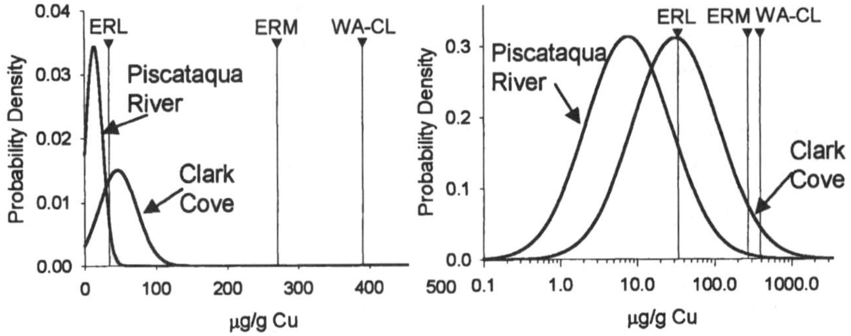

Figure 5 – *Probability of exceeding sediment benchmarks for copper assuming a normal (left) or lognormal distribution (right).*

from contaminant sources on the island to the estuary. The number of seep samples was limited and there was no information on seeps located in the reference area. The seeps were rapidly diluted upon entering the river so the increased risk was worst case.

Sediment –The higher probability of exceeding multiple sediment benchmarks in the reference area (Figure 4) was due to wider distributions and higher correlations between the PAH compounds calculated for the reference area than for Clark Cove (MESO 2000). Exposure calculated from porewater may be more accurate than exposures estimated from bulk sediment chemistry because binding phases of the sediment that control chemical bioavailability are taken into account (Di Toro et al. 1990, 1991). The benchmarks for porewater exposure were based on sediment quality criteria and amphipod toxicity (Table 1), which are appropriate for protection of benthic organisms.

Mussel Tissue Residues – The mussel tissue data were used to evaluate two routes of exposure, trophic transfer through dietary uptake by black ducks and bioaccumulation to estimate surface water (or sediment) exposure levels. Mussel tissue concentrations are a function of the exposure condition (Nelson 1990, Bergen et al. 1993) and can be used to infer the exposure levels to other marine organisms. Although direct harm to mussels was not widely evident in the data from the estuary, their ability to accumulate contaminants and their stationary lifestyle results in accumulation of contaminants that can be used to evaluate exposure to other ecological receptors. It was assumed that mussel tissue concentrations were at steady state; that exposure conditions were constant; that the chemicals bioaccumulated were directly proportional to exposure levels; and that chemical exposure to other organisms was similar to the chemical exposure to mussels.

Higher risk of an effect from Pb bioaccumulation was simulated for the reference area than for Clark Cove (Figure 3, Table 3). However, there was more risk of exceeding multiple benchmarks in mussel tissue for Clark Cove than the reference area (Figure 4). This was because the exposure levels for DDT, tDDx, Hg, DDD, and DDE were all higher for Clark Cove and there was a high correlation among DDT and its metabolites.

Risk to Sea Urchins – The cause and effect models developed between Pb exposure and effects to sea urchins (Figure 2) provide a means to evaluate the probability of an effect from Pb exposure. Because the effect distributions for larval development, fertilization, and fecundity are far to the right of the exposure distributions (Figure 3) there was little risk to those endpoints (Table 3). Higher sensitivity to Pb exposure for adult female survival and sea urchin population growth rate increased risk, but because the slope of the response curves for adult survival and population growth rate was much flatter than the other endpoints (Figure 2), the magnitude of the response was less. Further work is needed to evaluate the significance of these results.

Risk Drivers

The accumulation of contaminants in depositional areas of the lower estuary is controlled by the sources of chemical inputs, transport pathways, and assimilation processes. Over time these processes, will redistribute and mix pollutants and contribute to the ambient pollution levels present in the estuary. Although arbitrary, an incremental increase in risk greater than or equal to 0.05 is a strong indication that contaminant levels were elevated above ambient levels. Thus a meaningful improvement in the ecological condition of the estuary could be achieved if clean up efforts focused on reducing exposure to the risk drivers.

Uncertainty

It was assumed that the exposure data from reference locations in the Piscataqua River represented ambient conditions. Although other sources of contamination in the estuary could increase ambient exposure and risk, the risk assessment was concerned with quantifying the incremental risk that could be linked to the shipyard. The incremental risk calculated for Clark Cove is the increased likelihood that a receptor could be exposed to potentially harmful concentrations beyond what would occur from ambient exposure. Many assumptions in selecting benchmark concentrations, measuring exposure conditions, and estimating probability distributions had to be made. These assumptions applied to both the areas of concern and reference areas. By comparing the difference between reference and areas of concern, risks were evaluated on a relative basis.

There was uncertainty in assuming that the data conformed to lognormal distributions. In some cases, the raw data did not conform well to either a normal or lognormal distribution. The distributions are a result of the number of samples, frequency of detection, and range of concentrations. Outliers, inappropriate sampling design, and analytical interferences can bias estimates of μ and σ. By assuming that the data came from a lognormal distribution, the parameters of the distribution are less influenced by outliers. Nevertheless, small sample sizes ($n < 30$) could unduly influence the shape of distribution. The "worst case" is included by assuming that the data are lognormally distributed (Figure 5).

There was also uncertainty in selecting benchmarks and effect levels. The benchmarks are a result of what is available in the literature and can be improved, as more knowledge becomes available. Assuming that it is just as detrimental to exceed one benchmark as another (uniform sensitivity and protectiveness), the simulation of exceeding multiple benchmarks estimated the probability of more than one stressor acting simultaneously. The high number of positive correlations between stressors suggests that a location that is contaminated with one pollutant is also likely to be contaminated with other pollutants.

Conclusion

The chemicals most likely responsible for the low ecological risk in Clark Cove were Cr, Ni, Cu, and DDD from sediment exposure and DDD and DDT from mussel data. For the shore seeps, Cu, Pb, Ni, and Zn had a high probability (P>0.2) of exceeding chronic water quality criteria. Given that ecological risk is present, the analysis presented in this paper is useful for identifying the chemicals most likely responsible for the risk. In the case of remediation or restoration, attention to risk drivers will help identify sources of risk, help reduce the ambient concentrations within the estuary, and assure that problems, if corrected, will make an improvement in the ecological condition of the estuary.

Acknowledgment

A cooperative research and monitoring agreement between the U. S. Navy and the U. S. EPA supported this work. The conclusions are the views of the authors and are not official policy of the U. S. Navy or U. S. EPA. Mention of trade names does not constitute an endorsement or recommendation for use. This is contribution number 00-025 of the U.S. EPA, National Health, and Environmental Effects Research Laboratory, Atlantic Ecology Division, Narragansett, RI.

References

Bergen, B. J., Nelson, W. G. and Pruell R. J., 1993, "The Bioaccumulation of PCB Congeners by Blue Mussels (*Mytilus edulis*) in New Bedford Harbor, MA," *Environmental Toxicology and Chemistry*, Vol. 12, No 9, pp. 1671-1681.

Boese, B. L., Lee, H., II, and Echols, S., 1997, "Evaluation of a First-Order Model for the Prediction of the Bioaccumulation of PCBs and DDT from Sediment into the Marine Deposit-Feeding Clam *Macoma nasuta*," *Environmental Toxicology and Chemistry* Vol. 16, No.7, pp. 1545-1553.

Bruce, R. and Versteeg, D., 1992, "A Statistical Procedure for Modeling Continuous Toxicity Data," *Environmental Toxicology and Chemistry*, Vol. 11, pp. 1485-94.

Di Toro, D., Mahony, J., Hansen, D., Scott, K. J., Hicks, M., Mayr, S., and Redmond M., 1990, "The Toxicity of Cadmium in Sediments: The Role of Acid Volatile Sulfide," *Environmental Toxicology and Chemistry* Vol. 9, No. 6, pp. 1487-1502.

Di Toro, D., Zarba, C., Hansen, D., Berry, W., Swartz, R., Cowan, C., Pavlou, S., Allen, H., Thomas, N., and Paquin, P., 1991, "Technical Basis for Establishing Sediment Quality Criteria for Nonionic Organic Chemicals Using Equilibrium Partitioning," *Environmental Toxicology and Chemistry*, Vol. 10, No. 6, pp. 1541-83.

Eisler, R., 1987, *Polycyclic Aromatic Hydrocarbon Hazards to Fish, Wildlife, and Invertebrates: A Synoptic Review*, Biological Report 85(1.11), Contaminant Hazard Reviews Report No. 11, Fish and Wildlife Service, Laurel, MD.

Gilbert, R. O., 1987, *Statistical Methods for Environmental Pollution Monitoring*, Van Nostrand Reinhold Company, Inc., New York, NY.

Ginn, T. C. and Pastorok, R. A., 1992, "Assessment and Management of Contaminated Sediments in Puget Sound," *Sediment Toxicity Assessment*, Lewis Publishers, Boca Raton, Florida, pp. 379-401.

Gleason, T., Munns, W. R. Jr., and D. Nacci, 2000, "Projecting Population-Level Response of Purple Sea Urchins to Lead Contamination for an Estuarine Ecological Risk Assessment," *Journal of Aquatic Ecosystem Stress and Recovery*, Vol. 7, pp. 177-185.

Johnston R. K., Munns, W. R. Jr., Mills, L.J., Short, F.T., and Walker H.A. (eds), 1994, *Estuarine Ecological Risk Assessment for Portsmouth Naval Shipyard, Kittery, Maine: Phase I: Problem Formulation*, Naval Command Control and Ocean Surveillance Center, Technical Report 1627, San Diego, CA.

Long, E. R., MacDonald, D. D., Smith, S. L., and Calder F. D., 1995, "Incidence of Adverse Biological Effects Within the Ranges of Chemical Concentrations in Marine and Estuarine Sediments," *Environmental Management*, Vol. 19, pp. 81-97.

Marine Environmental Support Office, 2000, *Estuarine Ecological Risk Assessment for Portsmouth Naval Shipyard, Final Report*, Vol. I and II, Space and Naval Warfare Systems Center, San Diego, CA.

Nacci, D., Cayula, S., Tracey, G., Gleason, T., Serbst, J., and Munns, W. R. Jr., 1994, *An Assessment of Exposure-Response Data from the Estuarine Ecological Risk Assessment Case Study for Portsmouth Naval Shipyard*, Naval Command, Control and Ocean Surveillance Center, San Diego, CA.

Nacci, D., Serbst, J., Gleason, T., Cayula, S., Thursby, G., Johnston, R. K., and Munns, W. R. Jr., 2000, "Biological Responses of the Sea Urchin, *Arbacia puntulata*, to Lead Contamination for an Estuarine Ecological Risk Assessment," *Journal of Aquatic Ecosystem Stress and Recovery*, Vol. 7, pp. 187-199.

Nelson, W. G., 1990, "Use of the Blue Mussel, *Mytilus edulis*, in Water Quality Toxicity Testing and *in situ* Marine Biological Monitoring," *Aquatic Toxicology and Risk Assessment*, Vol. 13, ASTM STP 1096, American Society for Testing and Materials, Philadelphia, PA., pp. 167-175.

National Oceanic and Atmospheric Administration, 1991, *Second Summary of Data on Chemical Contaminants in Sediments from the National Status and Trends Program*, Technical Memorandum NOS OMA 59, Rockville, MD.

Patton, J. and Dieter, M., 1980, "Effect of Petroleum Hydrocarbons on Hepatic Function in the Duck," *Comparative Biochemistry and Physiology*, Vol. 65C, pp. 33-36.

Pruell, R. J., Lake, J. L., Davis, W., and Quinn, J. G., 1986, "Uptake and Depuration of Organic Contaminants by Blue Mussels (*Mytilus edulis*) Exposed to Environmentally Contaminated Sediment," *Marine Biology*, Vol. 91, pp. 497-507.

Sample, B., Opresko, D., and Suter, G., 1996, *Toxicological Benchmarks for Wildlife: 1996 Revision*. ER/TM-86/R3, Oak Ridge National Laboratory, Oak Ridge, TN.

Shafer, E. W., Jr., Bowles, W. A., and Hurlbut, J., 1983, "The Acute Oral Toxicity, Repellency, and Hazard Potential of 998 Chemicals to One or More Species of Wild and Domestic Birds," *Archives of Environmental Contamination and Toxicology*, Vol. 12, pp. 355-382.

Sokal, R., and Rohlf, F., 1995, *Biometry*, W. H. Freeman and Company, New York, NY.

Swartz, R., Schults, D. W., Ozretich, R. J. Lamberson, J. O. Cole, F. A., DeWitt, T. H., Redmond, M.S., Ferraro, S.P., 1995, "ΣPAH: A Model to Predict the Toxicity of Polynuclear Aromatic Hydrocarbon Mixtures in Field-Collected Sediments," *Environmental Toxicology and Chemistry*, Vol. 14, No. 11, pp. 1977-1987.

Thomann, R. V., Mahony, J. D., and Mueller, R., 1995, "Steady-State Model of Biota Sediment Accumulation Factor for Metals in Two Marine Bivalves," *Environmental Toxicology and Chemistry*, Vol. 14, No. 11, pp. 1989-1998.

U.S. EPA, 1993a, *Technical Basis for Deriving Sediment Quality Criteria for Nonionic Organic Contaminants for the Protection of Benthic Organisms Using Equilibrium Partitioning*, EPA-822-R-93-011, Office of Water, U.S. EPA, Washington, DC.

U.S. EPA, 1993b, Wildlife Exposure Factors Handbook, Volume I, EPA/600/R-93/187a, Office of Research and Development, U.S. EPA, Washington, DC.

U.S. EPA, 1994, *Ambient Aquatic Life Water Quality Criteria for: Phenantherene*, EPA/822/R-88100, Office of Water, U.S. EPA, Washington, DC.

U.S. EPA, 1998, *Guidelines for Ecological Risk Assessment*, EPA/630/R-95/002F, April 1998, Final, Risk Assessment Forum, U.S. EPA, Washington, DC.

U.S. EPA, 1999, *National Recommended Water Quality Criteria–Correction*, EPA 822-Z-99-001, April 1999, Office of Water, U.S. EPA, Washington, DC.

Van Fleet, J. F., 1982, "Amounts of twelve elements required to induce selenium-vitamin E deficiency in ducklings," *American Journal of Veterinary Reseach*, Vol. 43, pp. 851-857.

Paul B. Tchounwou,[1] Barbara A. Wilson,[1] and Ali B. Ishaque[1]

Embryotoxicity of Arsenic Trioxide and Atrazine to Japanese Medaka (*Oryzias latipes*), and Cytotoxicity to Human Liver Carcinoma Cells ($HepG_2$)

Reference: Tchounwou, P. B., Wilson, B. A., and Ishaque, A. B. "**Embryotoxicity of Arsenic Trioxide and Atrazine to Japanese Medaka (*Oryzias latipes*), and Cytotoxicity to Human Liver Carcinoma Cells ($HepG_2$),**" *Environmental Toxicology and Risk Assessment: Science, Policy, and Standardization – Implications for Environmental Decisions: Tenth Volume, ASTM STP 1403*, B. M. Greenberg, R. N. Hull, M. H. Roberts, Jr., and R. W. Gensemer, Eds., American Society for Testing and Materials, West Conshohocken, PA, 2001.

Abstract: We investigated the acute toxicity of arsenic trioxide and atrazine, singly and in combination, to Japanese medaka embryos, and the cytotoxicity of these chemicals to human liver carcinoma cell lines ($HepG_2$). Two day-old embryos were exposed to serial concentrations of arsenic, atrazine, and a mixture of the two, following a 96-hrs static renewal test protocol. The *in vitro* bioassay was performed by exposing $HepG_2$ cells to arsenic and atrazine, and measuring the activity of lactate dehydrogenase using a spectrophotometer at 340 nm, after 48 hrs of incubation at 37°C and 5% CO_2. Results of the embryo bioassay indicated a concentration-response relationship with respect to chemical toxicity. Upon 96 hrs of exposure, the NOAEL, LOAEL, LC_{50}, and LC_{95} of arsenic were 0.07 (0.04-0.09), 0.15 (0.10-0.18), 0.23 (0.21-0.26), and 0.32 (0.28-0.41) mg/L, respectively. No significant differences ($p > 0.05$) in LC_{50} values were found between 24 and 96 hrs of exposure, indicating that arsenic is a fast acting chemical, with most acute poisoning occurring within 24 hrs of exposure. Within the range of concentrations tested, atrazine was found to be non-toxic to embryos, even at its maximum solubility of 200 mg/L in 2% DMSO. The mixture of arsenic with 100 mg/L atrazine resulted in a 96hrs-LC_{50} of 0.28 (0.26-0.31) mg/L, indicating a combined toxic effect that is simply additive or slightly antagonistic. The cytotoxicity assay yielded a LC_{50} value of 11.94 (8.8-15.1) mg/L for arsenic. Under the test conditions, the LC_{50} of atrazine was greater than 100 mg/L, and could not be computed with certainty due to its poor solubility in the test medium.

Keywords: embryotoxicity, cytotoxicity, arsenic, atrazine, *Oryzias latipes*, $HepG_2$ cells

---

[1] Associate professor and director, Environmental Science Ph.D. Program; Assistant professor, Department of Biology; and Post-doctoral research associate, Environmental Toxicology Research Laboratory, respectively, School of Science and Technology, Jackson State University, Jackson, MS 39217

Arsenic is a metalloid and exists in the earth's crust. Its sources as an environmental contaminant are mainly from natural phenomena such as erosion and volcanoes. Natural levels in soil are usually between 1 to 40 mg/kg. Anthropogenic activities such as metal smelting, coal combustion, and industrial production of arsenic-containing pesticides, pharmaceuticals, and other byproducts could significantly augment these levels. More than 80% of arsenic compounds are used to manufacture products with agricultural applications such as insecticides, herbicides, fungicides, algicides, sheep dips, wood preservatives, dyestuffs, and medicines for the eradication of tapeworms in sheep and cattle (NAS 1977). Arsenic compounds have been used for at least a century in the treatment of syphilis, yaws, amoebic dysentery, and trypanosomiasis. Arsenical drugs are still used in treating certain tropical diseases such as African sleeping sickness and amoebic dysentery, and in veterinary medicine to treat parasitic diseases, including filariasis in dogs and black head in turkeys and chickens (NAS 1977). During the period 1200 to 1650, it was used extremely in homicides (NRCC 1978).

In the environment, arsenic may be transported by wind or water erosion of small particles, or by leaching into rainfall or snowmelt. Transport and partitioning of arsenic in water depends upon the chemical form of arsenic and on interactions with other materials present. Soluble forms move with the water and may be carried long distances through rivers, while insoluble forms may be absorbed from water onto soils or sediments, especially clays, irons, aluminum hydroxides, manganese compounds, and organic materials (U.S. EPA 1982). Bioconcentration of arsenic occurs in aquatic organisms, primarily algae and lower invertebrates. In water, arsenic can undergo a series of transformations, including oxido-reduction reactions, ligand exchange, and biotransformation (U.S. EPA 1982). In a contaminated river, sediments can contain substantial amounts of arsenic that are predominantly mobile during water-sediments interactions. Factors influencing the fate of arsenicals in water include the oxido-reduction potential, pH, metal sulfide and sulfide ion concentration, iron concentrations, temperature, salinity, distribution and composition of the biota. The mobility of arsenic in these sediments is affected by the physical and chemical forms of the arsenic species as well as by environmental conditions (Mock and Wai 1994).

In the United States, the primary source of arsenic in humans is through food, mainly ingested from fish and shellfish which amounts to about 50 ug/d on the average (Borum and Abernathy 1994). Several epidemiological studies have demonstrated that arsenic is a known human carcinogen (IARC 1987, IRIS 1992). It has been implicated in the etiology of skin cancer, as well as several internal cancers involving the lung, the bladder and the liver (Tseng et al. 1968, Chen et al. 1985, 1992). The general health effects associated with arsenic exposure include cardiovascular and peripheral vascular disease, developmental abnormalities, neurologic and neurobehavioral disorders, diabetes, hearing loss, portal fibrosis of the liver, lung fibrosis, hematologic disorders, and carcinoma (Tchounwou et al. 1999, Tchounwou 2000).

Atrazine, on the other hand, is a xenobiotic, and it is one of the most heavily used herbicides in Mississippi and the United States as a whole. It is used mainly in corn and sorghum farms in the Mississippi Delta where most of the agricultural activities are performed. Atrazine may be released into the environment through effluent discharge from manufacturing facilities, and through its use as herbicide. In the United States, monitoring studies of surface waters as well as ground waters have shown widespread detection of triazine herbicides including atrazine (Coupe et al. 1998, Squillace et al. 1993). Surface waters collected from 149 sites in 122 Mid-western river basins indicated that 52% of the sites exceeded the United States Environmental Protection Agency (U.S. EPA)'s maximum contaminant level (MCL) of 3 ug/L for atrazine (Thurman et al. 1991).

Atrazine can be absorbed into the blood stream through oral, dermal, and inhalation exposure. The U.S. EPA considers atrazine as a systemic toxicant that has a potential of causing a variety of adverse health effects including: congestion of the heart, lungs and kidneys, hypotension, antidiuresis, muscle spasms, weight loss, bradycardia, and adrenal degeneration (Hallenbeck and Cummingham 1985). Death has been reported in studies with laboratory animals following exposure to high doses of atrazine (U.S. EPA 1988). Upon chronic exposure, atrazine also has the potential of causing weight loss, cardiovascular damage, retinal degeneration, and cancer (U.S. EPA 1999). Atrazine is considered as a possible human carcinogen (Group C) based on evidence of induction of mammary gland tumors in laboratory animals (U.S. EPA 1999).

Arsenic-containing compounds such as monosodium methanearsonate (MSMA) and disodium metahanearsonate (DMSA) have been and are still being used as herbicides in conjunction with atrazine, to control unwanted weeds in several agricultural areas of the Mississippi Delta. MSMA is also currently used by the Mississippi Department of Transportation to control vegetation along highways and rights of way. Therefore, it is highly expected that occupational co-exposure to arsenic and atrazine is likely to occur in several communities where both chemicals are applied.

Aquatic organisms have become important as surrogate species for toxicological testing of materials that may have adverse biological effects in humans. They can also provide direct information about the impact of pollutants on the health of the aquatic ecosystem as it relates to resident species (Helmstetter et al. 1996). The advantages of using the Japanese medaka (*Oryzias latipes*) as a model test organism (system) for screening toxicity and carcinogenicity of chemicals has been reported in literature (Helmstetter et al. 1996, Tchounwou et al. 2000). In this research, we investigated the acute toxicity of arsenic and atrazine, singly and in combination, to Japanese medaka embryos, and the cytotoxicity of these two chemicals to human liver carcinoma cells.

Materials and Methods

Chemicals

Arsenic trioxide (As_2O_3) - Lot No. 97313-24, with an active ingredient of 100% arsenic in 10% nitric acid was purchased from Fisher Scientific in Houston, Texas. Atrazine (2-choro-4-ethylamino-6-isopropylamino-s-triazine) - Lot No. 207-62B, with an active ingredient of 98% was purchased from Chem Service Inc. in West Chester, Pensylvania. Magnesium sulfate ($Mg\ SO_4.7H_20$) - Lot No. M18143, potassium chloride (KCl) - Lot No. M32613, calcium chloride ($CaCl_2$) - Lot No. L51333, sodium chloride (NaCl) - Lot No. M29358, and dimethyl sulfoxide (DMSO) - Lot No. 9224-01, were purchased from J.T. Baker in Phillipsburg, Pennsylvania.

Test Media

Synthetic water was used as medium for maintaining embryos. This medium was prepared by putting 960 mL of deionized water into a 1 L capacity volumetric flask, and adding 10 mL of each of the following solutions: NaCl (125 g/L), $MgSO_4.7H_20$ (20.4g/L), KCl (3.75g/L), and $CaCl_2$ (5g/L). The medium was used as solvent for arsenic dilutions, while 2% DMSO was used as a co-solvent for atrazine. Dulbecco's Modified Eagle's Minimal Essential Medium (DMEM) – Lot No. 1016511 was purchased from Life Technologies in Grand Island, New York.

Embryo Bioassays

Two day-old embryos of the Japanese medaka (*Oryzias latipes*) were purchased from the Gulf Coast Research Laboratory in Ocean Springs, Mississippi. Upon arrival at the laboratory the eggs/embryos were evaluated under a dissecting microscope to ensure successful fertilization. Unfertilized eggs that lacked a raised vitelline membrane (i.e., appearance of the previtelline space) were discarded and the remaining fertilized eggs were placed in glass petri dishes (100 mm x 15 mm) containing 40 mL of embryo-rearing solution or chemical solution, at a density of 20 eggs per dish.

A preliminary screening was carried out to determine the appropriate testing range of concentrations for each chemical. This task was done according to the standard QA/QC test protocol described by Johnson and Finley (1980) and by the U.S. EPA (1985). The dishes were maintained at room temperature. The 96-hrs static renewal bioassay was employed. The embryos were exposed to different concentrations of arsenic and atrazine, singly or in combination (serial dilutions of arsenic in 100 ppm atrazine). Two percent DMSO was used as co-solvent for atrazine. Each compound was tested at five different concentrations including controls (0, 0.1, 0.2, 0.3, and 0.4 mg As/L; and 0, 50, 100, 150, and 200 mg atrazine/L). Control embryos were cultured simultaneously with the experimental embryos under identical conditions. The experiments were done in duplicate and repeated once. Eggs/embryos were evaluated daily under the dissecting microscope for mortality. All eggs found to be dead were counted and discarded to avoid possible fungal or bacteria contamination of the remaining eggs in the dish. The test media were also renewed with freshly prepared solutions, to maintain chemical concentrations in the test containers. Criteria for embryo viability included: presence of heartbeat, presence of an intact pericardial sac, and the presence of circulating blood.

The percentages of mortality were calculated. The chemical concentrations effecting 50% mortality of embryos (LC_{50}) and their 95% confidence limits were computed using the U.S. EPA Probit Analysis Computer Program Version 3.0. The other toxic end points estimated include the no observed adverse effect levels (NOAEL), the lowest observed adverse effect levels (LOAEL), and the 95% effect level (LC95). The NOAELs were taken as halves of the LOAELs representing 1% reductions in the viability of embryos.

In Vitro Cell Bioassays

Frozen human liver carcinoma cell lines ($HepG_2$) – ID No. HB-8065 were purchased from the American Type Culture Collection (ATCC) in Manassas, Virginia. Upon arrival in the laboratory, cells were stored in liquid nitrogen until use. They were next thawed by gentle agitation of their containers (vials) for 2 minutes in a water bath at 37 °C. After thawing, the content of each vial was transferred to a 75 cm^2 tissue culture flask, diluted with DMEM supplemented with 10% fetal bovine serum (FBS) and 1% streptomycin and penicillin, and incubated for 24 hours at 37 °C in a 5%CO_2 incubator to allow the cells to grow, and form a monolayer in the flask. Cells grown to 90-100% confluence were washed with phosphate buffer saline (PBS), trypsinized with 10 mL of 0.25% (w/v) trypsin-0.03% w/v) EDTA, diluted and counted using a Beckman Z2 Coulter Counter, and seeded (10^5 cells/well) in 6-well tissue culture plates.

Seeded plates were incubated for 24 hrs at 37 °C in a 5%CO_2 incubator, followed by a replacement of the old medium by a fresh one containing the appropriate amount of the test chemicals: 0, 10, 20, 30 and 40 mg As/L; and 0, 25, 50, 75 and 100 mg atrazine/L. They were then re-incubated for 48 hrs, after which time, the medium was collected for LDH analysis using a Perkin Elmer UV/Vis spectrophotometer with the wavelength set at 340 nm. Triton X-100 was used as a positive control representing 100% cell death. The percentages of cell death for each chemical at a given concentration were derived by comparing the lactate dehydrogenase LDH activities (oxidation of NADH to NAD in the presence of pyruvate, with the formation of lactate) to that of Triton X-100 (100% cell death).

Results

Table 1 shows the summary of toxicological data obtained from acute exposure of Japanese medaka embryos to arsenic trioxide. These data show a concentration - response relationship with respect to arsenic toxicity. Upon 96 hrs of exposure, arsenic concentrations with corresponding fudicial limits of 0.07 (0.05-0.09), 0.15 (0.10-0.18), 0.23 (0.21-0.28), and 0.32 (0.28-0.41) mg/L were recorded for NOAEL, LOAEL, LC_{50}, and LC_{95}, respectively. No significant differences ($p > 0.05$) in LC_{50} values, and slopes of dose-response curves, were found between 24 and 96 hrs of exposure, indicating that arsenic is a fast acting chemical, with most acute poisoning occurring within 24 hrs of exposure (Figure 1).

Atrazine was found to be non-toxic to the Japanese medaka embryos, within the range of concentrations tested, even at its maximum solubility of 200 mg/L in 2% DMSO. The mixture of arsenic with 100 mg/L atrazine resulted in a 96 hrs-LC_{50} of 0.28 (0.26-0.31) mg/L. This LC_{50} was slightly higher than that obtained for arsenic alone (0.23 mg/L), indicating a combined toxic effect that was simply additive or slightly antagonistic (Figure 2).

The cytotoxicity test resulted in a concentration-response relationship with respect to arsenic effect on $HepG_2$ cells. The 48 hrs-EC_{50} was computed to be 11.90 (8.80 - 15.10) mg/L (Figure 3). Similar to the embryo bioassay, the test with atrazine did not show any acute toxicity to $HepG_2$ cells within the range of tested concentrations.

TABLE 1—*Summary of toxicological data obtained from the embryo bioassay after 96 hrs exposure to arsenic trioxide.*

Parameter (mg/L)*	24 hours	48 hours	72 hours	96 hours
NOAEL*	0.08 (0.05-0.09)	0.07 (0.04-0.09)	0.07 (0.04-0.09)	0.07 (0.05-0.09)
LOAEL*	0.15 (0.09-0.18)	0.13 (0.08-0.17)	0.13 (0.08-0.17)	0.15 (0.10-0.18)
LC_{50}*	0.27 (0.24-0.30)	0.24 (0.21-0.30)	0.24 (0.21-0.30)	0.23 (0.21-0.28)
LC_{95}*	0.41 (0.35-0.55)	0.36 (0.31-0.47)	0.36 (0.31-0.47)	0.32 (0.28-0.41)
Slope	8.85 (5.32-12.39)	9.41 (5.53-13.29)	9.41 (5.53-13.29)	12.31 (7.15-17.47)

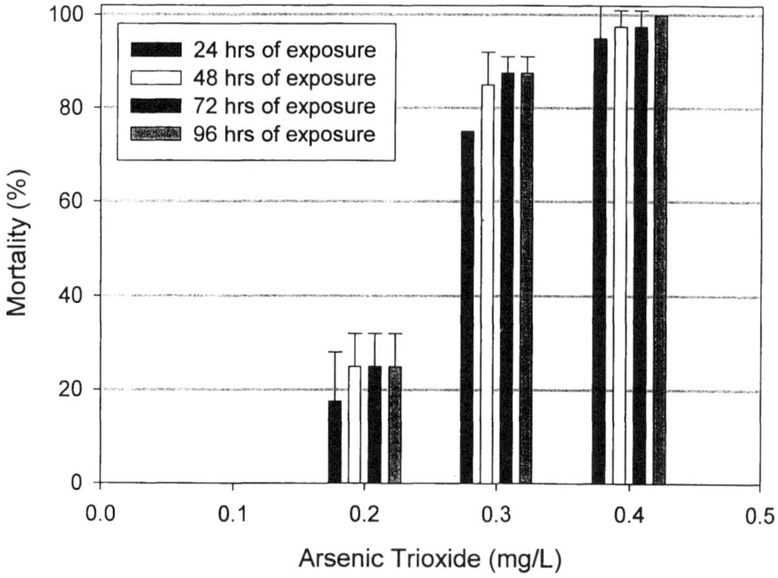

FIG. 1—*Toxic effects of arsenic trioxide to the Japanese medaka embryos.*

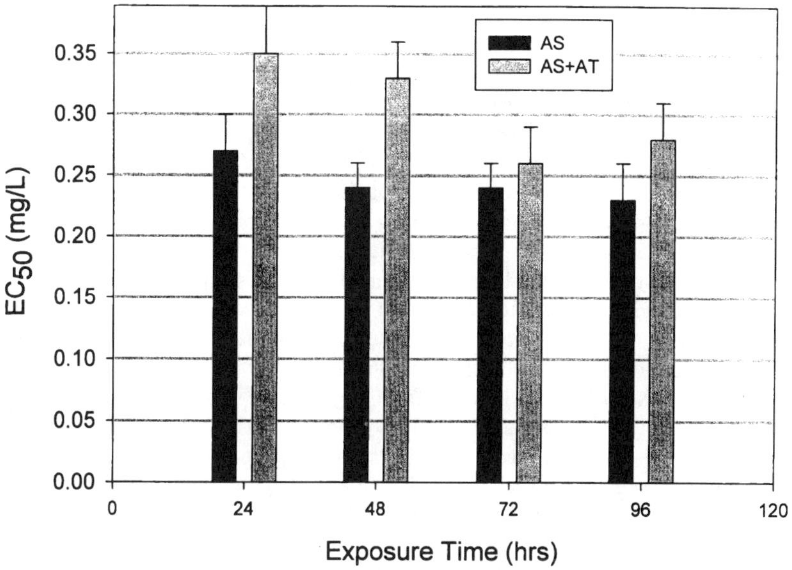

FIG. 2—*LC_{50}s resulting from exposure of Japanese medaka embryos to arsenic (AS), and a mixture of arsenic with 100 ppm of atrazine (AS+AT).*

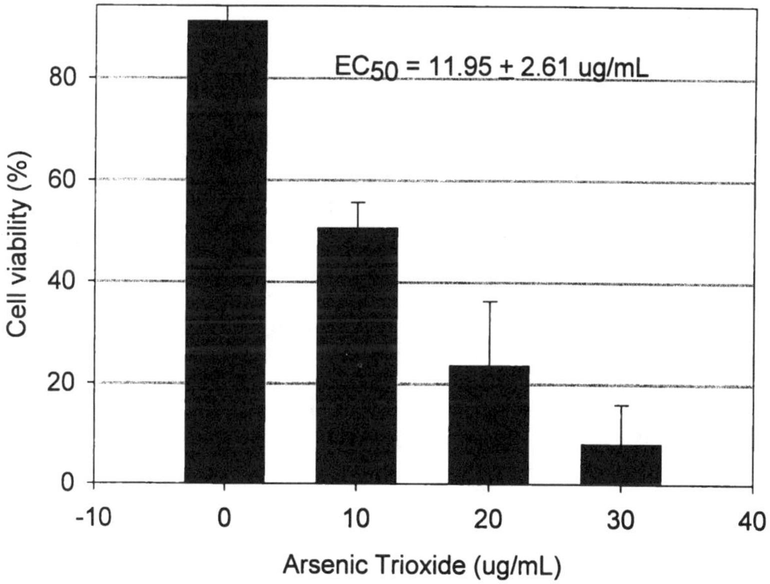

FIG. 3—*Cytotoxicity of arsenic to human liver carcinoma cells ($HepG_2$).*

Discussion

This study demonstrated that arsenic is acutely toxic to Japanese medaka embryos, and human hepatocytes. In both species, the toxic potency was concentration-dependent. The Japanese medaka eggs/embryos were more sensitive to arsenic toxicity (LC_{50} = 0.28 mg/L) than the human hepatocytes (EC_{50} = 11.95 mg/L). Difference in sensitivity could be attributed to several factors including the biological difference, and the test conditions (use of reconstituted water as solvent in embryo bioassay versus use of Eagle's minimum essential medium in cell bioassay; this may influence the bioavailability of arsenic). The cytotoxicity test was based on the loss of cell membrane integrity as a result of chemical assault. Lactate dehydrogenase is a cytoplasmic enzyme, which is released into the cell culture medium after the cell membrane has been disrupted. Its concentration in this medium is proportional to the level of cell death.

Many case reports of death in humans from ingestion of high doses of arsenic have been reported. A fatal dose of arsenic trioxide is probably in the 200 to 300 mg range, yet a dose as low as 10 to 20 mg has been life threatening, and recovery from 10 g has occurred (Schoolmeester and White 1980). Symptoms of acute intoxication usually occur within 30 minutes of ingestion, but may be delayed if arsenic is taken with food. In nearly all cases, the most immediate effects are severe nausea and vomiting, colicky abdominal pain, profuse diarrhea with rice stools, and gastrointestinal hemorrhage; death may ensue from fluid loss and circulatory collapse. Drowsiness and confusion are also seen along the development of psychosis, which is associated with paranoid delusions, hallucinations, and delirium. Finally, seizures, coma, and death, usually from shock may ensue. If death does not occur in the first 24 hours from irreversible circulatory insufficiency, then over the next several days death may result from hepatic or renal failure (Gordy 1994, Saady et al. 1989).

Previous research has pointed out that the mechanism by which arsenic exerts its toxic effect is through impairment of cellular respiration by the inhibition of various mitochondrial enzymes, and the uncoupling of oxidative phosphorylation. Most toxicity of arsenic results from its ability to interact with sulphydryl groups of proteins and enzymes, and to substitute phosphorous in a variety of biochemical reactions (ATSDR 1993). Experimentally, arsenic compounds are fetotoxic and teratogenic in mice, rats, and hamsters. The common developmental effects seen include malformations of the brain, urogenital organs, skeleton, ear, as well as small or missing eyes (Fan 1996). There are also several epidemiological studies reporting an association between exposure to inorganic arsenic and increased risk of adverse developmental effects such as congenital malformations, low birth weight, and spontaneous abortion (Nordstorm et al. 1979a, 1979b, Aschengran et al. 1989).

Different species of arsenic have different degrees of toxicity, with arsine and the trivalent forms causing the most injury. In addition to the exposure route, and the arsenic species involved, the toxicity also depends on the exposure dose, frequency, duration, and the biological species, as well as on individual susceptibilities, genetic and nutritional factors (ATSDR 1993, Tchounwou et al. 1999).

Because of its high potential to cause adverse effects in exposed persons, a number of regulations and guidelines have been established for various inorganic and organic forms of arsenic by international, federal, and state agencies. The International Agency for

Research on Cancer classifies arsenic in Group 1 – known human carcinogens (IARC 1987). The permissible limit for arsenic in drinking water has been fixed at 50 ug/L (U.S. EPA 1987). The World Health Organization's tolerable daily intake for inorganic arsenic is 2 ug/kg body weight (WHO 1984). The action level for arsenic in the air is 5 ug/m^3. The permissible exposure limit-total weighted average (PEL-TWA) is 10 ug/m^3 for inorganic arsenicals, and 500 ug/m^3 for organic arsenicals (OSHA 1989). The criterion for irrigation waste is 100 ug/L (Train 1979). Tolerances for residues in agricultural products/commodities vary from 0.35 ppm to 3.5 ppm. The oral reference dose (RfD) is $3x10^{-4}$ mg/kg/day, and the cancer potency factor is 15 $(mg/kg/day)^{-1}$ for inhalation, and 1.75 $(mg/kg/day)^{-1}$ for ingestion (IRIS 1992, Tchounwou et al. 1996, 1999).

Atrazine was found to be non toxic to Japanese medaka embryos within the range of concentrations tested, even at its maximum solubility of 200 mg/L in 2% DMSO. A similar conclusion was made from the test evaluating the effect of atrazine on the viability of human liver carcinoma cells ($HepG_2$). These results were in agreement with those of previous studies indicating that the acute toxicity of atrazine to vertebrate animals, and fish in particular, is very low compared to that of other freshwater organisms such as phytoplankton, macrophytes, benthic invertebrates, and zooplankton (Solomon et al. 1996).

In the fish bioassay, the mixture of arsenic trioxide in100 mg/L atrazine resulted in a 96 hrs-LC_{50} of 0.28 mg/L. This LC_{50} was slightly higher than that obtained for arsenic trioxide alone (0.23mg/L). Treating atrazine as a synergist, the synergistic ratio (SR – LC_{50} of arsenic alone divided by the LC_{50} of arsenic in the mixture with atrazine) was calculated. The SR is a measure of the effectiveness of the synergist (Walker et al. 1996). When there is synergism, the SR is greater than 1. The SR obtained for this study was 0.82, suggesting an antagonistic effect between arsenic trioxide and atrazine. A similar conclusion was drawn from bioassays using adult fish of the same species (Tchounwou et al. 2000). Based on the Marking's method of assessment (Marking 1980), a negative value of additive index was correlated with the sum of toxic action, indicating a reduction in toxicity from the mixture of arsenic and atrazine. This also confirms the antagonistic mechanism suggested above. Findings of this study are in agreement with publications from some studies suggesting that the toxicity of many pesticide mixtures to freshwater organisms is rarely greater than additive (Marking and Maulk 1975, Marking 1985, Abdelghani et al. 1997). Moreover, Naddy et al. (1995) evaluated the toxicity of selected metals to *Ceriodaphnia dubia*, and reported that arsenic and molybdenum in binary combination appear to be strongly antagonistic in their combined toxicity.

Conclusions

Findings from this study indicate that acute exposure to arsenic trioxide significantly reduced the viability of both Japanese medaka embryos, and human liver carcinoma cells. In both test systems, a strong concentration-response relationship was observed. A time-response analysis suggested that arsenic trioxide is a fast acting chemical whose acute toxicity is expressed shortly after exposure (24 hrs) to fish. Atrazine, on the other hand, showed a relatively low toxicity to human liver cells. Also, this herbicide was found to be non-toxic to Japanese medaka embryos. The mixture of arsenic trioxide and atrazine resulted in a combined toxic effect that was simply additive, or slightly antagonistic.

Based on the results of this research, further studies are underway to assess the sublethal effects of arsenic and atrazine on the embryonic development in the Japanese medaka fish, and the induction of stress genes and/or transcriptional factors in $HepG_2$ cells. Future research will provide valuable information on the developmental toxicity, and the potential mechanisms by which arsenic trioxide and atrazine exert toxicity at the molecular level.

Acknowledgments

This project was carried out as part of research initiatives of the Jackson State University Center for Environmental Health - RCMI, financially supported by a grant (No.1G12RR13459) from the National Institutes of Health. We thank Dr. Abdul K. Mohamed, dean of the School of Science and Technology, and the members of Internal and External Advisory Boards, for their technical support and advice on this research project.

References

Abdelghani, A.A., Tchounwou, P.B., Anderson, A.C., Sujono, H., Heyer, L.R., and Monkiedje, A., 1997, "Toxicity Evaluation of Single and Chemical mixtures of Roundup, Garlon-3A, 2, 4-D, and Syndets Surfactant to Channel Catfish (*Ictalurus punctatus*), Bluegill Sunfish (*Lepomis macrochirus*), and Crawfish (*Procambarus spp.*)," *Environmental Toxicology and Water Quality,* Vol. 12, pp. 237-243.

Aschengran, A., Zierler, S., and Cohen, A., 1989, "Quality of Community Drinking Water and the Occurrence of Spontaneous Abortion," *Archives of Environmental Health,* Vol. 44, pp. 283-290.

ATSDR., 1993, *Toxicological Profile for Arsenic. TP-92/09.* Agency for Toxic Substances and Disease Registry, Center for Disease Control, Atlanta, Georgia.

Borum, D.R., and Abernathy, C.O., 1994, Human Oral Exposure to Inorganic Arsenic. In W.R., Chappell, C.O. Abernathy and C.R. Cothern, eds., *Arsenic Exposure and Health*, Science and Technology Press, Northwood, UK., pp. 119-128.

Chen, C.J., Chuang, Y.C., Lin, T.M., Wu, H.Y., 1985, "Malignant Neoplasms among Residents of a Blackfoot Disease Endemic Area in Taiwan: High-Arsenic Artesian Well Water and Cancers," *Cancer Research,* Vol. 45, pp. 5895-5899.

Chen, C.J., Chen, C.W., Wu M.M., and Kuo T-L.,1992, "Cancer Potential in Liver, Lung, Bladder and Kidney due to Ingested Inorganic Arsenic in Drinking Water," *British Journal of Cancer*, Vol. 66, pp. 888-892.

Coupe, R.H., Thurman, E.M., and Zimmerman, L.R., 1998., "Relation of Usage to the Occurrence of Cotton and Rice Herbicides in Three Streams of the Mississippi Delta," *Environmental Science and Technology*, Vol. 32, pp 3673-3680.

Fan, AM., 1996, Assessment of Metals in Drinking Water with Specific References to Lead, Copper, Arsenic, and Selenium. In L.W. Chan, L. Magos, T. Suzuki, eds. *Toxicology of Metals*. Lewis Publishers - CRC Press, Boca Raton, Florida, pp. 39-53.

Gordby, M.S., 1994. Arsenic in Human Medicine. In J.O. Nriagu, Ed., *Arsenic in the Environment, Part II: Human Health and Ecosystem Effects*. John Wiley & Sons, Inc., pp. 1-16.

Hallenbeck, W.H., and Cummingham, B., 1985, Pesticides and Human Health. Springer-Verlag. New York, NY.

Helmstetter, M.F., Maccubbin, A.E., and Alden, R.W., 1996, The Medaka Embryo-Larval Assay: An *in vivo* Assay for Toxicity, Teratogenicity, and Carcinogenicity. In G.K. Ostrander, ed. *Techniques in Aquatic Toxicology*. Boca Raton, FL. Lewis Publishers. pp. 93-124.

IARC, 1987, *Monographs on the Evaluation of Carcinogenic Risks of Chemicals to Humans. Supplement F. Overall Evaluation of Carcinogenicity*. International Agency for Research on Cancer., World Health Organization. Lyon, France., pp. 29-57.

IRIS, 1992, *Integrated Risk Information System*. United States Environmental Protection Agency. Washington, DC.

Johnson, W.W., and Finley, M.T., 1980, *Handbook of Acute Toxicity of Chemicals to Fish and Aquatic Invertebrates. Resource Publication No. 137*. Wildlife and Fisheries Services. U.S. Department of the Interior. Washington, DC.

Marking, L.L., 1980, Method for Assessing Additive Toxicity of Chemical Mixtures. In , F.L. Mayerand, and J.L. Hamelink, eds. *Aquatic Toxicology and Hazard Evaluation*. American Society for Testing and Materials. Philadelphia, PA. pp. 99-108.

Marking, L.L., and Maulk, W.L., 1975, "Toxicity of Paired Mixtures of Candidate Forest Insecticides to Rainbow Trout," *Bulletin of Environmental Contamination and Toxicology*, Vol. 13, pp. 518-523.

Marking, L.L., 1985, Toxicity of Chemical Mixtures. In G. Rand, and S. Petrocelli, eds. *Fundamentals of Aquatic Toxicology*. Hemisphere Publishing Corporation. Washington DC., pp. 164-176.

Mock, W.M., and Wai, C.M., 1994, Mobilization of Arsenic in Contaminated Waters. In J.O. Nriagu, ed. *Arsenic in the Environment, Part 1: Cycling and Characterization*. John Wiley & Sons, Inc. New York, NY, 99-117.

Naddy, R.B., LaPoint, T.W., and Klaine S.J., 1995, "Toxicity of Arsenic, Molybdenum and Selenium Combinations to *Ceriodaphnia dubia*," *Environmental Toxicology and Chemistry*, Vol. 14, No. 2, pp329-336.

NAS, 1977, *Arsenic*. National Academy of Science. Washington DC.

Nordstorm, S., Beckman, L., and Nordenson, I., 1979a, "Occupational and Environmental Risks in and around a Smelter in Northern Sweden. V. Spontaneous Abortion among Female Employees and Decreased Birth Weight in their Offspring," *Hereditas* , Vol. 90, pp. 291-296.

Nordstorm, S., Beckman, L., and Nordenson, I., 1979b, "Occupational and Environmental Risks in and around a Smelter in Northern Sweden: VI. Congenital Malformations, " *Hereditas*, Vol. 90, pp. 297-302.

NRCC, 1978, Effects of Arsenic in the Environment. National Research Council of Canada. *National Research Council of Canada Publication*, pp.1-349.

OSHA., 1989, Occupational Safety and Health Administration. *Federal Register,* Vol. 54, pp. 2332-2335.

Saady, J.J., Blanke, R.V., and Pollis, A., 1989, "Estimation of the Body Burden of Arsenic in a Child Fatally Poisoned by Arsenic Weed Killer," *Journal of Analytical Toxicology*, Vol. 13, pp. 310-312.

Schoolmeester, W.L., and White, D.R., 1980, "Arsenic Poisoning," *Southern Medical Journal*, Vol. 73, pp. 198-208.

Squillace, P.J., Thurman, E.M., and Furlong, E.T., 1993, "Ground Water as a Non Point Source for Atrazine and Deethyl Atrazine in a River during Base Flow Conditions," *Water Resources Research*, Vol. 29, No. 6, pp. 1719-1729.

Solomon, K.R., Baker, D.B., Richards, R.P., Dixon, K.R., Klaine, S.J., LaPoint, T.W., Kendall, R.J., Weisskopf, C.P., Giddings, J.M., Giesy, J.P., Hall, L.W., and Williams, W.M., 1996, "Ecological Risk Assessment of Atrazine in North American Surface Waters," *Environmental Toxicology and Chemistry*, Vol. 15, No. 1, pp. 31-76.

Tchounwou, P.B., Abdelghani, A.A., Pramar, Y.V., Heyer, L.R., and Steward, C.M. 1996, "Assessment of Potential Health Risks Associated with Ingesting Heavy Metals in Fish Collected from a Hazardous-Waste Contaminated Wetland in Louisiana, USA,"*Reviews on Environmental Health*, Vol. 11, No. 4, pp.191-203.

Tchounwou, P.B., Wilson, B., and Ishaque, A. 1999, "Important Considerations in the Development of Public Health Advisories for Arsenic and Arsenic-Containing Compounds in Drinking Water," *Reviews on Environmental Health,* Vol. 24, No. 4, pp. 211-229.

Tchounwou, P.B., 2000, "Health Risk Assessment and Management of Arsenic and other Toxic and Hazardous Metals in Drinking Water," *Metal Ions in Biology and Medicine,* Vol. 6, pp. 21-23.

Tchounwou, P.B., Wilson, B., Ishaque, A., and Sutton, D., 2000, "Toxicity Evaluation of Arsenic Trioxide, and Atrazine to Three Developmental Stages of Japanese Medaka (*Oryzias latipes*)," *Metal Ions in Biology and Medicine,* Vol. 6, pp. 18-20.

Thurman, E.M., Goolsby, D.A., Meyer, M.T., and Kolpin, D.W., 1991, "Herbicides in Surface Waters of the Midwestern United States: The Effects of Spring flush." *Environmental Science and Technology*, Vol. 25, pp. 1794-1796.

Tseng, W.P., Chu, H.M., How, S.W., Fong, J.M., Lin, C.S., and Yeh, S., 1968, "Prevalence of Skin Cancer in an Endemic Area of Chronic Arsenicism in Taiwan," *Journal of the National Cancer Institute,* Vol. 40, pp. 453-463.

U.S. EPA, 1982, *An Exposure and Risk Assessment for Arsenic. EPA 440/4-85-005.* EPA Office of Water Regulations and Standards. Washington DC.

U.S. EPA, 1985, "National Primary Drinking Water Regulations." *Federal Register*, Vol. 50, pp. 46931- 47022.

U.S. EPA, 1987, *Special Report on Ingested Inorganic Arsenic: Skin Cancer and Nutritional Essentiality. Risk Assessment Forum.* United States Environmental Protection Agency. Washington DC.

U.S. EPA, 1988, *Atrazine Health Advisory.* Office of Drinking Water. United States Environmental Protection Agency. Washington DC.

U.S. EPA, 1999, *Drinking Water and Health: Technical Fact Sheet on Atrazine.* United States Environmental Protection Agency. Washington DC. On line at: http://www.epa.gov/OGWDW/dwh/t-soc/atrazine.html.

Walker, C.H., Hopkin, S.P., Sibly, R.M., and Peakall, D.B., 1996, Interactive Effects of Pollutants. In *Principles of Ecotoxicology*. Taylor and Francis Publishers. London, Great Britain, pp. 165-173.

WHO, 1984, *Guidelines for Drinking Water Quality.* World Health Organization, Geneva, Switzerland.

Carsten H. Baehr[1] and Clifford Habig[2]

Statistical Evaluation of the UTAB Database for Use in Terrestrial Nontarget Organism Probabilistic Risk Assessments

Reference: Baehr, C. H., and Habig, C., "**Statistical Evaluation of the UTAB Database for Use in Terrestrial Nontarget Organism Probabilistic Risk Assessments,**" *Environmental Toxicology and Risk Assessment: Science, Policy, and Standardization – Implications for Environmental Decisions: Tenth Volume, ASTM STP 1403,* B. M. Greenberg, R. N. Hull, M. H. Roberts, Jr., and R. W. Gensemer, Eds., American Society for Testing and Materials, West Conshohocken, PA, 2001.

Abstract

This paper provides a statistical analysis of the UTAB database (uptake/ accumulation, translocation, adhesion, and biotransformation). This database contains extensive data on organic chemicals and heavy metals in vascular plants. Data from the UTAB database are currently used by the U.S. Environmental Protection Agency (EPA) and pesticide registrants for conducting deterministic risk assessments of pesticide residues in the food chain of wildlife for pesticide registration. The primary purpose for this detailed analysis of UTAB data was to develop models for the distribution of pesticide residues in plant feed items so that these residue distributions can be used in probabilistic risk assessments for wildlife. Relevant data were grouped into the four feed item categories used by EPA for wildlife risk assessment. The data were analyzed statistically and percentiles were calculated. Results were compared to the currently used deterministic maximum and typical residue predictions of the U.S. EPA residue nomogram. More importantly, log normal and exponential distribution models were developed from the analysis, allowing simulation of typical and extreme dietary exposure scenarios in a probabilistic manner. These models can be used in Monte Carlo simulations to generate joint probability functions for a more probabilistic approach to wildlife risk assessment.

Keywords: probabilistic risk assessment, pesticide residues, UTAB Database

Introduction

Responsibility for assessing the risk of pesticides, and regulating pesticides has resided with the U.S. Environmental Protection Agency U.S. EPA) since 1970 under the Federal Insecticide, Fungicide, and Rodenticide Act (FIFRA).

[1] Master of Environmental Management, Nicholas School of the Environment, Duke University, Box 90328, Durham, NC, 27708.

[2] Director, Environmental Practice, Novigen Sciences, Inc.,
1730 Rhode Island Avenue, NW, Suite 1100, Washington, D.C. 20036.

An ecological risk assessment is carried out as part of the review process for pesticide registration to determine the potential risk that a particular pesticide use may pose to nontarget organisms. An ecological risk assessment estimates the probability or likelihood of an undesirable event (U.S. EPA 1992). For pesticides, the risk assessment estimates whether adverse effects to nontarget organisms, such as wildlife, would be expected to occur with labeled use of the pesticide (U.S. EPA 1997).

Recognizing that there are multiple methods for ecological risk assessment, the Environmental Fate and Effects Division (EFED) of EPA currently uses a deterministic quotient approach. This method compares an expected environmental concentration (EEC) of a pesticide to a toxicity effect endpoint (e.g. LC_{50} or no-observed effect concentration), resulting in a risk quotient (U.S. EPA 1986). Generally, the risk quotient represents a conservative, protective evaluation of the potential for adverse effects to nontarget organisms from pesticide use.

The risk quotient method provides a first tier, or screening level analysis, as to whether a pesticide use can be considered safe, but the procedure does not provide sufficient information on the magnitude or probability of effects, nor does it address uncertainty and variability in the estimates (ECOFRAM 1999). However, current EPA risk evaluations for terrestrial organisms (primarily birds and small mammals) stop with this screening level analysis because adequate tools for refining screening level assessments that suggest unacceptable risk are widely unavailable. In a review of EPA-EFED's risk assessment procedures, the Scientific Advisory Panel (SAP) recommended that EFED move from its current deterministic assessment to a more probabilistic approach to refine ecological risk assessments and provide decision makers with additional information concerning magnitude and likelihood of adverse effects, and the associated uncertainty (U.S. EPA 1997).

Probabilistic risk assessment is capable of addressing most complex applications across many different fields (ECOFRAM 1999). The Monte Carlo approach, which is one way of approaching probabilistic risk assessment, can be generally defined as a computer-based method of analysis that uses statistical sampling techniques to obtain a probabilistic approximation to the solution of a mathematical equation or model (U.S. EPA 1997). Using this approach, it is highly likely that the spectrum of outputs provides a good representation of the true output distribution (Cox and Baybutt 1981).

However, to use probabilistic methods for assessing risk to terrestrial organisms, several changes are necessary, with the main obstacle to overcome being the lack of supporting data (ECOFRAM 1999). Today, EFED's terrestrial risk assessments mainly focus on birds and small mammals, and consider dietary exposure as the major route of exposure. The underlying variable to estimating dose to an organism is pesticide residue on plant and insect feed items available to that organism. Currently, residues on plant feed items are estimated using a terrestrial residue nomogram, based on an analysis of residues on different types of plants immediately following pesticide application (Hoerger and Kenaga 1972, Kenaga 1973). The U.S. EPA used the results of the Hoerger and Kenaga (1972) analysis to develop a criteria paper including a nomogram for estimating exposure to nontarget species. This nomogram represents EFED's standard method for estimating the exposure of birds and small mammals for risk assessment. The original nomogram contained estimated maximum and typical (mean) residues for six different categories of plant feed items. The maximum and typical nomogram estimates were re-evaluated using a larger database (UTAB; uptake/ accumulation, translocation, adhesion, and biotransformation) that compiled literature reports of pesticide residues in plants (Fletcher et al. 1994). This re-evaluation resulted in a recommendation that the original six plant feed item categories suggested by Hoerger and Kenaga (1972) be condensed to four categories (short grass, long grass, forage and leafy crops, and seeds and fruit) by combining some of the original categories. This re-evaluation also resulted in a recommendation to increase the maximum estimated residue values for the forage-leafy crop and seed-fruit categories, along with some changes in the typical (mean) estimated residues. These recommendations have been incorporated into the current deterministic terrestrial organism risk assessment procedures used by EFED.

The UTAB database contains sufficient pesticide residue data to address the requirement for adequate data to undertake a probabilistic analysis. However, previous analysis of UTAB has been relatively limited. A primary focus of the analysis by Fletcher et al (1994) was to ensure that the maximum residue estimates used by EFED for risk assessment are equal to at least 95% of the residue values in UTAB for each crop category. Therefore, the UTAB database has been used only to provide point estimates for deterministic risk assessments. The available database has never been statistically evaluated for key data distribution properties.

This paper enhances the use of the UTAB database for risk assessment by providing a basis for probabilistic risk assessments for nontarget terrestrial organisms. Residue distribution models were developed from the database for typical and extreme exposure scenarios for each feed item category. These distribution models can be used instead of the current point estimates to estimate wildlife dietary exposures. Advances to more probabilistic risk assessments require this type of analysis because models of residue distributions represent a core component of a probabilistic assessment of potential dietary exposure of wildlife arising from a particular pesticide use.

Materials and Methods

Pesticide residue data for vascular plants were drawn from the the UTAB database, originally developed by the University of Oklahoma. (Nellessen and Fletcher 1992, Nellessen and Fletcher 1993). UTAB is comprised of more than 42 000 records, on approximately 1 047 organic chemicals, falling into 34 different chemical classes, and 21 heavy metals. The encoded information pertains to 294 genera of vascular plant species, falling into 95 families. The data records are derived from approximately 2 100 papers published in the scientific literature in the years from 1926 to 1987.

The UTAB data primarily consist of pesticide product residues on agricultural crops at different times following application. Overall, most available data refer to insecticides and herbicides, with a lesser number to fungicide compounds (Nellessen and Fletcher 1993). Among the insecticides, the organophosphorous class of is the most abundant, whereas for herbicides and fungicides the data are evenly distributed among several different classes of chemicals.

The UTAB database was screened for experimental conditions and data expressions as described in previous studies examining pesticide residue levels (Hoerger and Kenaga, 1972; Kenaga, 1973; Fletcher, et al., 1994). Only field trial studies reporting residue values in parts per million (ppm) wetweight following a single pesticide spray application, were used. Data records from studies carried out under different experimental conditions were not included. Data from experiments treating crops post harvest were also excluded. Application rates ranged from 0.05 to 11 lbs/acre (A), with most pesticides being sprayed at rates in the range of 0.5-2.0 lbs/A.

All relevant pesticide residue data for day zero (immediately following application up to 12 h) and day one (12 h post application up to 36 h) following chemical application, were divided into four feed item categories (Fletcher et al. 1994). The four categories are short grass, long grass, leafy crops and forage, and fruits and seeds. Combined day zero and day one residue data records are summarized according to plant category and plant species (Table 1).

Table 1 – *Distribution records by plant category and species.*

Plant Category and Species	Number of Records
Short Grass	
Bermuda Grass (*Cynodon dactylon*)	41
2 other grass species	3
Long Grass	
Corn (*Zea mays*)	23
Ryegrass (*Lolium perenne*)	4
2 other species	4
Leafy Crops and Forage	
Alfalfa (*Medicago sativa*)	35
Tobacco (*Nicotiana tabacum*)	21
Lettuce (*Lactuca virosa*)	20
Cauliflower (*Brassica oleracea*)	16
Pea (*Pisum sativum*)	15
30 other species	109
Fruits and Seeds	
Tomato (*Lycopersicum esculentum*)	13
Orange (*Citrus sinensis*)	11
Okra (*Hibiscus esculentus*)	11
Strawberry (*Fragaria virginianis*)	10
Green Bean (*Phaseolus vulgaris*)	9
27 other species	102
Total	447

All chemicals evaluated were used as either insecticides or herbicides (Thompson 1993). Organophosphates (247 records) constitute the largest number of data records among insecticides, followed by diphenyl compounds (98), cyclo compounds (55), carbamates (30) and pyrethroids (2). Heterocyclic nitrogen derivatives (5) make up the largest number of data records among the herbicides, followed by carbothiolates (4), phenoxy compounds (4) and organochlorines (2). Data on dinitroanalines, nitrites, amides, acetamides, analides, carbamates and urea compounds are not available through the UTAB database.

The correlation of data obtained from the UTAB database was carried out as described by Hoerger and Kenaga (1972). The amount of pesticide applied (dosage) was standardized to a unit area of cropland (pounds per acre (lbs/A). Residues (ppm) from a unit dosage (RUDs) were calculated by dividing residue reported by the application rate used in a particular study. This method of standardization assumes that residues following application of a pesticide to a given plant surface area are directly proportional to dosage; all influencing factors such as mode of application, experimental and field variables are assumed similar, and run-off from the plant is assumed insignificant.

Statistics

Descriptive Statistics – Insecticide and herbicide RUD data for day zero and day one following application were statistically described, including the mean, median, minimum, maximum and standard deviation. In addition, upper tail 90th, 95th, 98th and 99th percentiles were calculated directly from the sample data by linear interpolation. It should be noted that linear approximation results in percentiles that are very sensitive to extremely high values, especially when the number of data points towards the upper extremes is limited.

Model Distributions – Distributions for simulating feed item residues on days zero and one following application were developed for each of the four feed item categories. The log normal distribution was used to simulate the data set for typical residue scenarios, based on the phenomena that many processes in the natural environment are random product processes, including environmental concentrations of chemicals (Ott 1995).

For each of the four feed item categories, optimal log normal parameters were estimated and distributions were fit for day zero and day one RUD values. Distribution parameter values were estimated using the maximum likelihood estimation (MLE) method (Ott 1995). In general, MLE estimates the most likely parameters of a given distribution from the number of n observations. For log normal distributions, MLE determines optimal values for the parameters μ and σ.

The MLE approach requires the logarithm of each observation, so difficulties may arise if an observation is zero. To overcome this problem, all data records for each feed item category were empirically grouped into intervals of equal length (k), according to Sturges' rule (Hamburg 1996) (1)

$$k = 1 + 3.3\log_{10}(n) \qquad (1)$$

where n equals the number of data points. Percentage probability and quantile-quantile probability plots were graphed to visualize the process, plotting the cumulative probability of the input data versus the fitted cumulative distribution.

While several goodness-of-fit tests are available for evaluating the fit of the model distribution to the sample data, the Shapiro-Wilks test was selected, as recommended by the U.S. EPA, to assess the fitted distributions' acceptability (U.S. EPA 1997). Test statistics are compared to standard values, with the appropriate number of degrees of freedom at a given level of significance ($\alpha = 0.05$), and p-values were derived.

Adverse effects of environmental contamination are often associated with high concentrations, so the assessor's interest typically focuses on the upper tail of distributions. Overall, log normal distributions often do not adequately estimate the upper extremes of a sample distribution, and many sample distributions behave as though they are exponential after a certain point towards the more extreme values (Ott 1995). In fact, the exponential model provides better estimates than other available distributions (e.g., Weibull) (Breimann et al. 1995), and thus is most suitable for simulating high end residue values or extreme scenarios. However, exponential models do not necessarily fit complete distributions well, even though they can help refine tail analysis (Lambert et al. 1994, Ott 1995).

The exponential method was used to fit exponential distributions to the extreme upper RUD values of each of the four feed item category distributions. The method provides a simple, robust and fairly general method to assess environmental data probabilistically (Ott 1995). Essentially, the tail exponential method utilizes the MLE approach to estimate optimal scale parameters (θ) for single-parameter exponential models for values above a particular cutoff cumulative (f_c) frequency. For these data sets, the cutoff frequency (f_c) used was the 90th percentile ($f_c = 0.9$), as calculated by linear interpolation, or three highest RUD values within a particular group of data.

Applying the Developed Models

An example probabilistic analysis, using Monte Carlo methodology, is provided. Details on the Monte Carlo approach, including advantages and disadvantages, are provided elsewhere (Cox and Baybutt 1981, Ott 1995).

A pesticide residue distribution was directly simulated using the developed probabilistic models. The resulting output was then used to estimate of the total amount of pesticide residue ingested by the species of interest. In the example, an avian species is assumed to feed exclusively on plant material immediately following a single pesticide spray application of 1 lb active ingredient (a.i.)/A. The example assumed that the particular species' diet typically consists of 23% leafy crops and forage and 77% fruits and seeds.

Total pesticide residue in the diet was calculated using a joint probability model in Monte Carlo analyses. Typical residue dietary exposure scenarios (0% to 90%) were simulated using the log normal model. Extreme dietary exposure scenarios (upper 10%) were simulated using the exponential model.

Typical and extreme scenarios were estimated by simulating 10 000 trials for both the leafy crops and forage, and fruits and seeds feed item categories. The distributions for each feed item category were combined in a manner that reflected the dietary contribution of each feed item category, resulting in joint typical or extreme dietary exposure probability models. In this example, the leafy crops and forage category contributed 23% and the fruits and seeds category 77% to each joint probability model.

Results

A total of 447 data records encoded in the UTAB database, taken from 73 papers published in the scientific literature, were used in this analysis. Overall, the study includes a total of 55 pesticides, of which 49 are insecticides and 6 are herbicides, and a total of 64 different plant species, including crops, grass and legume species (Table 1). The data included 259 data records for day zero following application and 188 data records for day one following application. Most of these records fall into the leafy crops and forage or fruits and seeds feed item categories, while a lesser number of records are grouped into the short and long grass feed item categories.

Descriptive Statistics

Summary statistics, including number of records, minimum, mean, median, maximum and standard deviation, for all pesticide RUD records are provided for days zero and one following pesticide application (Table 2).

Mean and median values RUD values for days zero and one following pesticide application are highest in the short grass category, followed by the leafy corps and forage, long grass, and fruits and seeds categories. In all four categories day zero mean and median values are higher than day one values. The wide range of residue values for each category reflects the high variability of pesticide residues found on numerous plant species under various environmental conditions.

Table 2 – *Pesticide day zero and day one RUD summary statistics (ppm wetweight).*

Parameter	Short Grass	Long Grass	Leafy Crops and Forage	Fruits and Seeds
		Day Zero Following Pesticide Application		
Number of Records	22	12	140	85
Minimum:	0.00	6.67	0.00	0.00
Mean:	57.26	15.11	43.05	3.81
Median:	51.69	13.23	23.51	2.03
Maximum:	169.84	28.62	376.71	34.26
Std Deviation:	41.87	7.18	63.42	5.43
		Day One Following Pesticide Application		
Number of Records	22	19	76	71
Minimum:	16.50	0.07	0.00	0.00
Mean:	41.80	10.99	33.79	2.00
Median:	37.61	10.00	14.75	1.20
Maximum:	111.00	60.67	356.00	11.09
Std Deviation:	25.03	13.75	53.87	2.22

Frequency histograms for feed item category RUD values clearly show that most chemical residue values are aggregated towards the median and lower end of the chemical residue spectrum, with fewer residue values towards the upper tail. Logarithmic transformation yields distributions more normal in shape.

The 90th, 95th, 98th and 99th percentiles were calculated using linear interpolation for all four feed item categories for both days zero and one following pesticide application (Table 3). These percentiles show a marked decrease in day one residue concentrations compared to day zero values for all feed item categories except the long grass category (Table 3). This discrepancy at upper percentiles in the long grass category results from a single outlier (thiodan, RUD = 60.67), as determined in a boxplot graph.

Table 3 – *RUD percentiles for day zero and one and U.S. EPA nomogram values (ppm wetweight).*

Percentile	90	95	98	99	Maximum U.S. EPA Values	Typical U.S. EPA Values
		Day Zero Following Pesticide Application				
Short Grass	99.27	112.62	137.54	146.33	240	85
Long Grass	22.49	23.64	24.03	24.16	110	36
Leafy Crops and Forage	92.80	142.92	271.12	340.14	135	45
Fruits and Seeds	7.45	11.55	20.34	28.34	15	7
		Day One Following Pesticide Application				
Short Grass	60.56	88.43	96.56	98.98	-	-
Long Grass	15.58	23.56	42.21	48.43	-	-
Leafy Crops and Forage	78.61	117.02	184.10	242.30	-	-
Fruits and Seeds	4.18	5.53	9.09	10.60	-	-

Comparison to U.S. EPA Nomogram Estimates

The calculated statistical means and percentiles for day zero following application were compared to corresponding currently used point estimates of typical (mean) and maximum residues from the U.S. EPA nomogram (Table 3). The estimated day zero 95th percentiles and statistical means compared to U.S. EPA nomogram predictions are shown in Figure 1.

Linearly derived 99th percentile estimates for the short grass and long grass feed item categories are substantially lower than the currently used nomogram maximum residue estimates for these categories. For the leafy crops and forage category, the maximum U.S. EPA nomogram estimate falls between the 90th and 95th percentile as estimated by linear interpolation. For the fruits and seeds category, the maximum EPA nomogram estimate falls in between the statically derived 95th and 98th percentiles. Mean residue estimates derived from these distributions are generally lower than corresponding typical residue estimates based on EPA's revised nomogram (Tables 2, 3).

Model Distributions

The log normal distribution was selected as the candidate probability model for all feed item categories for days zero and one following application. In general, log normal processes are processes in which the variable of interest results from the product of many independent variables multiplied together (Ott 1995). Chemical residues present on crops following pesticide application are influenced by a number of factors, including the chemical's environmental fate properties, rate and mode of application, meteorological conditions, sampling procedures, and methods of chemical extraction and analysis.

Log normal distributions were fit for both the day zero and day one feed item categories. Log normal distribution parameters derived for μ and σ are summarized (Table 4). The Shapiro-Wilks test, considered the most powerful goodness-of-fit test, was used to evaluate the assumption that the data fit a log normal distribution (D'Agostino 1986). Test statistics, indicating the accuracy of the fit, and derived *p*-

values are presented in Table 5. A low *p*-value indicates that the current sample is highly unlikely and the fit should therefore be rejected. In contrast, a high *p*-value indicates that the sample is likely and would be repeated, and thus the fit should not be rejected. In this study all fitted distributions with *p*-values <0.05 were rejected; all distributions with *p*-values >0.05 were not rejected.

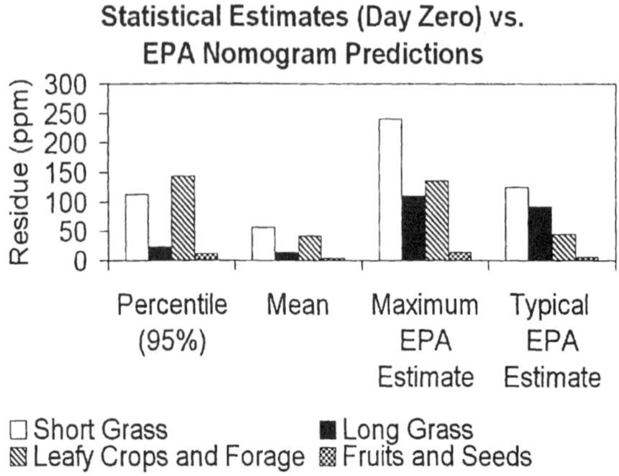

Figure 1 – *Statistically derived day zero percentiles vs. U.S. EPA nomogram estimates.*

Resulting parametric fits for day zero are most accurate for the long grass and fruits and seeds feed categories, while log normal fits for the short grass and leafy crops and forage RUD data are less accurate. The best fit for day one is for the short grass category. The main cause for rejection of a particular distribution by the goodness-of-fit tests is due to discrepancies at the extreme upper tail of the distributions, determined from corresponding percentile-percentile and quantile-quantile plots (not shown).

Table 4 – *Log normal model and extreme tail (exponential) model parameters.*

Feed Item Category	μ	σ	θ (90% cutoff)
	Day Zero Following Pesticide Application		
Short Grass	3.39	2.21	134.61
Long Grass	2.61	0.448	25.28
Leafy Crops and Forage	2.28	1.91	196.62
Fruits and Seeds	0.675	1.25	15.71
	Day One Following Pesticide Application		
Short Grass	3.59	0.526	91.93
Long Grass	1.15	2.17	32.98
Leafy Crops and Forage	2.48	1.94	179.40
Fruits and Seeds	-0.0004	1.57	6.79

Table 5 – *Shapiro-Wilks goodness-of-fit test results for log normal model for day zero and day one.*

Results	Short Grass	Long Grass	Leafy Crops and Forage	Fruits and Seeds
		Day Zero Following Pesticide Application		
Test Statistic W	0.5315	0.9698	0.7398	0.979
p-value	<0.0001	0.8582	0	0.5261
Result	Reject	Do not reject	Reject	Do not reject
		Day One Following Pesticide Application		
Test Statistic W	0.9563	0.803424	0.8499	0.8856
p-value	0.4141	0.0009	<0.0001	<0.0001
Result	Do not reject	Reject	Reject	Reject

Log normal probability distributions used to model RUD distributions for the four feed categories on days zero and one adequately simulate typical exposure scenarios. However, in cases of an inaccurate fit, they do not provide good estimates of upper extreme tails, and the inaccuracy increases towards the more extreme values. A property of log normal distributions is that extreme upper tail observations are often overestimates (Ott 1995). Therefore, using log normal models displaying an inaccurate fit for estimation of upper tail pesticide residues would yield extremely high, unrealistic values.

Because of the problems with the fit of log normal distributions at the upper tails, exponential distributions were used to provide refined estimates for extremely high RUD values and a more accurate representation of extreme exposure scenarios. The cutoff cumulative frequencies for switching to an exponential distribution corresponded to the 90th percentile. Calculated scale parameters (θ) for switching to the exponential distribution for all four feed item categories are presented in Table 4.

Probability Model Results vs. U.S. EPA Nomogram Estimates

The probability (P) of exceeding maximum or typical deterministic EPA nomogram values using Monte Carlo model simulations for all day zero feed item categories was examined using the exponential model for the upper tails and the log-normal model for the remainder of the distribution (Table 6). The derived models generally simulate conservative plant residue estimates because, except for the long grass category, the chance of exceeding the EPA nomogram estimates with a simulation are relatively high.

Table 6 – *Day zero model comparisons to U.S. EPA nomogram estimates.*

	Probability (P) Of Exceeding EPA Nomogram Estimates	
Feed Item Category	Maximum Residue Estimate Exponential Model Used	Typical Residue Estimate Log Normal Model Used
Short Grass	0.17	0.26
Long Grass	0.01	0.00
Leafy Crops and Forage	0.50	0.25
Fruits and Seeds	0.38	0.37

For example, the probability of exceeding the short grass maximum U.S. EPA nomogram estimate (240 ppm) is $P = 0.17$, indicating a 17% chance that residues estimated with the model will be higher than the maximum EPA estimate.

Example Results

The results of simulations for a typical exposure scenario (log normal model) and an extreme exposure scenario (exponential model) are graphically displayed in Figure 2. The mean and median dietary residues are 12.65 ppm and 5.47 ppm, respectively, as estimated from the log normal model. Extreme upper percentiles are 66.64 ppm, 80.22 ppm and 91.28 ppm and 109.87 ppm for the 90th, 95th, 97.5th and 100th percentiles, respectively as estimated from the tail exponential model. These values are based on Monte Carlo simulations for a diet consisting of 23% leafy crops and forage, and 77% fruits and seeds using the day zero distributions for these feed item categories.

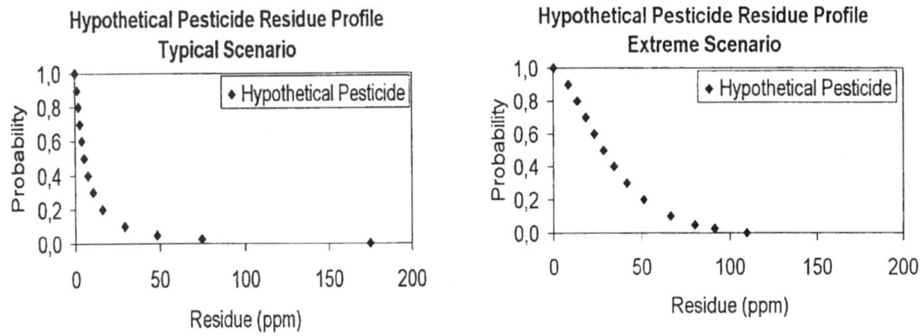

Figure 2 a, b – *Typical (log normal model) and extreme case (exponential model) hypothetical pesticide residue profiles.*

Discussion

The general model for estimating risk of pesticides to nontarget species is outlined by the U.S. EPA (U.S. EPA 1986). The model applies to deterministic as well as probabilistic approaches, with the main difference being that the probabilistic methods require descriptions of variables as probability density functions (pdfs), instead of using point estimates. Results yield output distributions, describing the probability and magnitude of effects, in contrast to a simple index values. The U.S. EPA and pesticide registrants currently use RUD values based on the revised U.S. EPA food-chain nomogram (Fletcher et al, 1994) to estimate pesticide residues on wildlife feed item items immediately following pesticide application to a crop. The current approach to terrestrial wildlife risk assessment uses deterministic, point estimates of RUD values for dietary exposure, and generally focuses on maximum (extreme) residue exposure scenarios.

Similar point estimates of RUD values for dietary exposure are commonly used to estimate acute and longer-term (subchronic) exposure.

Data records available in UTAB are drawn from numerous scientific studies and include numerous plant-chemical combinations and diverse environmental conditions (weather) found across the United States. These data are representative of a broad spectrum of plant types, pesticide application methods, and environmental conditions, and therefore can be considered applicable to agricultural conditions across the United States. Consistent with the current EPA-EFED approach to terrestrial organism risk assessment, the data records were grouped into four feed item categories for analysis. The feed item categories are short grass, long grass, leafy crops and forage and fruits and seeds. Using these categories, EPA-EFED estimates residues on insect feed items as being similar either to residue estimates for leafy crops and forage (small insects) or fruits and seeds (large insects).

This study presents the first thorough statistical analysis of data encoded in the UTAB database. Previous work with the UTAB database has primarily focused on ensuring that pesticide residues estimated using the EPA nomogram maximum residue estimates for each feed item category were greater than at least 95% of the residue values in UTAB. In this study, statistical descriptions, including upper end percentiles (90th to 99th), are provided for all pesticide data records for day zero and day one following application. Histograms reveal that for each of the feed item categories the data are skewed to the right, and log normal transformation yields distributions more normal in shape (not shown). The percentile information places the currently used EPA-EFED maximum residue point estimates for each feed item category in perspective relative to the distribution of pesticide residue data in UTAB for each feed item category. The currently used standard RUD point estimates for the short grass and long grass categories are above the 99th percentile of residues for these categories, while the maximum RUD values for leafy crops and forage, and fruits and seeds, correspond to the 90th – 95th percentile, and 95th – 98th percentile, respectively.

In previous work with the UTAB database, RUD values for days zero and one following application were combined (Fletcher et al 1994), resulting in a larger sample size for evaluating the accuracy of the EPA nomogram estimates. However, in this study day zero and day one data were analyzed separately; results indicated that day one RUD values, particularly at the upper end percentiles for all feed item categories, show a marked decrease compared to the day zero RUD values, except for the highest percentiles in the long grass category. This discrepancy with the long grass category was traced to a single outlier residue value for the pesticide thiodan. Because this analysis indicated that day zero RUD values were generally higher than day one values, pesticide residue simulations were based on the day zero models to maintain more conservative residue estimates.

The major advance of this analysis of the UTAB database compared to previous work is that distribution models for simulating pesticide residues on wildlife feed items have been developed. These models permit probabilistic use of the pesticide residue data in UTAB instead of being limited to point estimates of wildlife dietary exposure. To estimate exposure in a more probabilistic risk assessment approach, point estimates need to be replaced by appropriate probability density functions (pdfs), which capture the natural variability and uncertainty associated with measurement error and lack of knowledge about the biological or chemical system in question. Model exposure pdfs should reflect parameter variability over space and time, such as heterogeneity of residues throughout different locations, and degradation. Residue distributions were developed for all four feed item categories for days zero and one following pesticide application. The log normal distribution was the initial candidate distribution for simulating the pesticide residue distributions. However, the Shapiro-Wilks goodness of fit test indicated that using the log normal distribution to simulate the extreme exposure scenarios resulted in inaccurate fits for most of the feed item categories for days zero and one. Therefore use of the log normal distribution model would often result in unrealistically high residue estimates for upper percentile, extreme exposure scenarios. To correct this inaccuracy, exponential distributions were fit to the upper tail RUD values for each feed item category, using the 90th percentile as the cutoff cumulative frequency. The exponential distributions provide more sound representations of the extreme exposure scenarios. Overall, optimal results are obtained by simulating typical dietary exposure scenarios using log normal distributions and extreme dietary exposure scenarios using a tail exponential model.

These residue distribution models can be used in higher tier risk assessments for birds and small mammals to provide a probabilistic estimate of dietary exposure. For example, these distributions can be used in Monte Carlo analyses for refinement of exposure estimates for animals belonging to different dietary guilds, and thus ingesting varying percentages of feed items from the available feed item categories.

Recommendations

The EPA nomogram is a simple device that is primarily used to estimate maximum potential residues in the food chain of wildlife. Originally, the nomogram was developed as an interim tool for estimating pesticide residues on wildlife feed items, with the intention of having actual residue data for a pesticide replace the nomogram estimates as these residue data became available (Hoerger and Kenaga 1972, Kenaga 1973). However, the nomogram is now routinely used by EPA-EFED and pesticide registrants to provide point estimates of pesticide residues on wildlife feed items. Although the nomogram was originally developed to estimate pesticide residues immediately following application (Hoerger and Kenaga 1972, Kenaga 1973), nomogram estimates of pesticide residues are now also routinely applied to estimates of subchronic dietary exposure as well as acute dietary exposure.

Currently, the nomogram provides only point estimates of pesticide residues in feed items for use in deterministic risk assessments. In order to progress to a more probabilistic risk assessment for wildlife, distribution models of dietary exposure are necessary to provide exposure pdfs. The models presented in this report provide the risk assessor with the tools to conduct higher tier, probabilistic exposure assessments for wildlife belonging to various feeding guilds. This permits a risk assessor to focus on species whose feeding habits place them at potentially high risk for a given pesticide use.

Although developing the distribution models with the UTAB data for both typical and extreme dietary exposure scenarios provides the basis for conducting probabilistic risk assessments with these data, it should be noted that much of the underlying data in UTAB was developed in the 1950s, 1960s, and 1970s. Since then, extensive residue data have been generated by pesticide registrants, often following good laboratory practices (GLPs). Therefore, an opportunity exists to update and expand the underlying database supporting these distribution models.

Probabilistic risk assessment is still relatively uncommon with regards to assessing the impact of pesticide application and residue concentrations in wildlife feed items. The applicability and use of the models presented here should be evaluated with specifically planned and conducted sensitivity analyses and risk assessment research.

References

Breimann, L., Stone, C. J., and Gins, J. D., 1995, " Further Development of New Methods for Estimating Tail Probabilities and Extreme Value Distributions," Technology Service Corp., Santa Monica, CA, TSC-PD-A234-1 (January 1981). In: Ott, W., 1995, *Environmental Statistics and Data Analysis*, CRC Press, Boca Raton.

Cox, D. C., and Baybutt, P., 1981, "Methods for Uncertainty Analysis: A Comparative Survey," *Risk Analysis*, Vol. 1, No. 4, pp. 251-258.

D'Agostino, R.B., and Stephens, M. A., *Goodness-Of-Fit Techniques*, Marcel Dekker, Inc., New York.

Ecological Committee on FIFRA Risk Assessment Methods (ECOFRAM), 1999, "ECOFRAM Terrestrial Draft Report," URL: http://www.epa.gov/oppefed1/ecorisk/terrreprot.pdf.

Fletcher, J. S., Nellessen, J. E., and Pfleeger, T.G., 1994, "Literature Review and Evaluation of the EPA Food-Chain (Kenaga) Nomogram, An Instrument For Estimating Pesticide Residues on Plants," *Environmental Toxicology and Chemistry*, Vol. 13, No. 9, pp. 1383-1391.

Hamburg, M, 1996, *Statistical Analysis for Decision Making*, Harcourt Brace Jovanovich, New York.

Hoerger, F. D., and Kenaga, E. E, 1972, "Pesticide Residues on Plants Correlation of Representative Data as a Basis for Estimation of Their Magnitude in the Environment," *Environmental Quality*, Vol. I, Academic Press, New York.

Kenaga, E. E, 1973, "Factors to be Considered in the Evaluation of the Toxicity of Pesticides to Birds in Their Environment," *Environmental Quality and Safety*, Vol. II, Academic Press, New York.

Lambert, J. H., Matalas, N. C., Ling, C. W., Haimes, Y. Y., and Li, D., 1994, "Selection of Probability Distributions in Characterizing Risk of Extreme Events," *Risk Analysis*, Vol. 14, No. 5, pp. 731-742.

Nellessen, J. E., and Fletcher, J. S., 1992, "UTAB: A Computer Database on Residues of Xenobiotic Organic Chemicals and Heavy Metals in Plants," *Journal of Chemical Information and Computer Science*, Vol. 32, No. 2, pp. 144-148.

Nellessen, J. E., and Fletcher, J. S., 1993, "Assessment of Published Literature Pertaining to the Uptake/Accumulation, Translocation, Adhesion and Biotransformation of Organic Chemicals by Vascular Plants," *Environmental Toxicology and Chemistry*, Vol. 12, pp. 2045-2052.

Ott, W., 1995, *Environmental Statistics and Data Analysis*, Lewis Publishers, Boca Raton.

Thompson, W. T., 1993, *Agricultural Chemicals*, Vols. 1 to 4, Thompson Publishing, Davis.

U.S. EPA, 1986, "Hazard Evaluation Division Standard Evaluation Procedure: Ecological Risk Assessment," EPA-540/9-85-001.

U.S. EPA Risk Assessment Forum, 1992, "Framework for Ecological Risk Assessment," EPA/630/R-92/001

U.S. EPA, 1997, "Guiding Principles for Monte Carlo Analysis," EPA/630/R-97/001.

U.S. EPA Environmental Fate and Effects Division (EFED), 1997, "EFED's Summary of the SAP Review of Ecological Risk Assessment Methodologies," URL: http://www.epa.gov/oppefed1/ecorisk/efedsum.htm, U.S. EPA.

ASTM STANDARDS AND THEIR APPLICATIONS

Jerry C. Smrchek[1] and Maurice Zeeman[1]

Harmonization of Test Methods Between the U.S. EPA (OPPTS) and the Organization for Economic Cooperation and Development (OECD): General Overview of Recent Activities with Emphasis on Aquatic and Sediment Methods

---

Reference: Smrchek, J. C. and Zeeman, M., "**Harmonization of Test Methods Between the U.S. EPA (OPPTS) and the Organization for Economic Cooperation and Development (OECD): General Overview of Recent Activities with Emphasis on Aquatic and Sediment Methods,**" *Environmental Toxicology and Risk Assessment: Science, Policy, and Standardization - Implication for Environmental Decisions: Tenth Volume, ASTM STP 1403,* B. M. Greenberg, R. N. Hull, M. H. Roberts, Jr., and R. W. Gensemer, Eds., American Society for Testing and Materials, West Conshohocken, PA, 2001.

Abstract: A description of ecological effects harmonization activities occurring since 1990, within the U.S. EPA's Office of Prevention, Pesticides, and Toxic Substances (OPPTS), and occurring between OPPTS and OECD was presented at the ASTM Eighth Symposium on Environmental Toxicology and Risk Assessment in 1998. This presentation was subsequently published (Smrchek and Morcock 1999). Recently, there has been a great increase in harmonization activities between OPPTS and OECD. Many additional activities are currently ongoing in five test method areas: physical chemical properties (e.g., K_{ow} methods), effects on biotic systems (ecological effects, e.g., *Lemna* growth inhibition, covered elsewhere), fate (degradation and accumulation, e.g., aerobic and anaerobic biodegradation), health effects, and in special activities such as in method development and testing of endocrine disruptors (e.g., avian reproduction, fish whole life cycle). The goal remains as before: to harmonize OPPTS guidelines (eventually to be published final as parts 810-885 in volume 40 of the U.S. Code of Federal Regulations) and test guidance with OECD so as to avoid unnecessary and duplicative testing of those chemicals marketed on a world wide basis, to increase efficiency, save test animals, and to reduce nontariff barriers to trade. The latest harmonization activities and results achieved, with a specific emphasis on aquatic and sediment methods are presented. ASTM has played and must continue to play an important part in the U.S. role in the development of these OECD tests. Recent activities include revision of OECD Test

---

[1]Senior Biologist, Existing Chemicals Assessment Branch, and U.S. National Coordinator for OECD Test Guidelines Program, respectively, Risk Assessment Division (Mail Code 7403), Office of Pollution Prevention and Toxics, Office of Prevention, Pesticides, and Toxic Substances, US Environmental Protection Agency, Ariel Rios Building, 1200 Pennsylvania Avenue N. W., Washington, DC, 20460.

Guideline No. 202, *Daphnia* sp., Acute Immobilisation Test; development of a new oligochaete reproduction test; two chironomid sediment tests (spiked water and spiked sediment); an oligochaete bioaccumulation test; and a guidance document on Aquatic Toxicity Testing of Difficult Substances and Mixtures. Challenges and potential problems for effective harmonization continue to be present. These can be categorized into internal within the U.S. EPA and external to the agency. The former include having adequate available resources, redistribution and changes in workloads to accommodate OECD work, continual education to demonstrate the advantages of harmonization, and obtaining continued support in an environment of budget constraints. External aspects include challenges from the public, the problem of incurring continuing harmonization costs by U.S. industry, accommodating voluntary standards organizations such as ASTM, and difficulties in developing a "U.S. position" on OECD test guidelines. There also continue to be difficulties (not unexpected) in coordination, communication, and cooperation in expert panels and among participating OECD member countries. Several principles for effective harmonization in updating existing OECD test guidelines or in developing new test guidelines are discussed.

Keywords: harmonization, aquatic and sediment effects test methods, U.S. EPA, OPPTS, OPPT, OECD.

At the ASTM Eighth Symposium on Environmental Toxicology and Risk Assessment in 1998, a presentation was made and subsequently published (Smrchek and Morcock 1999) on the process of harmonizing test guidelines both within OPPTS (as series 810-885 draft guidelines appearing in 1996) and between OPPTS and OECD. High priority tests that need to be developed as harmonized OECD ecological effects test guidelines were listed, and OPPTS involvement in these activities was described. The advantages of harmonization also were discussed, as well as the results, with examples, of harmonization achieved up to April 1998 (updated to February 1999, in Smrchek and Morcock 1999). Finally, issues, challenges, and potential problems preventing progress in harmonization were listed and discussed. This publication should be consulted as information presented there will not be repeated here. It will serve to complement the present paper.

Since early 1999, the pace of harmonization between OPPTS and OECD has increased considerably (see below) and will continue at a high level for the next several years as work proceeds and is completed on increased numbers of new or updated existing test guidelines. Here we present additional, current (as of August 2000) information on harmonization (or standardization) efforts involving both organizations. Aquatic and sediment effects test methods are emphasized and discussed here.

Overview of OPPTS/OECD Harmonization

Harmonization and Standardization Defined

We use the term "harmonization" interchangeably with "standardization." The former may be a more general term denoting the process of standardization undertaken by OECD with its 29 member countries. Both terms denote that a consensus among all interested parties be achieved by following written, well-defined, transparent procedures. The harmonization process in OECD is for all intents a standardization process; it can include or use any test method from any of the OECD member countries that has been developed and standardized (and recommended by regulators) by a particular country. This method(s) can then serve as the basis for an OECD test guideline. For example, an OPPTS ecological effects test method that has been developed and harmonized between the Office of Pollution Prevention and Toxics (OPPT) and the Office of Pesticide Programs (OPP) can serve as a background document or basis for development of a similar harmonized OECD test guideline. These harmonized OPPTS test methods are used by OPPT as agency specified standards for developing test data from actions taken under the Toxic Substances Control Act of 1976 (Section 4). The next step is the harmonized OECD guideline used in place of, or replacing, a country-specific guideline. Procedures for effective implementation of these substitutions or replacements are under development. This is especially important when there are differences between both guidelines.

Use of Voluntary Consensus Standards

In carrying out its TSCA mandated activities, OPPT also makes use of voluntary consensus technical standards from organizations such as ASTM and the International Organization for Standardization (ISO). This use is required by Office of Management and Budget OMB Circular A-119, "Federal Participation in the Development and Use of Voluntary Standards." The latter, first issued in 1982 and later revised in 1993, is codified as provision 12(d) of the Technology Transfer Improvements Act of 1995, Public Law Number 104-113 (Kono 1996). A final revision to Circular A-119 was published in the Federal Register (Volume 63, No. 33, pp. 8545-8558) on February 19, 1998 (Kono 1998).

In following the circular, the meaning of the word "use" is critical. It is defined in the 1998 Federal Register notice and is dependent on the practicality, adequacy, feasibility, efficiency, usefulness, and consistency of the standards activity in relation to agency program needs or mission. Implementation may range, for example, from simply citing by reference, an ASTM standard in an OPPT test method or regulation, to incorporating in whole or in part, procedural details or large portions of methods from an ASTM published standard (Annual Book of Standards, Section 11 Water and Environmental Technology, Vol. 11.05 Biological Effects and Environmental Fate; Biotechnology; Pesticides) in an OPPTS test guideline.

The OECD Process

The current process of test guideline development, harmonization, or standardization in OECD is shown (Figure 1, modified from the flow diagram presented in OECD 1995).

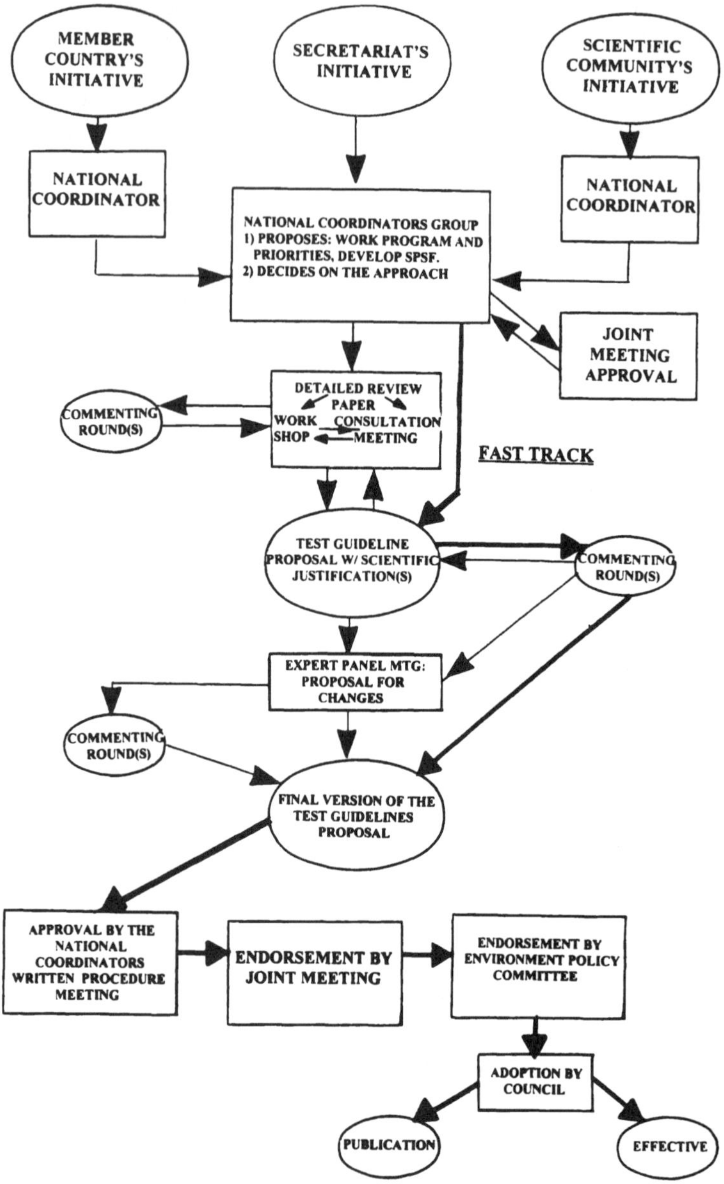

Figure 1 - *The OECD test guideline development process. Modified from OECD (1995). "Commenting rounds" include member countries, BIAC (Business and Industry Advisory Committee), and scientific societies, as appropriate. "Joint meetings" are meetings of the Chemicals Group and Management Committee, Special Program On the Control of Chemicals, an oversight group for the Test Guidelines Program. Bold arrows denote a Fast Track procedure where a detailed review paper (see text) is not prepared.*

The National Coordinators from each OECD member country have a central role in this process because they submit national proposals for new test guidelines or for updates/revisions to existing guidelines and serve as centers for distribution of OECD documents. They also provide nationally agreed or country-specific comments (e.g., a U.S. Position) on documents sent by the OECD Secretariat. National coordinators also work to set priorities for test guideline activities. The OECD Secretariat in Paris serves as the structural support for the test guidelines program.

Proposals for new or updated test guidelines can be made from several sources: the member country, the international scientific community, industry, a non-governmental organization, or the OECD Secretariat (OECD 1995). A Standard Project Submission Form (SPSF) is completed for each current guidelines project and for each proposed activity. It serves to standardize the process by listing the same information for each project, including the anticipated end product, the country or group taking the lead for the activity, a proposed work plan, and a justification for why the activity should be started. Each proposal is given a priority (high, medium, low).

A detailed review paper can be prepared by the lead for the activity. The "state-of-the-art" is extensively discussed with reference to the test guideline proposal. Existing methods are reviewed, data gaps identified, a need for the new or updated test guideline is made, and the relationship between the proposed and existing tests, including possibilities and limitations of use, is discussed. Alternatively, a draft test guideline proposal may be prepared directly (fast track procedure), without completing a detailed review paper (Fig. 1). The detailed review paper or draft guideline proposal is circulated among member countries for comment.

At this stage in the process a workshop may be conducted to discuss issues associated with the proposal, experts may be consulted, or an expert panel established. One or more meetings may then be held to discuss the proposal and proceed with revising the current test guideline or writing a new test guideline. It is here that U.S. experts (e.g., scientists from academia, the testing community, the regulatory community, and from national standards organizations such as ASTM) nominated by the national coordinators become involved in reviewing documents and serving on expert panels. The experts bring to the process their expertise and experience in specific test methods they use or are familiar with; it is here that consensus building and harmonization occurs. Often, round-robin or ring-tests are conducted to determine the repeatability and reproducibility of the draft test guideline (Environment Agency 1999). Also assessed is the extent to which the test method can be performed and if the validity criteria of the method can be met. Quality control criteria for test accuracy and precision are derived, so that the performance of the test can be assessed. Ideally, after several commenting rounds, revisions, and additional expert meetings, the final product is a harmonized draft new OECD test guideline or a harmonized updated draft existing test guideline.

The harmonized new or updated draft test guideline is approved by the expert panel and is then passed on to the Secretariat. The latter formats the draft into the OECD test guideline format and sends it to each national coordinator for commenting, revision, more commenting as needed, and eventual approval, after all member country-specific objections have been resolved. In the United States the national coordinator has developed a mailing list of recipients from other EPA offices, other government offices,

ASTM, industry, the public, and testing laboratories for each OECD document. A specific group of experts may need to be identified to review a particular draft test guideline.

After comments are received, each national coordinator develops a country-specific position (e.g., a U.S. position) on each comment made by country-specific reviewers sent the draft. Eventually, after several commenting rounds, much discussion, resolution of differences and objections, and consensus building, the draft new test guideline or updated existing test guideline is approved by all member countries. The test guideline is then formally approved, endorsed, and adopted by the OECD; it is added as an addendum to the complete OECD Guidelines for the Testing of Chemicals available for purchase from OECD.

Existing test guidelines may also be deleted. This would be due, for example, to development of new and better techniques, changes in acceptance or use of the guideline, or a duplication of some sort.

OECD Test Guidelines

The complete set of OECD test guidelines consists of four sections: Section 1- Physical Chemical properties, Section 2- Effects on Biotic Systems, Section 3- Degradation and Accumulation, and Section 4- Health Effects. All of these guidelines cannot be listed here, however, titles can be viewed at the OECD web site, http://www.oecd.org/, or the test guidelines web site, http://www.oecd.org/ehs/test/testlist.htm. As of early March 2000, a total of 93 test guidelines have been adopted by OECD (18 in ecological effects and bioaccumulation), and a total of 30 draft test guidelines or draft new test guidelines are listed. The four sections above correspond to the four areas (plus one on Special Activities- see below) where harmonization activities are occurring.

Unlike ASTM, OECD test guidelines do not have to be reapproved every four to five years, but they can be updated at any time, provided a strong scientific rationale can be made by the country, or organization taking the lead for the updating.

Table 1 lists the adopted and draft OECD Section 2 test guidelines, currently totaling 11, that are considered to be harmonized with OPPTS since the harmonization program was initiated by OPPTS in 1990 (Smrchek and Morcock 1999). Activity in this area has increased and the program has become more efficient. On an annual basis, more test guideline documents were produced from 1995 to 1999 than were produced in 1982 through 1994. Since 1998, seven new test guidelines have been adopted, one is ready for adoption and addition to the year 2000 addendum, and six draft test guidelines are currently undergoing review by OECD member countries.

Harmonization Efforts and Results

Aquatic (Non-plant) and Sediment Test Methods

Recent activities have involved several existing aquatic (non-plant) OECD test guidelines. Harmonized test guideline No. 202, *Daphnia* sp., Acute Immobilisation Test is being slightly revised, i.e., test period was increased from 24 to 48 hours, and is based in large part on OPPTS harmonized draft test guideline 850.1010, Aquatic Invertebrate Toxicity Test, Freshwater Daphnids. It was commented on in Fall 1999 and, barring any major objections, is ready for approval, endorsement, and adoption by OECD.

Table 1 - *Adopted and draft OECD Section 2 (Effects on Biotic Systems) Test guidelines harmonized with OPPTS since 1990. List current as of August 2000.*

Test Guideline No.	Guideline Title	Date of Adoption As An Original Or As An Updated Version. Also Date of Draft
203	Fish, Acute Toxicity Test	July 17, 1992 (Updated)
210	Fish, Early-Life Stage Toxicity Test	July 17, 1992
211	Daphnia magna Reproduction Test	September 21, 1998
212	Fish, Short-term Toxicity Test on Embryo and Sac-Fry Stages	September 21, 1998
213	Honeybees, Acute Oral Toxicity Test	September 21, 1998
214	Honeybees, Acute Contact Toxicity Test	September 21, 1998
215	Fish, Juvenile Growth Test	January 21, 2000
216	Soil Microorganisms, Nitrogen Transformation Test	January 21, 2000
217	Soil Microorganisms, Carbon Transformation Test	January 21, 2000
202	Daphnia sp., Acute Immobilisation Test	Draft (Updated) Guideline, July 1999 draft
305	Bioconcentration: Flow-through Fish Test	June 14, 1996 (Updated)

The harmonized guidelines No. 211, *Daphnia magna* Reproduction Test; No. 212, Fish, Short-term Toxicity Test on Embryo and Sac-fry Stages; No. 213, Honeybees, Acute Oral Toxicity Test; and No. 214, Honeybees, Acute Contact Toxicity Test, were adopted in September 1998. Harmonized test guideline No. 215, Fish, Juvenile Growth Test, was finally adopted by OECD in January 2000, after several lengthy commenting rounds.

In development of new sediment toxicity tests there has also been increased activity. Revised drafts of proposed new test guideline No. 218, Sediment-Water Chironomid Toxicity Test Using Spiked Sediment; and No. 219, Sediment-Water Chironomid Toxicty Test Using Spiked Water were received in February 2000 for another round of commenting. As the U.S. comments (April 2000) on these drafts were again extensive (as they were for the first draft reviewed in summer 1998), resolution of objections and eventual adoption by OECD is not expected in the near term.

In early March 2000, proposed new test guideline No. 220, *Enchytraeidae* Reproduction Test, was received for a second round of commenting. It had first been commented on in Fall 1999.

A workshop was held in April 1999 on "Bioaccumulation: Sediment Test Using Benthic Oligochaetes," convened by the German Federal Environmental Agency (UBA) and organized by ECT Oekotoxikologie GmbH. A draft guideline of this test, written in the OECD format, was prepared for this meeting and commented on by US experts. It is expected that this document will be submitted to OECD in the year 2000 as a proposed new test guideline.

Other aquatic harmonization activities by OECD involve development of a Guidance Document on Aquatic Toxicity Testing of Difficult Substances and Mixtures. This document is important because it will give advice and suggestions on testing chemicals that are poorly water soluble, volatile, easily degradable in toxicity test systems, adsorb or form complexes, and are colored, hydrophobic, or ionized. The revised draft was reviewed in Winter 2000; it is not clear at this time if this document will be ready for OECD approval, endorsement, and adoption in the year 2000.

Special Activities

In November 1996, activity on chemicals that may be endocrine disruptors (or disrupters) was initiated by the OECD. The focus of this work is to provide information on member-country activities for these chemicals, develop appropriate test guidelines and, where possible, to harmonize hazard/risk procedures. Within the test guidelines program, a Task Force on Endocrine Disrupter Testing and Assessment (EDTA) was established. New and enhanced guidelines are to be identified and prioritized, for example, avian reproduction and fish whole life cycle tests. A harmonized testing strategy is to be eventually developed. The EDTA has discussed what screening and definitive tests are available for non-mammalian test species, using existing OECD tests, and what future test guideline development work is needed for fish, birds, reptiles, amphibians, and aquatic invertebrates. Existing test methods from member countries could serve as a basis for some OECD harmonized guideline development.

This work complements the US EPA's Endocrine Disruptor Screening Program (EDSP) proposed in late 1998, as recommended by the Endocrine Disruptor Screening and Testing Advisory Committee (EDSTAC). Tests and screens proposed by this program must be standardized and validated before they can be used for regulatory purposes. Tests and screens of international interest are being examined by the OECD Task Force described above.

Harmonization Problems and Mechanisms for Improvement

Problems Internal to U.S. EPA

Effective harmonization activities involves the expenditure of resources that could always be spent elsewhere in the agency. OPPTS policy in the past has been that this work is important, and we believe that this is still true. Thus, adequate support must continue to be provided, and sufficient time must continue to be made available to accomplish these activities. Also, sufficient resources must be made available and must continue on a regular basis. If needed, workloads are redistributed to accommodate increases in OECD work. Periodic briefing of agency personnel should continue to occur to reinforce the advantages of harmonization to the agency, especially when turnover in management occurs. There must also be regular communication between different agency individuals involved in various harmonization activities to increase coordination and efficient use of agency resources.

Problems External to U.S. EPA

The agency continues to face challenges from the public, for example, on animal welfare issues such as the number of test animals used in a harmonized toxicity test. Frequently, animal welfare groups believe the number of animals used is excessive. The agency is very aware of this criticism and must balance the number of test animals used, against an increased probability of having to repeat the test if not enough animals were used to conduct a scientifically valid test. In the end, repeating tests may result in more test animals being used than if a higher number had been used in initial testing.

There is a continual dialog between the US chemical industry and OPPTS over whether costly testing with harmonized test methods should be required, and if so, how many tests. Often a compromise is reached between a company or group of companies and OPPTS on testing issues.

There are also challenges from voluntary consensus standards organizations, where use of a particular test method is advocated (to the exclusion of others). When commenting on controversial aspects of an OECD test guideline, where there may be differences of opinion, it is a challenge to develop a U.S. position from divergent comments and opinions.

The almost continual process of test guideline development/updating can cause problems. For example, a national standard may be heavily relied upon in developing a harmonized international test guideline. This development at the international level may take several years to complete, especially if it is difficult to harmonize due to divergent opinions or controversial issues. By the time an international test guideline is finally completed, the national standard on which it is based, may have been revised and changed greatly. As a result, the international test guideline may not be widely used and may become obsolete sooner than expected.

Another problem is how to address differences between a member country test guideline and an OECD test guideline. The extent of differences between both guidelines is important. Supposedly, these differences have to be accepted by the member country because it is assumed that all objections regarding the OECD test guideline will have been resolved in the harmonization process. However, this does not always occur, especially for issues that are difficult to resolve satisfactorily for all countries by compromise. Due to these divergences, it may be very difficult to harmonize some guidelines.

There are other problems that were discussed previously (Smrchek and Morcock 1999), including duplicative testing if a chemical is marketed in several different countries to satisfy different regulatory requirements, lack of specificity in the test method, distinct differences on aspects of the method, and inconsistencies between standards. The goal of harmonization must be to lessen, minimize, or eliminate these problems.

The OECD recently identified other concerns associated with harmonization and the test guidelines program (OECD 1999). The process was concluded to be too slow even with an increased number of member country experts involved in the process. The review process and consensus building structure of the test guidelines program allows for extensive commenting and almost unlimited scientific and technical input from member countries. Several commenting rounds may result and thus, it may take 5 or more years for consensus to be reached and the guideline completed. This problem is especially important because of the need for timely, internationally acceptable test guidelines and the importance of harmonization to industry and government.

OECD believes work priorities are insufficiently defined such that the process is not transparent and is based too much on *ad hoc* decisions. New, well-defined criteria developed for the SPSF by OECD may solve this problem.

The role of the national coordinators in the development of harmonized new test guidelines and updating of existing test guidelines is crucial to the success of the OECD test guidelines program. Sufficient resources must continue to be made available to each national coordinator, and a sufficient commitment must continue in order to effectively carry out this role. Coordination among commenters and commenting groups within a country must be sufficient to represent adequately the country and the position of the country in the OECD test guidelines program. Also, maintaining national networks of experts willing to serve on panels and to review documents is vital to the success of the program. Consistency at the national level in commenting is important, even though experts may unavoidably change on the panels from time to time. Discussions concerning the same aspects of a test guideline should not occur repeatedly when new experts come into the process.

The issue of whether or not to conduct round-robin or ring-testing for every new test guideline is important, as well as when to conduct this testing in guideline development.

It seems important to determine whether or not a new test guideline can be conducted and if it will result in obtaining valid test results with a minimum of repeat testing. Repeatability and reproducibility information on the test guideline is important to have available. However, round-robin studies may add several years to the time it takes for a new test guideline to be developed, for example with test guideline No. 211, Daphnia magna Reproduction Test, or only one to two years as occurred in the development of the new *Lemna* inhibition test.

Other problems include policy aspects that may enter into what is essentially a technical activity of test guideline development, causing delays that are unrelated to scientific or technical disagreements. Originally, the test guidelines program was focused on working only with industrial chemicals. In recent years pesticides, biocides, polymers, and other different chemicals have been added. Also, the program has expanded to cover special topics such as endocrine disruptors (discussed earlier). Discussion has involved whether or not chemical specific test guidelines should be developed.

The OECD, with approval by the national coordinators, made recommendations for improvement of the process (OECD 1999). These included better defining each project by developing the SPSF, establishing criteria for priority setting, establishing *ad hoc* expert groups to reduce the number of commenting rounds, and generally streamlining the process (Figure 1) where ever possible.

Discussion and Conclusions

Principles for An Effective (OPPTS/OECD) Harmonization Process

There are several principles that may be useful in effectively updating existing OECD test guidelines or developing new test guidelines in the harmonization process. This process may be relatively efficient and productive, or agonizingly difficult.

1) Transparency: The complete process, including information flow and written documents such as meeting minutes and responses to member country comments, must be open, transparent, and written in sufficient detail (especially if controversial aspects of methods are being discussed) to obtain an understanding of why a decision was made. This information must be available for comment.

2) Role of the chairperson: The chairperson of the expert panel involved with developing a new harmonized test guideline or updating an existing test guideline is very important to the effectiveness of the harmonization process. This person must be flexible, must communicate with each panel member on a regular basis, must be receptive to all viewpoints, and must conduct all expert panel activities in a transparent manner.

3) Commitment: Attendance by member country experts at all panel meetings is desirable and necessary. Often it is difficult to capture in meeting minutes everything that was said at a meeting or the basis for certain decisions that were made. On the other hand, the meeting minutes must be written in enough detail so that attendance at all meetings is not completely mandatory due to unforeseen circumstances.

4) Timeliness: All documents from an expert panel must be sent to all panel members in a timely manner.

5) Consistency: The same experts should be involved in a test guideline activity, from beginning to completion, if at all possible.

Harmonization: The Future

It is always difficult to speculate into the future, nevertheless we make an attempt here and discuss several possible trends.

1) Increasing use of technology in communication and information transfer. The worldwide web has revolutionized information transfer; for example, documents can be received from the OECD Secretariat with a minimum of delay. It may be possible to participate in expert panel meetings, from one's desk, by linking countries around the world together. This would allow for increased participation and involvement by countries and companies that in the past could not attend meetings. Geographic representation would also probably be increased.

2) Continuing trend of decreased emphasis on standards development at the national level, with an increased emphasis on international standards development and harmonization. Since increased economic activities are occurring on a worldwide basis, the global view continues to be considered important, and because of the advantages of harmonization (Smrchek and Morcock 1999) the view will remain that international harmonization should continue.

3) Related to this is the increase in development of regional standards, e.g., harmonization activities in the United States related to the North American Free Trade Agreement (NAFTA).

4) Continuing efforts in finding ways to decrease the time taken to develop an international standard, with resulting savings in resources.

5) When consensus within an expert panel cannot be achieved, due to major disagreements, perhaps a set of test guidelines, representing different levels of consensus within the expert panel and within OECD could be developed. This is similar to what has occurred in ISO.

6) The most obvious future trend is continued development of new harmonized test guidelines, along with identifying and developing priorities for future new test guidelines.

This paper, along with those of Petrie (in this volume) and Smrchek and Morcock (1999) have attempted to give the reader a more-or-less complete picture of U.S. EPA (OPPTS) harmonization efforts with OECD since 1990.

Acknowledgments

The authors would like to thank Chris Ingersoll, Columbia Environmental Research Center, U.S. Geological Survey, Columbia, MO, and Mark Hinman, Exxon Biomedical Sciences, Inc., East Millstone, NJ, for asking us to participate and present the contents of this paper at a session on "ASTM Standards and Their Application," held at the ASTM 2000 meeting in Toronto, Ontario, Canada. Thanks are also extended to Marie-Chantal Huet, Environmental Health and Safety Division, Environment Directorate, OECD, who offered useful comments. She is a tireless, dedicated scientist and good friend, whom we have worked with effectively over the past several years in test guideline development and updating as well as on various harmonization issues.

Disclaimer

This document has been reviewed by the Office of Pollution Prevention and Toxics, U.S. Environmental Protection Agency, and is approved for publication. Approval neither signifies that the contents necessarily reflect the views and policies of the Agency nor does mention of tradenames or commercial products constitute endorsement or recommendation for use.

References

Environment Agency (UK), 1999, *The OECD* Lemna *Growth Inhibition Test, Development and Ring-Testing of Draft OECD Test Guideline,* Research and Development Technical Report EMA 003, Environment Agency, Bristol, UK.

Kono, K, 1996, "OMB A-119 Becomes Law," *ASTM Standardization News,* Vol. 24, No. 5, pp. 40-42.

Kono, K, 1998, "OMB A-119 Revised," *ASTM Standardization News,* Vol. 26, No. 6, pp. 19-21.

OECD, 1995, *Guidance Document For the Development of OECD Test Guidelines For Testing of Chemicals,* Environment Monograph No. 76, OECD, Paris, France. (Available from the OECD Secretariat, Paris)

OECD, 1999, *Output of the Test Guidelines Programme: How To Do More,* ENV/JM(99)6, April 12, 1999, OECD, Paris, France. (Available from the OECD Secretariat)

Smrchek, J. C. and Morcock, R. E, 1999, "Harmonization of Ecological Effects Test Methods Between the U.S. EPA (OPPTS) and the Organization for Economic Cooperation and Development (OECD): Description, Results, and Current Activities," *Environmental Toxicology and Risk Assessment: Standardization of Biomarkers for Endocrine Disruption and Environmental Assessment: Eighth Volume, ASTM STP 1364*, D. S. Henshel, M. C. Black, and M. C. Harrass, Eds., American Society for Testing and materials, West Conshohocken, PA, pp. 473-490.

Richard C. Petrie[1]

HARMONIZATION OF PLANT TOXICITY TESTS

Reference: Petrie, R. C. "**Harmonization of Plant Toxicity Tests,**" *Environmental Toxicology and Risk Assessment: Science, Policy, and Standardization - Implications for Environmental Decisions: Tenth Volume, ASTM STP 1403*, B. M. Greenberg, R. N. Hull, M. H. Roberts, Jr., and R. W. Gensemer, Eds., American Society for Testing and Materials, West Conshohocken, PA, 2001.

Abstract: The Environmental Protection Agency (EPA) Office of Pesticide Programs (OPP) is participating in Organization For Economic Cooperation and Development (OECD) workgroups to update OECD guidelines number 201 (aquatic algal toxicity), number 208 (terrestrial plant toxicity), and to develop a new yet unnumbered guideline for the aquatic macrophyte *Lemna spp.* The EPA participants have presented the 850 series EPA guidelines and existing American Society for Testing and Materials (ASTM) guidelines to the OECD workgroups for their consideration. Under the existing North Atlantic Free Trade Agreement (NAFTA), the EPA is harmonizing plant toxicity tests and nontarget plant risk assessment methods with the Pest Management Regulatory Agency (PMRA), Canada. A pesticide regulatory workshop was recently held at the EPA to share information with Mexican government pesticide regulators. The OECD guidelines are focusing on pesticide and toxic substances, whereas NAFTA harmonization efforts to date are primarily for methods used to evaluate pesticides. While some of the plant tests are similar for toxic substances and pesticides, statutes and risk assessment methods are different.

Keywords: harmonization, plant toxicity, OECD, USEPA.

Introduction

The harmonization of plant toxicity tests and risk assessment methods within the Environmental Protection Agency (EPA), with our neighbors to the North and South, and with the world is ongoing. Harmonization of plant toxicity tests within the EPA began as an apples to oranges process. The two EPA program offices that require plant toxicity tests, the Office of Pollution Prevention and Toxics (OPPT) and the OPP operate under two different Federal statutes. The OPPT is responsible for regulation of toxic substances under the Toxic Substances Control Act (TSCA) and the Pollution Prevention Act (PPA).

---

[1] Senior Agronomist, Environmental Hazard Branch, Environmental Fate and Effects Division (7507C), Office of Pesticide Programs, Office of Pollution Prevention and Toxics, U.S. Environmental Protection Agency, Ariel Rios Building, 1200 Pennsylvania Avenue, N.W., Washington, D.C. 20460.

The OPP is responsible for regulation under the Federal Insecticide, Fungicide, and Rodenticide Act (FIFRA) as amended, food additive aspects of the Food and Drug Administration (FDA), and the Food Quality Protection Act (FQPA). Each program identified similarities and differences among these environmental statutes as they relate to plant toxicity testing. Those plant test guidelines that were unique to a given program office were identified as such so that harmonization of similar guidelines could proceed. The EPA harmonized guidelines for ecological testing were presented to the FIFRA Scientific Advisory Panel (SAP) in 1996 and the draft published in the Federal Register shortly thereafter.

Regardless of the type of test, harmonization with other countries or nations is difficult. A clear, concise plan must be developed and adhered to. Poor communication and political resistance must be overcome at all levels. Lack of planning for travel expenses and personnel time commitment can seriously reduce the ability to reach consensus. Research money must be set aside in order to generate baseline data, assess existing data bases, and conduct round-robin testing. New technology such as E-mail and conference calls have helped to reduce the time required to review and comment on documents, however, accommodation must be made for the extra time and effort needed. New technology, however, cannot replace the benefit of face-to-face interaction.

The NAFTA fosters communication and cooperation with our neighbors to the North and the South. In the spirit of NAFTA the Office of Pesticide Programs (OPP) and the Pest Management Regulatory Agency (PMRA) have identified areas of testing and risk assessment that can be harmonized in order to improve review consistency. One of these areas is non-target plant toxicity testing and risk assessment methods. Similarities and differences in soils, climate, flora, fauna, crops, pesticide application methods farming practices need evaluation and consideration in our assessment.

Types Of Environmental Standards Developed/Needed

The large volume of herbicides, desiccants, defoliants and other phytotoxicants that are used each year in the United States dictates the need for sophisticated plant toxicity tests that will be predictive of their phytotoxic potential (Aspelin and Grube 1999). Some factors that may vary considerably when comparing the United States with other countries include different plant species, the importance of aerial pesticide application for pest control, pesticide formulation differences, soil type differences, and climatic differences.

The FIFRA SAP and other state and regional EPA offices have criticized our existing plant toxicity screen for not including reproductive endpoints, and for not including a greater spectrum of plant types (ferns, perennials, non-crop native plants). While the majority of phytotoxicants are used to control weeds in agricultural row crops, millions of pounds are also used each year in non-crop sites such as forestry and rights-of-way which can result in high potential for nontarget plant exposure to pesticide residues (Aspelin and Grube 1999). The OPP also evaluates the potential for exposure and adverse effects to endangered or threatened plant species. As of December, 1998, there were 706 plants listed as endangered or threatened. Of these, 672 are flowering plants, 26 are ferns and allies, 6 are conifers, and 2 are lichens (USFWS 1998).

Current plant toxicity tests are grouped into 2 broad categories, aquatic and terrestrial.

There are two broad categories of plant toxicity tests, aquatic and terrestrial. Of the aquatic plants, the OPP currently tests five species. The five aquatic plants currently tested are the freshwater green microalgae *Pseudokershneria subcapitata* formerly known as *Selenastrum capricornutum* (Hindak 1990), the freshwater diatom microalgae *Navicula pelliculosa*, the freshwater blue-green cyanobacteria *Anabaena flos-aquae*, the marine diatom microalgae *Skeketonema costatum*, and the freshwater floating aquatic macrophyte *Lemna gibba*. The microalgae tests are four days in duration and the floating aquatic macrophyte test is seven days in duration.

The EPA, OPP does not require the routine testing of many classes of aquatic plants such as red and brown microalgae, marine macroalgae, emerged-rooted macrophytes, floating broadleaf macrophytes, and submersed-rooted macrophytes. Microcosm, mesocosm, and limnocorral multiple species tests are not routinely conducted for the majority of pesticide registrations but can be requested on a case-by-case basis.

Terrestrial plant toxicity tests currently required for registration of known phytotoxicants having outdoor uses include only early growth tests. The two required tests are seedling emergence and vegetative vigor. Both tests are 14-28 days in duration depending on the mode of action of the test pesticide. The OPP currently requires that 10 plants be included in each test. Corn, soybean and a root crop such as carrot or radish are required species in all tests. The remaining test species are typically crop plants such as oat, wheat, ryegrass, sugarbeet, canola, tomato, onion, cabbage, lettuce, or cucumber. Edge-of-field tests are occasionally required on a case-by-case basis to evaluate movement of residues from the field to non-target plants.

Plant Test Standards in Need of Further Development Include Aquatic and Terrestrial, both Laboratory and Field.

Aquatic Plants

Test standards specific to the culturing and testing of individual aquatic plant species similar to ASTM Test Method for Algal Growth Potential Testing with *Selenastrum capricornutum* (D3978-80), ASTM Test Method for Conducting Static Toxicity Tests with *Lemna gibba* G3 (E1415-91), and ASTM Test Method for Conducting Toxicity Tests with Bioluminescent Dinoflagellates (E1924-97) are needed for the aquatic microalgae and Cyanobacteria: blue-green (*Cyanobacteria*), diatoms (*Bacillariophyceae*), yellow-green (*Xanthophyceae*), golden-brown (*Chrysophyceae*), and red (*Rhodophyceae*).

Possible modifications to E1415-91 (*Lemna gibba)* and the ASTM Test Method for

Conducting Renewal Phytotoxicity Tests with Freshwater Emergent Macrophytes (E1841-96) might include the addition of foliar drift simulation tests (application of test chemical to the plant foliage). The 14 day emergent macrophyte test E1841-96 might also be modified to include the entire plant life cycle.

Terrestrial Plants

Early growth tests for terrestrial plants include seed germination, seedling emergence (early seedling growth), and vegetative vigor. The OPP has generally waived the routine submission of seed germination tests. Seed germination is a specific endpoint captured in the seedling emergence (early seedling growth) test. No ASTM vegetative vigor (application of test material to plant foliage) test is yet available for greenhouse early plant growth or to assess reproductive endpoints in the greenhouse or field.

Future modifications to the ASTM Test Method for Conducting Terrestrial Plant Toxicity Tests (E 1963-98) might include the consideration of key ecological plant species more representative of plants utilized for food and shelter by fish and wildlife. Herbicides are extensively used for vegetation control in non-crop areas such as forest clear-cuts, and power line and highway rights-of-way (Aspelin and Grube 1999). Plant test species representative of endangered/threatened plants should also be considered when assessing test species selection. Inclusion of key plant species representative of distinct eco-regions of the U.S.,Canada, and Mexico in our test strategies would allow consideration of effects on plants other than food crops. Any testing scheme should include biennial and perennial plants as well.

A laboratory single species life-cycle test and a woody plant toxicity test are addressed in E 1963-98, (Annex A3 and Annex A4, respectively).

Aquatic and Terrestrial Plants

Standards in need of development for both aquatic and terrestrial plants include foliar soil toxicity tests (simulate airborne soil particles), bioassay plants for residue monitoring and field studies, field tests study design, methods, and analysis (species, community, ecosystem), reproductive tests (single and multiple exposures, multiple toxicants), testing difficult substances (volatility, solubility, pH, photosensitivity), to support deterministic and probabilistic risk assessments.

The Standardization Process in The Office Of Pesticide Programs for Non-Target Plant Tests

Our harmonization efforts to date have been considerable, and will likely increase in the future. Harmonization of plant toxicity tests can occur at many levels: within the EPA, with other federal agencies, within our hemisphere (NAFTA), and outside our hemisphere (OECD countries and others). An offshoot of test harmonization is cooperation with regard to test data acceptance criteria. A final benefit of harmonization may be understanding and acceptance of risk assessment methods and procedures.

Harmonization Efforts To Date

EPA Program Office

Harmonization among EPA program offices began in 1994 and ended in 1996 with the publication of the Office of Pollution Prevention and Toxic Substances Test Guidelines, *Series 850 - Ecological Effects Test Guidelines*: Group D - Nontarget Plants Test Guidelines: 850.4000 - 850.4800, Group E - Toxicity to Microorganisms Test Guidelines: 850.5100 - 850.5400. These draft guidelines are located on the EPA web page.

Other U.S. Government Regulatory Agencies

Harmonization of plant test guidelines with other government agencies is not required. In 1994 the government agency FDA was contacted because of their past interest in plant toxicity testing. While the Food and Drug Administration required the submission of plant toxicity data prior to 1994, they have not required it since.

NAFTA Countries

Harmonization of plant tests with other NAFTA countries is ongoing. The Canadian Pest Management Regulatory Agency (PMRA) and our office are in the process of identifying similarities, differences, and areas in need of update in our testing requirements and risk assessment methods. A review of the literature and all available plant test methods will also be conducted. Mexican pesticide officials are interested in harmonization. A pesticide regulatory workshop was held at the EPA in March to familiarize ourselves with each other's regulatory programs and data requirements. Harmonization efforts within the Americas allows us a broader understanding of soil, climatic, and plant species differences and the need for guideline flexibility to account for these differences.

European Countries

Harmonization of plant tests with OECD is ongoing. The OECD contact for these guidelines is Marie-Chantal Huet. Limited descriptions of OECD projects are as follows:

OECD 201 - Aquatic plant test guideline for freshwater and marine microalgae is ongoing. Two workgroup meetings have been completed in Oslo, Norway, one in 1997 and one in 1999. It is expected that this guideline will be updated to include 3 additional types of plants: blue-green cyanobacteria, freshwater diatom, and a marine diatom.

OECD 208 - Terrestrial plant test guideline for early growth tests: seedling emergence and vegetative vigor. Two workgroup meetings, in 1997 and 1999, have been held in Paris, France. This guideline update is expected to add an early plant growth vegetative vigor test and increase the choice of test species. The updated guideline is hoped to be useful for toxic chemical and pesticide screens.

OECD *Lemna sp.* - Floating aquatic macrophyte test of 7 day duration. Two workgroup meetings were held, one in Ispra, Italy in 1997 and a second meeting in Medmenham, England in 1998. This is a new OECD guideline undergoing OECD member country review.

Problems Caused by the Lack of Harmonization

Some problems of the lack of harmonization can include the expenditure of additional agency resources to review European studies (Ex. green algae, EPA four day study length vs OECD three day study), and poor communications among scientists and other regulatory agencies regarding tests, test methods, and risk assessments.

Some problems with harmonization can include trying to satisfy different laws and statutes that have different requirements, needs, and capabilities (Ex. TOSCA vs FIFRA). Many of our guidelines are "unique" to a given program and are labeled as such.

Other problems can include different pesticide application methods (Ex. In the U.S. aerial application is used to a great extent vs Europe), different climates, soil types, and geographies (Ex. Warm season plants in S. U.S. vs cool season plants in Canada). Many of these issues go unresolved due to the scarcity of research funding to generate baseline data.

How Can We Improve Harmonization

A few suggestions to improve harmonization include the following::

Research

Extensive baseline research is needed to progress beyond our limited screening tests that may have little or no relevance to the field. Surrogate species analysis research is needed to assess Canadian vs U.S. vs S. American plant types that could serve as non-crop test surrogates within our hemisphere, the relationship of early plant growth effects to latent reproductive growth effects, greenhouse vs field ratio, and annual vs biennial vs perennial plant testing in the greenhouse and the field. Plant life cycle tests in the greenhouse and field are only minimally developed. Research that evaluates long range transport of pesticide residues, and resulting effects on plant growth is needed.

Time and Money

Scientists must convince their supervisors that harmonization is time consuming and costly, and that these efforts require an unending dedication to harmonization throughout a large portion of the year. Long term planning is required on the part of all participants so that budget allocations can be made well in advance. ASTM and OECD standard setting priorities may be different than those of the Agency or other member countries and may require many high level meetings to resolve.

Frequent Workshops

Frequent workshops at least every five years are suggested to evaluate existing government guidelines and available ASTM and international test standards. Recommendations can then be made to improve existing standards and/or develop new ones.

Acknowledgment

The author would like to thank Chris Ingersoll, Columbia Environmental Research Center, U.S. Geological Survey, Columbia, MO and Mark Hinman, Exxon Biomedical Sciences, Inc., East Millstone, NJ for asking for my participation, and presentation of this paper at the ASTM session "ASTM Standards and Their Application", held at the ASTM 2000 meeting in Toronto, Ontario, Canada.

Disclaimer

This document has been reviewed by the Office of Pollution Prevention and Toxics, US Environmental Protection Agency, and is approved for publication. Approval neither signifies that the contents necessarily reflect the views and policies of the Agency nor does mention of trade names or commercial products constitute endorsement or recommendation for use.

References

Aspelin, A.L. and A.H. Grube, 1999, "Pesticide Industry Sales and Usage Data: 1996 and 1997 Market Estimates," EPA Website: www.epa.gov/oppbead/pestsales. Posted on web 1/25/00.

Hindak, F, 1990, *Biologicke Prace*, Vol 5, pp. 209.

USEPA, 1996, "OPPTS Harmonized Test Guidelines," Ecological Effects Test Guidelines, OPPTS 850 series, EPA 712-C-96-163, "Public Draft", Also on the EPA website: www.epa.gov/OPPTS_harmonized.

USFWS, 1999, "Endangered and Threatened Wildlife and Plants," U.S. Fish and Wildlife Service, 50CFR 17.11 and 17.12, pp. 1 to 54.

G. L. Stephenson,[1] N. C. Feisthauer,[2] N. Koper,[3] J. H. McCann,[4] and R. P. Scroggins[5]

The Influence of Four Types of Water on Seedling Emergence and Growth of Barley and the Toxic Interaction with Copper Sulfate

Reference: Stephenson, G. L., Feisthauer, N. C., Koper, N., McCann, J. H., and Scroggins, R. P., **"The Influence of Four Types of Water on Seedling Emergence and Growth of Barley and the Toxic Interaction with Copper Sulfate,"** *Environmental Toxicology and Risk Assessment: Science, Policy and Standardization – Implications for Environmental Decisions: Tenth Volume, ASTM STP 1403*, B. M. Greenberg, R. N. Hull, M. H. Roberts, Jr., and R. W. Gensemer, Eds., American Society for Testing and Materials, West Conshohocken, PA, 2001.

Abstract: One aspect of the development and validation of terrestrial plant toxicity test methods is to determine the influence of the type of water that is used to irrigate test plants on emergence and seedling growth, and on the toxicity of contaminants in soil. Acute screening and definitive plant seedling emergence and growth tests were conducted with barley in artificial soil. Seedlings were irrigated with tap, well, or deionized water, or a nutrient solution. The influence of water type was similar for both the acute screening and definitive plant tests. No effect of water type on seedling emergence was observed. Shoot growth was greater in barley watered with nutrient solution, but no difference was observed among other water types. Root length was not affected. Root mass was greater when plants were watered with the nutrient solution, but only if compared to plants watered with deionized water. Definitive plant toxicity tests that assessed the toxicity of copper sulfate to barley were conducted. Plants were irrigated with a nutrient solution or tap water. The toxicity of copper sulfate to seedling emergence was affected by water type. Copper sulfate was more toxic to barley when seedlings were watered with the nutrient solution. These results indicate that the type of water used to irrigate terrestrial test plants can influence contaminant toxicity and must be considered when generating or interpreting data.

Keywords: seed germination, seedling growth, toxicity test, water type, copper sulfate

[1] Ph. D. Candidate, University of Guelph, Guelph, Ontario, Canada N1G 2W1.

[2] Environmental Toxicologist, 361 Southgate Dr., ESG International, Inc., Guelph, Ontario, Canada, N1G 3M5.

[3] Ph. D. Candidate, Department of Renewable Resources, University of Alberta, Edmonton, Alberta, Canada, T6G 2M7.

[4] Environmental Guidelines Officer, National Guidelines and Standards Office, Environment Canada, Ottawa, Canada, K1A0H3.

[5] Manager, Method Development and Applications Section, Environment Canada, Ottawa, Ontario, Canada, K1A0H3.

Introduction

Environment Canada has undertaken a multi-year program to develop, validate and standardize terrestrial toxicity tests that can be used to assess the relative toxicity of soil contaminants to plants and invertebrates. The aim of this project is to develop tests that can be used for soil contaminant delineation, site-specific risk assessments, and to evaluate the efficacy of site remediation technologies. One aspect of the development and validation of the toxicity test methods using terrestrial plants is to determine the influence of the type of water used to irrigate test plants. It was hypothesized that the nature of the water itself could affect the emergence and growth of plants and influence the toxicity of contaminants used in seedling tests.

Artificial and field-collected natural soils are commonly used in terrestrial plant toxicity testing. An advantage of using the artificial soil is that it has a well-defined, uniform texture, and it can be easily formulated in the laboratory with physico-chemical properties that are consistent among batches. Artificial soil is also free of non-test organisms such as seeds and soil invertebrates that may be found in field-collected soils. A disadvantage of using artificial soil is that it is often low in nutrients, which can result in reduced vigor of test plants. Nutrient deficiency in test plants grown in artificial soil can be exacerbated by the type of water used for irrigation, especially nutrient-poor water such as deionized or distilled water. The length of the toxicity test can also be a factor. Nutrient deficiency may not manifest in plants during a seedling emergence or early growth test if the duration of the test is relatively short. However, seedlings used in longer-term definitive tests where irrigation water provides limited nutrients might exhaust seed and soil nutrient reserves and suffer from nutrient deficiency.

The type of irrigation water used in plant toxicity tests might also influence the toxicity of the compound being evaluated. If nutrient-poor water and soil are used, the health of test plants can be compromised and render the plants more sensitive to the toxicant. There could also be interactions between impurities in the irrigation water and the toxicant that might affect the toxicity of the contaminant. Copper sulfate ($CuSO_4$) was chosen as the test toxicant in this study because copper is a common soil contaminant and is also an essential micronutrient for most plant species and, depending on the concentration, it can elicit both stimulatory and inhibitory responses in plants.

With this in mind, the objectives of the research described in this paper were to 1) determine the effect of four different types of irrigation water on the seedling emergence and growth of a common test species, barley (*Hordeum vulgare*, var. Chapais), grown in artificial soil for short (acute screening) and longer (definitive) periods; and 2) determine the influence of two different types of water on the toxicity of copper sulfate to barley seedlings grown in an artificial soil for an extended period of time (definitive tests).

Materials and Methods

Experimental Design and Conditions

Acute screening and definitive plant tests were performed with barley between April and June 1999. All tests were conducted in environmentally controlled growth chambers, with simulated natural sunlight (fluorescent Vita-Lite® lighting) at an average light intensity of 400 μmoles/m^2/s, temperature of 24/16 $\pm$ 1°C (day/night, respectively) and photoperiod of 16 h light, 8 h dark. Test endpoints measured in all seedling tests included mortality (failure to emerge), shoot and root length, and shoot and root wet and dry mass. Soil pH and conductivity were measured at the beginning and end of each test.

The effect of water type on barley emergence and growth was studied (without a toxicant) in acute screening and definitive plant tests in artificial soil. Plants were watered with either deionized water (DI), municipal tap water (TW), raw well water (WW) or a nutrient solution (N). The acute screening test was conducted over 7 days and consisted of four treatments with 10 replicates per treatment, whereas, the 14-day definitive plant test consisted of four treatments, with 6 replicates per treatment.

The influence of water type on toxicity of copper sulfate to barley was studied in definitive tests where plants were watered with either tap water or a nutrient solution. Each definitive plant toxicity test consisted of 11 treatments and the copper sulfate exposure concentrations were 0, 500, 750, 1000, 1250, 1750, 2000, 4000, 6000, 8000 and 10 000 mg $CuSO_4$ / kg soil dry weight (d.w.). The test designs and methods were derived from Stephenson et al. (1997) and Environment Canada (1998).

Control Soils

An artificial soil was used for all experiments. The soil was formulated by combining silica sand (70%), kaolinite clay (20%) and sphagnum peat (10%) as dry constituents, and then carefully hydrating with deionized water while mixing. Calcium carbonate (30g per 1 kg peat) was added to buffer the pH to between 6.0 and 6.5. The artificial soil was a sandy soil with moderate organic content and relatively low cation exchange capacity. The physico-chemical characteristics of the artificial soil are listed in Table 1.

Table 1–*Physico-chemical characteristics of the formulated artificial soil.*

Total N (%)	0.05
P (mg/kg)	23
K (mg/kg)	22
Mg (mg/kg)	149
Ca (mg/kg)	1848
Na (mg/kg)	67
Na absorption ratio	0.57
Cation exchange capacity (Cmol +/kg)	18.5
Soil texture	fine sandy loam
Organic matter (%)	9
pH (units)	6.09
Conductivity (mS/cm)	0.3
Source	Formulated from constituents

Preparations of Test Soil and Test Units

In the toxicity tests, soil-spiking procedures began with the addition of anhydrous copper sulfate (97% purity, Fisher Scientific) to a quantity of deionized water sufficient to increase soil moisture content to 30 % (about 70-80% of the water holding capacity of the test soil). The chemical-water mixture was distributed evenly over the surface of a measured mass of soil and mixed with a mechanical mixer until homogeneous. The soil was partitioned by weight among treatment replicates; glass petri plates for acute tests and 1-L clear polypropylene containers for the definitive tests. The control soil (and treatment soils for the toxicant-free experiments) had no copper sulfate added to the deionized water, but otherwise they were treated in a manner identical to that of the other treatments with copper sulfate.

Pre-screened and pre-sorted seeds were pressed into the soil in a circular pattern, with four seeds in a circle around a fifth seed, to a depth that was twice that of the width of the seed. Soil was gently pressed over the seed. The soil was misted lightly with deionized water after planting. In acute tests, the petri dish, with 70 g test soil w.w., was placed into an inverted 1-L clear polypropylene container with the lid sealed; this constituted a test unit. In definitive tests, the 1-L polypropylene container filled with soil (485 g test soil w.w.) constituted the test unit. The lid remained closed until seedling emergence was observed later during the course of the experiment. Shortly after planting the seeds, test units were placed into an environmental chamber for the duration of the experiment. The test units were watered daily with either deionized water, tap water, well water, or a nutrient solution, depending upon the treatment. The physico-chemical characteristics of each of the water types are presented in Table 2.

Table 2–*Physico-chemical characteristics of the water types used to irrigate test units*[1].

Parameter	DW	TW	WW	N
Total salts (mmho/cm)	< 0.10	0.84	0.89	2.96
pH (units)	7.60	7.60	8.10	5.90
Total hardness (mg/L)	0.12	77.66	382.97	412.01
Total solids (%)	0.01	0.06	0.06	0.16
Nitrate N (mg/L)	< 0.50	1.00	< 0.50	221.00
P (mg/L)	< 0.10	< 0.10	< 0.10	191.50
K (mg/L)	< 0.10	0.64	1.03	259.50
Ca (mg/L)	< 0.10	21.71	92.92	93.79
Mg (mg/L)	< 0.10	5.68	36.66	41.98
Zn (mg/L)	0.01	0.02	0.01	0.80
Mn (mg/L)	0.01	0.01	0.01	0.66
Cu (mg/L)	0.01	0.03	0.01	0.85
Fe (mg/L)	0.01	0.01	0.01	1.45
B (mg/L)	0.03	0.04	0.05	0.33
Si (mg/L)	0.50	3.60	5.30	5.50
Na (mg/L)	0.53	146.80	28.60	41.79
Chloride (mg/L)	5.00	49.00	72.00	93.00
Sulfates (mg/L)	< 1.00	85.90	114.90	108.80
Bicarbonate (mg/L)	41.00	344.00	312.00	104.00

[1]DW deionized water,
TW tap water,
WW well water, and
N nutrient solution.

Test Unit Processing

At the end of the test, the test units were removed from the growth chamber and the visual response of the plants to copper sulfate was photographed before the test units were processed. Processing of the test units involved gently removing the soil adhering to the roots with water and measuring the shoot and root length and the shoot and root wet masses. Wet plant material was placed into a drying oven at 70°C for 48 hours, after which the dry shoot and root masses were determined.

Statistical Analyses

The results of the barley emergence and growth tests (toxicant-free) were analyzed using a univariate general linear model (SPSS, 1997) with water type as the main effect. Residuals generated by the model were visually assessed to verify assumptions of homoscedasticity and normality of the data (Draper and Smith 1981). Post-hoc Bonferroni's pairwise comparison tests were conducted following the analysis of variance (SPSS 1997). Emergence of barley exposed to copper sulfate was analyzed in the same manner as described except that a two-factor ANOVA was conducted (water type and $CuSO_4$ concentration as main effects). The ICp (inhibitory concentration that results in a specified percent effect) values for the $CuSO_4$ toxicity tests were determined with non-linear regression procedures (Stephenson et al. 2000).

Results and Discussion

Water type had no significant effect upon the emergence of barley in either the acute screening or definitive plant tests conducted in artificial soil (AS) without a toxicant ($p > 0.05$) (Figs. 1 and 2). The influence of water type on the growth of barley seedlings was the same in both the 7-day acute screening and the 14-day definitive plant tests. There were no statistical differences in shoot growth (length and wet/dry mass) among barley plants watered with deionized, tap, or well water. However, barley watered with nutrient solution had significantly greater

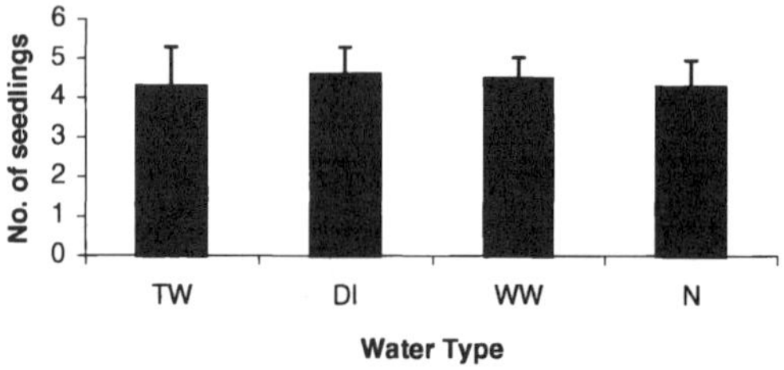

Figure 1–*The effect of irrigation water type on seedling emergence of barley in an acute screening test in artificial soil. Bars indicate standard deviation (n = 10). TW = tap water; DI = deionized water; WW = well water; N = nutrient solution.*

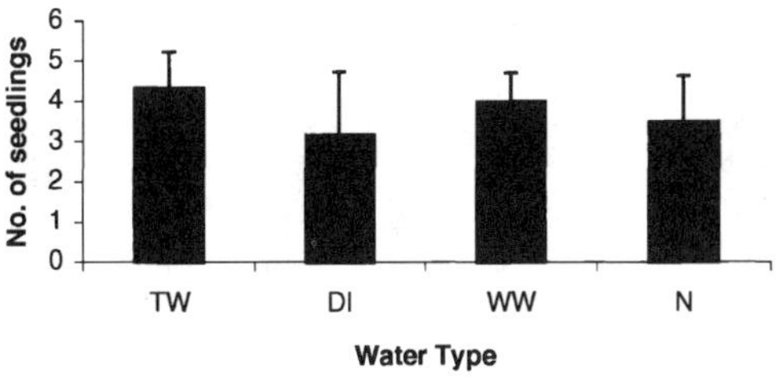

Figure 2–*The effect of irrigation water type on seedling emergence of barley in a definitive plant test in artificial soil. Bars indicate standard deviation (n = 6). TW = tap water; DI = deionized water; WW = well water; N = nutrient solution.*

shoot growth (length, wet/dry mass) than barley irrigated with the other three water types (Fig. 3A,B,C). There were no significant effects of water type on root length (Fig. 3D). Root wet and dry mass was significantly greater in barley plants watered with nutrient solution however, only when compared to that of barley watered with deionized water (Figs. 3E and 3F).

Despite the differences in the nutrient content of the tap, well, and deionized water (Table 1), there were no adverse (i.e., abnormalities or chlorosis) effects on seedling growth. It is possible that sufficient nutrient reserves in the seed endosperm and/or the artificial soil exist to compensate for differences in nutrient levels of the watering solutions. It is evident, however, that nutrient levels or availability in the artificial soil and seed reserves were not optimal, since barley seedlings responded positively to watering with the nutrient solution. The acute screening and definitive plant tests are relatively short (7 to 14 days) and, as a result, differences in seedling growth between tap, well, and deionized water might emerge once nutrient reserves are depleted for tests of longer duration. However, for seedling emergence and growth tests of short duration, tap, well, and deionized water are equally suitable for use.

The toxicity of copper sulfate to barley exposed in artificial soil was influenced by water type. There were significant main effects (e.g., water type) and interaction effects (e.g., copper sulfate concentration and water type) on the emergence of barley seedlings. Seedling emergence of barley watered with tap water and nutrient solution decreased with increasing copper sulfate concentrations. However, seedling emergence decreased at lower copper sulfate concentrations when barley was watered with nutrient solution than when barley was irrigated with tap water (Fig. 4).

The effect of copper sulfate on seedling growth was also influenced by the type of water used to irrigate the plants. Copper sulfate had a much greater toxic effect on barley shoot length, wet and dry mass when seedlings were watered with nutrient solution as compared to seedlings watered with tap water (Fig. 5). The effect of copper sulfate was also greater on root wet and dry masses when barley seedlings were watered with nutrient solution, although the effect was not as defined as that for barley shoots. Water type did not appear to affect the toxicity of copper sulfate to seedling root length (Fig. 6). The IC50s and IC20s for barley exposed to copper sulfate in artificial soil and irrigated with either tap water or nutrient solution are presented in Table 3. Barley seedlings watered with nutrient solution were more sensitive to copper sulfate than were seedlings watered with tap water.

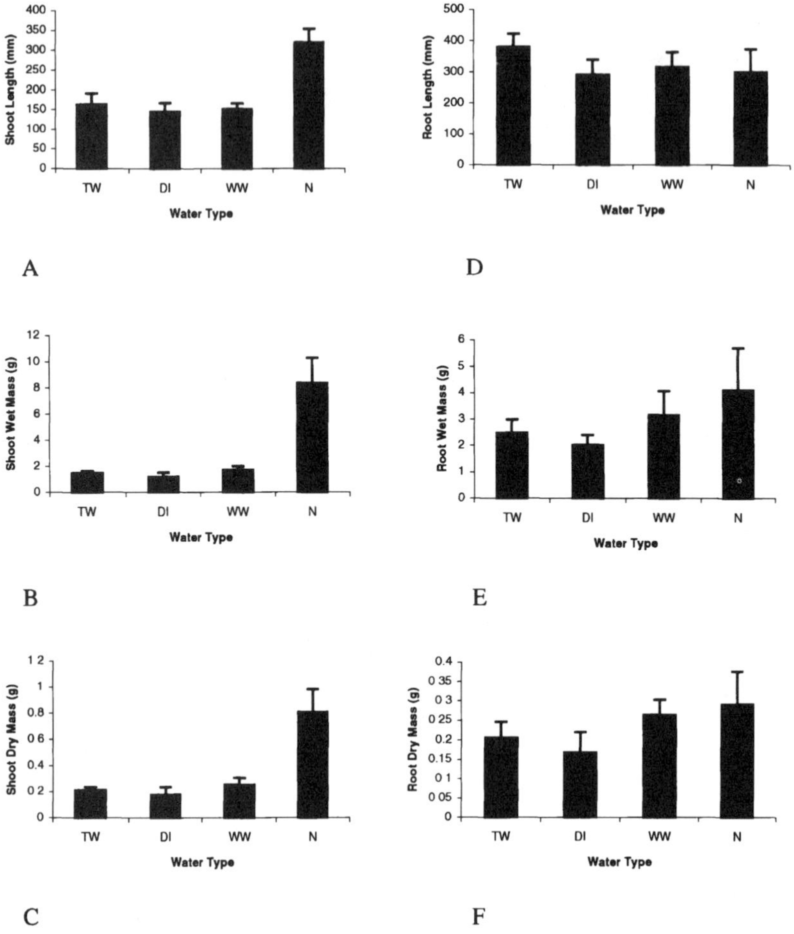

Figure 3(A-F)-*The effect of irrigation water type on seedling growth of barley in a definitive plant test in artificial soil. Bars indicate standard deviation (n = 6). TW = tap water; DI = deionized water; WW = well water; N = nutrient solution.*

Although slightly higher levels of copper were present in the nutrient solution as compared to the tap water (Table 2), it is unlikely that this sulfate would have enhanced the effect of copper sulfate on barley watered with the nutrient solution. The difference in total copper applied to the plants via watering was very small. The nutrient solution contained 0.85 mg/L of soluble copper as compared to the 0.03 mg/L in tap water.

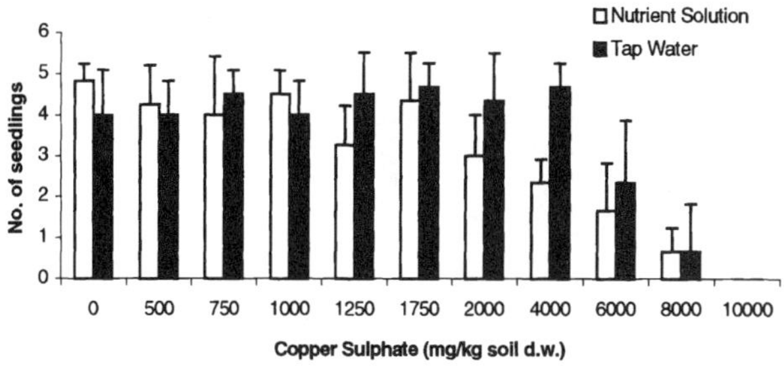

Figure 4–*Effect of copper sulfate concentration and irrigation water type on the emergence of barley seedlings. Bars indicate standard deviation of the mean (n = 6 - 3).*

During the course of a definitive test, all seedlings were watered with an estimated 500 mL of solution (nutrient or tap water). Seedlings watered with nutrient solution were therefore exposed to 0.41 mg more copper than seedlings watered with tap water. This difference in copper concentrations is likely too negligible to enhance the effect of copper sulfate on barley watered with nutrient solution. Instead, the difference in copper sulfate toxicity is likely the result of interactions with copper sulfate and the chemical components of the nutrient solution. The most likely reason for the enhanced toxicity of copper sulfate to barley when it was watered with nutrient solution was the differences in pH between the two water types (Table 2). Tap-water pH was 7.60 and that of the nutrient solution was 5.90. Soil has a maximum holding capacity for copper at neutral to slightly alkaline conditions (pH 6.7 – 7.8) (CCME, 1997). Below that pH, copper becomes more mobile, and hence more available for plant absorption. Soil pH at the end of the toxicity tests ranged from 7.57 to 4.28 and 5.88 to 4.05 for tap water and nutrient solution-watered test units, respectively.

Table 3–*Effect of irrigation water type*[1] *on the toxicity of copper sulfate to barley seedling growth. Values in brackets are the 95% confidence intervals.*

Endpoint	IC 50 (mg/kg soil d.w.)		IC 20 (mg/kg soil d.w.)	
	TW	N	TW	N
Shoot length	1841 (1427-2254)	1288 (1040-1536)	612 (378-845)	436 (247-627)
Shoot wet mass	1395 (958-1831)	363 (237-489)	387 (133-641)	55 (-18-128)
Shoot dry mass	2382 (1396-3368)	502 (325-679)	744 (146-1342)	90 (35-145)
Root length	840 (753-926)	961 (860-1062)	601 (794-708)	598 (464-732)
Root wet mass	1035 (918-1152)	639 (479-800)	830 (637-1023)	457 (243-671)
Root dry mass	1013 (767-1259)	754 (551-956)	505 (239-770)	543 (306-780)

[1] DW deionized water,
TW tap water,
WW well water, and
N nutrient solution.

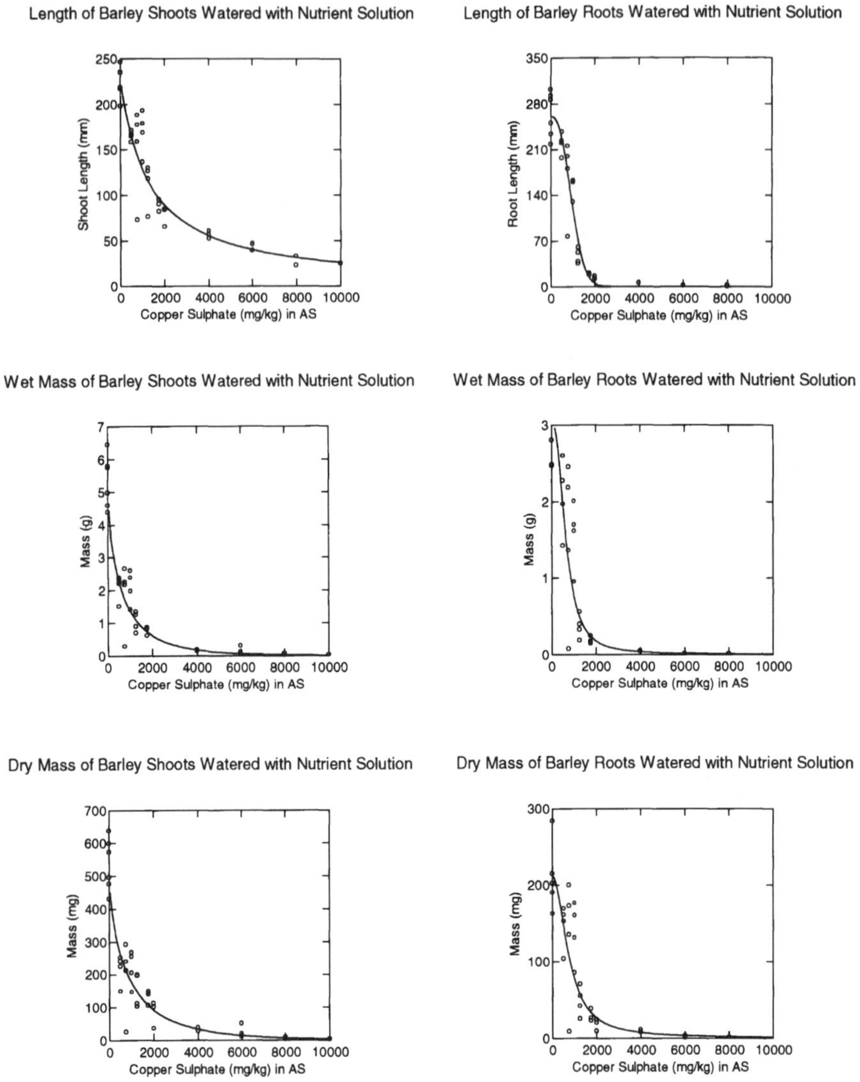

Figure 5-*The effect of longer term (definitive) exposure of copper sulfate to growth of barley in artificial soil when watered with nutrient solution.*

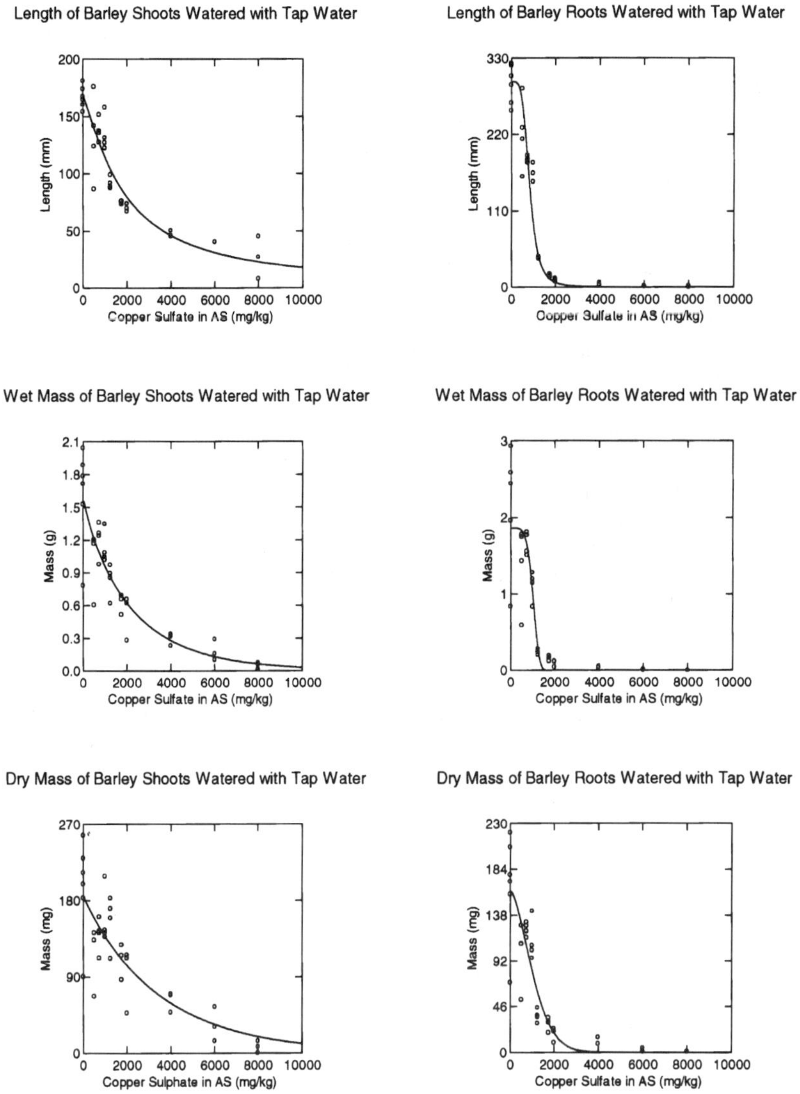

Figure 6–*The effect of longer term (definitive) exposure of copper sulfate to growth of barley in artificial soil when watered with tap water.*

The pH decreased with increasing copper sulfate concentrations regardless of water type used, probably because of the acidification of the sulfate component. However, the pH of nutrient-watered soils was lower at each exposure concentration relative to soils watered with tap water. It is evident that the pH of the watering solution influenced the pH of the test soil. This could have then resulted in an increase in uptake, and therefore toxicity, of copper in plants watered with the nutrient solution.

There are many terrestrial plant toxicity test methods described in the literature including the ASTM Standard Practice for Conducting Early Seedling Growth Tests (E 1598-94), the ASTM Standard Guide for Conducting Terrestrial Plant Toxicity Tests (E 1963-98) and the EPA Ecological Effects Test Guidelines (712-C-96-152, 153, 163, 363, and 364). While some standard methods recommend the use of a nutrient solution "if the soil medium is sand or a soil low in nutrients" (E 1598-94), others recommend against adding nutrients or soil amendments to short-term tests since "the amendments may interact with the toxicants and alter the toxicity response" (E 1963-98). Most terrestrial plant toxicity studies described in the literature only specify the type of irrigation water if a nutrient solution is used and, even then, few details are provided. However, the effect of irrigation water types on terrestrial plant toxicity can be substantial, and this aspect of toxicity testing should be carefully considered when generating or reviewing terrestrial plant toxicity data. The decision to irrigate with deionized water, tap water, or nutrient solution depends to a large extent on the purpose of the toxicity test. However, if a nutrient solution is selected as the irrigation water, there is the potential for an interaction with the toxicant.

Acknowledgments

This project is a joint effort of government, academia and private industry. The agencies and institutions providing the physical and financial resources include ESG International Inc., the Canadian Network of Toxicology Centres, University of Guelph and Environment Canada. We are grateful for their contributions and support. We thank J. Qiu, J.I. Princz, and N. Mackintosh for their technical assistance.

References

Canadian Council of Ministers of the Environment (CCME), 1997, *Recommended Canadian Soil Quality Guidelines.* March, 1997. CCME Documents c/o Manitoba Statutory Publications, 200 Vaughan Street, Winnipeg, Manitoba R3C 1T5.

Draper, N. R., and Smith, H., 1981, *Applied Regression Analysis,* Second edition, John Wiley & Sons, Toronto.

Environment Canada, 1998, *Development of Plant Toxicity Tests for Assessment of Contaminated Soils*. Prepared for: Method Development and Application Section, Environmental Technology Centre, Environment Canada, by: Aquaterra Environmental, Orton, Ontario, 75 pp.

Stephenson, G. L., Solomon, K. R., Hale, B., Greenberg, B. M., and Scroggins, R. P., 1997, "Development of Suitable Test Methods for Evaluating the Toxicity of Contaminated Soils to a Battery of Plant Species Relevant to Soil Environments in Canada," *Environmental Toxicology and Risk Assessment: Modeling and Risk Assessment (Sixth Volume), ASTM STP 1317*, F. J. Dwyer, T. R. Doane, and M. L. Hinman, Eds., American Society for Testing and Materials, West Conshohocken, PA, 1997, pp. 474-489.

Stephenson, G. L., Koper, N., Atkinson, G. F., Solomon, K. R., and Scroggins, R. P., 2000 , "Use of nonlinear regression techniques for describing concentration-response relationships for plant species exposed to contaminated site soil, " *Environmental Toxicology and Chemistry* Vol. 19, No. 12, pp. 229-242.

SPSS, 1997, *SYSTAT 7.0.1*, SPSS, Inc., 1800 Sherman Avenue, Evanston, Illinois.

BIOMONITORING OF SEDIMENTS AND AQUATIC SYSTEMS

Yousef S. El-Alawi,[1] D. George Dixon,[2] and Bruce M.Greenberg[2*]

Comparison of Short- and Long-Term Assays to Detect Toxicity of Anthracene to a Luminescent Bacteria

Reference: El-Alawi, Y. S., Dixon, D. G., and Greenberg, B. M. "**Comparison of Short- and Long-Term Assays to Detect Toxicity of Anthracene to Luminescent Bacteria,**" *Environmental Toxicology and Risk Assessment: Science, Policy, and Standardization - Implications for Environmental Decisions: Tenth Volume, ASTM STP 1403*, B. M. Greenberg, R. N. Hull, M. H. Roberts, Jr., and R. W. Gensemer, Eds., American Society for Testing and Materials, West Conshohocken, PA, 2001.

Abstract: Anthracene (ANT) toxicity increases significantly after exposure to simulated or natural sunlight. A simple, rapid method for monitoring the photoinduced short- and long–term toxicity of ANT and other PAHs has been developed. The assay is based on changes in the luminescence intensity and growth rate of *Vibrio fischeri*. Under suitable conditions, *V. fischeri* emits a constant amount of light as a metabolic by-product. After exposure to a toxicant, the light intensity can be diminished by an amount which is often proportional to the extent of toxicant impact. Generally, *V. fischeri* has been used in short-term (15-30 min) assays. However, this does not reveal the toxicity of all hazardous chemicals. In particular, we found ANT is not highly toxic in short-term (e.g. 15 minute) assays. As well, the prevalent phototoxicity of this compound was not revealed in a short-term assay. A long-term (e.g. 18 hour) test was developed that assesses the photoinduced toxicity of ANT.

Keywords: polycyclic aromatic hydrocarbons, anthracene, *V. fischeri*, luminescence intensity, photoinduced toxicity.

Introduction

Many intact and photomodified polycyclic aromatic hydrocarbons (PAHs) are present in aquatic environments (Huang et al. 1999). Anthracene (ANT) is ubiquitous in the environment primarily as a product of incomplete combustion of fossil fuels (Cook et al. 1983; Edwards 1983; Jacob et al. 1986). It has been identified in surface and drinking water, ambient air, exhaust emissions from internal combustion engines, tobacco smoke, smoked food, edible aquatic organisms, and in sediments (Edwards 1983; Cook et al. 1983; Jacob et al. 1986). As well, a large body of literature exists on the toxicity and

[1]Research assistant, and [2]Professors, respectively, Department of Biology, University of Waterloo, 200 University Ave. West, Waterloo, Ontario, Canada, N2L 3G1.
[*]Corresponding author email: greenber@sciborg.uwaterloo.ca

carcinogenicity of ANT (Jacob et al. 1986; Cook et al. 1983).

The phototoxic properties of PAHs are well studied in aquatic environments (Allred and Giesy 1985; Kagan et al. 1990, Krylov et al. 1997). These studies strongly suggest that there is a real hazard to aquatic ecosystems from photoinduced toxicity of PAHs (Kochevar et al. 1982; Allred and Giesy 1985; Kagan et al. 1990; Huang et al.1993, 1995; Mallakin et al. 1999). Previous work in our laboratory using ANT showed that toxicity is enhanced through photosensitization and photomodification reactions (Ren et al. 1994; Huang et al. 1993, 1995; Duxbury et al. 1997; Mallakin et al. 1999). In particular, several photoproducts are generated when ANT is exposed to simulated or natural solar radiation. The time frame for generation photoproducts is on the order of hours. Many of the photoproducts have significant toxic activity (Huang et al. 1995; Mallakin et al. 1999).

Several bioassays have been developed to test toxicity of PAHs and degradation products to aquatic organisms. This includes changes in growth, survival, metabolism, inhibition of enzymatic activities, and inhibition of photosynthetic and mitochondrial electron transport (Bulich and Isenberg 1981; Steinberg et al. 1995; Gensemer et al. 1998). Among these toxicity tests are bacterial luminescence assays, which are important tools in aquatic toxicology because they are rapid, simple and accurate (Bulich 1979; Curtis et al. 1982; Bulich and Isenberg 1981; Environment Canada 1993). The luminescent bacteria *Vibrio fischeri* has been used extensively in toxicity assessments (Environment Canada 1993; Steinberg et al. 1995). For instance it is used in the Microtox assay for a 15 minute test based on loss of luminescence (Environment Canada 1993; Steinberg et al. 1995). However, this assay could return false negatives for chemicals that act slowly or require time to be assimilated. For instance, ANT, which increases dramatically in toxicity following photomodification, did not induce a toxic response in the Microtox test (Kaiser and Devillers 1994). Thus, this study was conducted to help develop a toxicity test based on luminescence and growth inhibition for *V. fischeri*. ANT photoinduced toxicity was evaluated in this study. ANT was found to have high toxicity when there was a pre-incubation period in simulated solar radiation (SSR), allowing time for photooxidation of the compound.

Materials and Methods

Chemicals and Bacterial Strain

Anthracene was purchased in high purity (Sigma Chemical Co., St. Louis, MO). The strain of luminescent bacteria used for this study was *Vibrio fischeri* (strain NRRL B-11177), formally known as *Photobacterium phosphoreum*. It was obtained from the Midwest Area National Center for Agricultural Utilization Research (Peoria, IL).

Growth Media

Vibrio fischeri was cultured on a complex media containing: monobasic potassium phosphate (KH_2PO_4), 2.5 g/L; sodium chloride (NaCl), 30 g/L; magnesium sulfate ($MgSO_4.7H_2O$), 1 g/L; glycerol ($C_3H_8O_3$), 5 g/L; yeast extract, 1 g/L; peptone, 5 g/L; bactopeptamin, 1 g/L; and agar when required, 15 g/L. The final pH of the media was adjusted to 7.2 ± 0.1 with 10 M NaOH. The mixture was autoclaved at 121°C for 30 minutes. Minimal media was the above without glycerol, yeast extract, peptone, and bactopeptamin. Peptone and yeast extract were obtained from BDH Inc., Toronto, ON, and Bactopeptamin was obtained from Difco Laboratories, Detroit, MI. Stock cultures of *V. fischeri* were grown on agar plates and used for primary inoculation of liquid cultures. A spectrophotometer (Perlsin-Elrner, Mississauga, Ontario, CA) and Cytofluor 2350 fluorescence measurement system (Millipore Ltd., Mississauga, Ontario, Canada) were used to measure cell density and light output.

Growth Conditions

To generate a starter culture for toxicity tests, cells of *V. fischeri* were cultured in 100 mL of complex media with shaking at room temperature (20°C) for 24 hours. Two methods were used to follow *V. fischeri* growth (Fig. 1). The first type involved diluting cells from the starter culture into complex media. The second type involved diluting cells into minimal media (complex media without a reduced carbon source) for 8 hours, at which point the media was made complex by addition of the above reduced carbon sources. For the first type of test, 0.5 mL of actively growing starter cells in log-phase were harvested and put into 10 mL of complex media to give an approximate cell density of 0.2 OD to start the experiment. The diluted cells 0.5 mL were added to 0.5 mL complex media in the wells of a 48-well culture plate (Costar Safety Products, VWR Scientific Ltd, Toronto, ONT. Canada) and grown under darkness or SSR with shaking at 20°C for up to 28 hours. For the second type of experiment, 0.5 mL of *V. fischeri* cells from the starter culture were diluted into 10 mL of minimal media to give an approximate cell density of 0.2 OD to start the experiment. The diluted cells (0.5 mL) were added to 0.5 mL of minimal media in the wells of a 48-well culture plate. Cells were pre-incubated for 8 hours in minimal media in SSR or darkness at which point an equal volume of complex media with glycerol ($C_3H_8O_3$) at 10 g/L, yeast extract at 2 g/L, peptone at 10 g/L bactopeptamin at 2 g/L was added to each well in the culture plate. Cells were grown up to 28 hours. Cell density and luminescence intensity of the culture was measured every 4 hours. The cell density of the culture was measured with a spectrophotometer. The luminescence intensity of the *V. fischeri* was measured with a Cytofluor 2350 multi-well culture plate reader.

Short- and Long-Term Assays of Toxicity

The short-term toxicity test was based on inhibition of light production from luminescent bacteria incubated for 15 minutes under darkness or SSR. For the long-term toxicity test, inhibition of light production by the bacteria and inhibition of growth were used. In the latter case, toxicity was measured after 18 hours of growth of the bacteria (Fig. 1).

Short-Term Assay

The starter culture was diluted as above with complex or minimal media and twenty-four 500 μl aliquots of cells were added to a 48-well cell culture plate (Costar

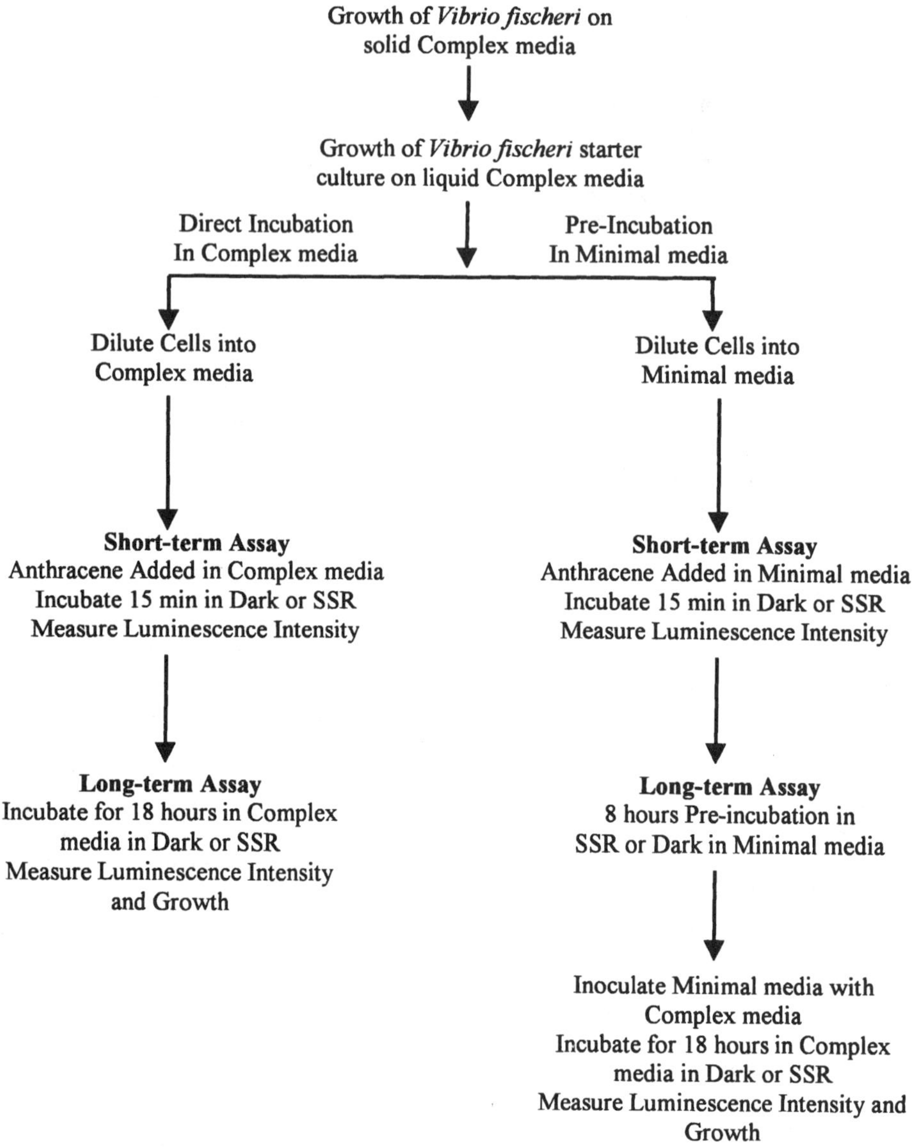

Fig. 1 Flow-chart for short- and long-term toxicity tests in complex media and minimal media.

Safety Products, VWR Scientific Ltd, Toronto, Ontario, Canada). After 5 minutes acclimatization in the 48-well cell culture plates, the luminescence intensity was measured. After the initial measurement of bacterial luminescence, the cells were dosed with ANT. Aliquots of 500 μL of the cell culture were combined with equal volumes of the test chemical in complex or minimal culture media. A dilution series of each chemical (nominal concentrations from 0.0625 mg/L to 4.0 mg/L plus the control) were added in a geometric series to the wells in triplicate. Stock solutions of ANT were prepared in dimethyl sulphoxide (DMSO) and added by 1000 fold dilution to the culture liquid media to give the specified concentration. The DMSO concentration of 0.1% does not affect luminescence or growth of *V. fischeri*. After dosing, the cells were incubated in darkness or SSR at room temperature for 15 minutes and the luminescence intensity was measured.

Long-Term Assay

After the short-term test was completed the multi-well culture plate was returned to the growth chamber. If the assay was in complex media, the cells were incubated for 18 hours in SSR or darkness at 20°C. Growth and luminescence were then determined as above. If the assay was in minimal media cells were incubated with the chemical in darkness or SSR at 20°C for 8 hours. After this pre-incubation, the media was made complex as above. The cells were then incubated for an additional 18 hours in SSR or darkness at 20°C. Toxicity was determined by inhibition of growth and luminescence.

RESULTS AND DISCUSSION

Growth and Luminescence Intensity

V. fischeri cells in log-phase growth diluted into complex media continued log-phase growth for more than 20 hours (Fig. 2). For these cells, luminescence showed a lag period of 8 hours, after which light output mirrored cell growth. Relative to darkness, there was no effect of SSR on growth of the cells. No growth was observed for cells cultured in minimal media and luminescence gradually dropped. After 8 hours incubation in minimal media, the cells shifted almost immediately into log-phase growth after transfer to complex media (Fig. 2). The growth rate was identical to that of cells placed directly in complex media. Luminescence recovered after an 8 hour lag period and then mirrored growth. There was no effect of SSR relative to darkness for these cells. This demonstrates that a pre-incubation for 8 hours in minimal media does not harm the *V. fischeri*.

Short-Term Effects of ANT on V. fischeri

In the short-term toxicity assay, *V. fischeri* was incubated with ANT in darkness and SSR to determine the toxicity (Table 1). The calculated EC50 of ANT in darkness in minimal media was 17.92 mg/L, which agrees well with published EC50 (20.8 mg/L) obtained using the Microtox assay (Jacobs et al. 1993). When the assay was performed using complex media no toxicity was observed (Table 1). The high reduced carbon content of the complex media could be limiting bioavailability of ANT. This is consistent

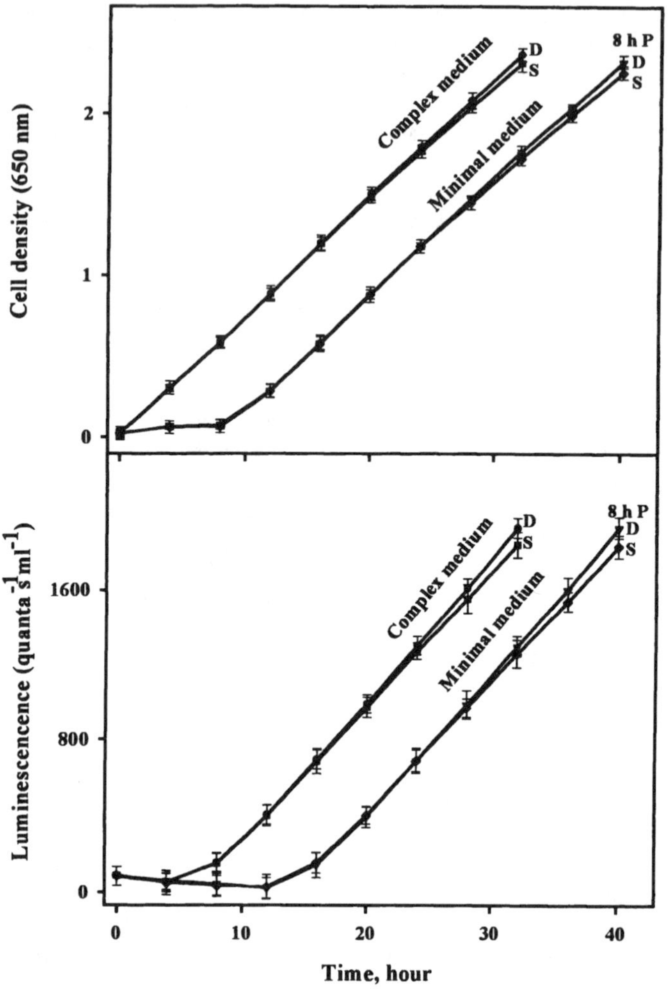

Fig. 2 Growth and luminescence intensity of Vibrio fischeri under darkness and SSR. Log-phase cells were diluted into complex or minimal media as described in material and methods. For cells initially placed into minimal media for 8 hours, the media was made complex as described in materials and methods. Error bars are ± 95 % confidence intervals.

with previous studies where humic acids were shown to ameliorate toxicity of PAHs (Oris et al. 1990; Gensemer et al. 1998). Conversely, the complex media could allow for healthier cells and thus tolerance to chemical stress.

Table 1 Calculated EC50s for short-term toxicity of ANT to V. fischeri, cultured in both complex and minimal media and under both darkness or SSR.

	EC50 mg L^{-1}	
Media	Dark	SSR
Complex Media	N/D	N/D
Minimal Media	17.92 ± 0.072	16.78 ± 0.088

Data are presented as EC50s in mg L^{-1} ± standard deviation, n = 6
N/D: No detectable effect.

To determine if short-term toxicity of ANT could be photoinduced, the assay was performed in SSR. No light effect was observed in complex or minimal media (Table 1). This is consistent with the mechanism of photoinduced toxicity of ANT, which depends in part on photooxidation of the chemical to more toxic forms (Huang et al. 1995; Mallakin et al. 1999).

Long-Term Effects of ANT on V. fischeri

The results for long-term toxicity measurements are given in Fig. 3 and Table 2. When the assay was carried out in complex media, ANT had little effect in darkness or SSR (Table 2). The SSR result was surprising because ANT is known to be highly phototoxic (Huang et al. 1995; Mallakin et al. 1999). It is possible that in complex media, the ANT is not sufficiently bioavailable and growth of the cells rapid enough to escape toxic effects.

To probe whether cell growth allowed escape from toxicity, the cells were pre-incubated with ANT in minimal media. First, *V. fischeri* was pre-incubated in minimal media for 8 hours in SSR to allow up-take and photooxidation of ANT. Toxicity was then assessed following 18 hours growth in complex media under SSR. This resulted in very high toxicity (EC50 = 0.13 mg L^{-1}, Fig. 3; Table 2). Second, *V. fischeri* was pre-incubated in darkness for 8 hours and then allowed to grow in darkness for 18 hours. This resulted in low toxicity (Fig. 3, Table 2). Third, *V. fischeri* was pre-incubated in minimal media for 8 hours in darkness followed by 18 hours growth in SSR in complex media or vice versa. Both of these treatments showed moderate toxicity (Fig. 3, Table 2), with the SSR pre-incubation followed by growth in dark being the more toxic of the two treatments.

This work shows that complex media can greatly limit ANT uptake by the bacteria. Importantly, the highest levels of toxicity were observed when the pre-incubation was carried out in SSR, indicating that photooxidation of ANT ($t_{1/2}$ = 2 hours in SSR) is important for bacterial toxicity. In this regard, the higher toxicity of an SSR pre-incubation followed by a dark incubation relative to a dark pre-incubation followed by an SSR incubation is striking. This implies that during the 8 hours pre-incubation in

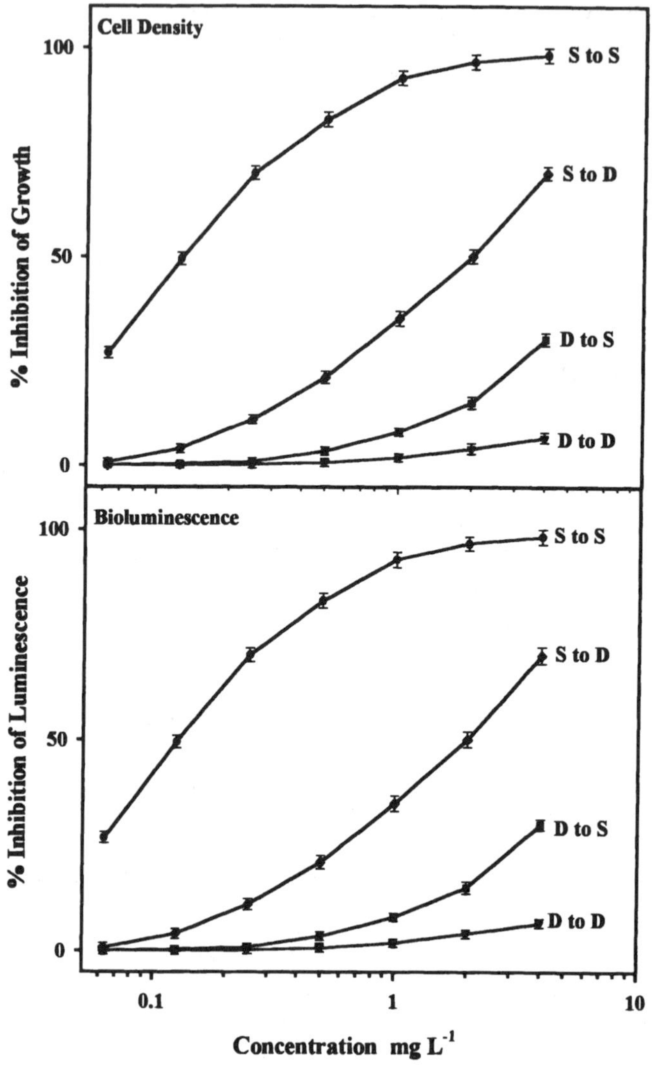

Fig. 3 Dose-response of V. fischeri to ANT. V. fischeri was exposed to a concentration series of anthracene as described in materials and methods. Bacterial response was measured as inhibition of growth and inhibition of luminescence, and plotted versus chemical concentration. Each data point represents an average of six replicates. Error bars are ± 95 % confidence intervals.

SSR, a good deal of photooxidation occurred. Once this happened toxicity no longer require SSR to be manifested.

Table 2 Calculated EC50s for V. fischeri after long-term exposure to ANT in complex and minimal media under darkness and SSR condition.

Pre-incubation in minimal media	Incubation in complex media	EC50, mg L^{-1}	
		% Luminescence inhibition	% Growth Inhibition
None	Dark	N/D	N/D
None	SSR	N/D	N/D
Dark	Dark	85.78 ± 0.097	84.88 ± 0.098
Dark	SSR	4.49 ± 0.082	4.11 ± 0.098
SSR	Dark	1.44 ± 0.062	1.38 ± 0.055
SSR	SSR	0.13 ± 0.052	0.12 ± 0.068

Data are presented as EC50s in mg L^{-1} ± standard deviation, n = 6
N/D: No detectable effect.

Conclusions

This study suggests that the *V. fischeri* assay can be adapted to screen for phototoxicants and/or slow acting contaminants. With the assays we have developed, it will be possible to compare toxicity due to photomodification or photosensitization. We note that our manipulations are environmentally relevant, as bacteria in natural conditions are often nutrient limited and therefore exposure to toxicants under sub-optimal growth conditions will be common. Under these sub-optimal growth conditions there is time for contaminant modification and assimilation.

Acknowledgments

We thank B. McConkey for his time and assistance with the data analysis. The authors acknowledge members of the Greenberg, Dixon and Bols laboratories for their fruitful discussions. This work is supported by the Canadian Network of Toxicology Centers (CNTC), and by the Natural Sciences and Engineering Research Council (NSERC).

References

Allred, P. M., and Giesy, J. P., 1985, "Solar Radiation Induced Toxicity of Anthracene in *Daphnia pulex*",Environ. Toxicol. Chem., Vol. 4, pp. 219-226.

Bulich, A. A., 1979, "Use of Luminescent Bacteria for Determining Toxicity in Aquatic Environment", Aquatic toxicology, Markings LL. Kimerie RA (eds). American

Society for Testing and Materials. Philadelphia, pp. 98-103.

Bulich, A. A., and Isenberg, D. L., 1981, "The use of the Luminescent Bacterial System for the Rapid Assessment of Aquatic Toxicity", *ISA Transactions*, Vol. 20, No.1, pp. 29-33.

Cook, R. H., Pierce, R. C., Eaton, P. B., Lao, R. C., Onuska, F. I., Payneand, J. F., and Vavasour , E., 1983, *"Polycyclic Aromatic Hydrocarbons in the Aquatic Environment; Formation, Sources, Fate and Effects on Aquatic Biota"*. National Research Council of Canada, Ottawa, ONT, Canada, NRCC 18981

Curtis, C. A., Lima, A., Lorano, S. J., and Veith, G. D., 1982, "Evaluation of a Bacterial Bioluminescence Bioassay as a Method for Predicting Acute Toxicity of Organic Chemical to Fish", Aquatic Toxicity and Hazard Assessment, Pearson JG, Foster RB, Bishop WE (eds.), STP 766. American Society for Testing and Materials. Philadelphia, pp. 170-178.

Duxbury, C. L., Dixon, D. G., and Greenberg, B. M., 1997, "Effects of Simulated Solar Radiation on the Bioaccumulation of Polycyclic Aromatic Hydrocarbons by the Duckweed *Lemna gibba*", Environ. Toxicol. Chem., Vol. 16, pp. 1739-1748.

Edwards, N. T., 1983, "Reviews and Analysis. Polycyclic Aromatic Hydrocarbons (PAHs) in the Terrestrial Environment", – a Review, J. Envirom. Qual., Vol. 12, pp. 427-441.

Environment Canada, 1993, "Toxicity Testing Using Luminescent Bacteria *Photobacterium phosphoreum*", Report EPA 1/RM/24, Environmental Protection Publications, Ottawa, ON, Canada, pp. 3-11

Gensemer, R. W., Dixon, D. G., and Greenberg, B. M., 1998, "Amelioration of the Photo-Induced Toxicity of Polycyclic Aromatic Hydrocarbons by a Commercial Humic Acid", Ecotoxical. Environ. Saf., Vol. 39, pp. 57-64

Huang, X. -D., Dixon, D. G., and Greenberg, B. M., 1993, " Impacts of UV Radiation and Photomodification on the Toxicity of PAHs to higher plant *Lemna gibba* (Duckweed)", Environ. Toxicol. Chem., Vol. 12, pp. 1007-1077.

Huang, X. -D., Dixon, D. G., and Greenberg, B. M., 1995, "Increased Polycyclic Aromatic Hydrocarbon Toxicity Following their Photomodification in Natural Sunlight: Impacts on the Duckweed *Lemna gibba* L. G-3", Ecotoxol. Environ. Saf., Vol. 32, pp. 194-200.

Huang, X. -D., Dixon, D. G., and Greenberg, B. M., 1999, "Occurrence and Hazards of Modified PAHs in the Environment", SETAC News (Learned Discourses), Vol. 19, No.6, pp. 15-16

Jacob, J., Karcher, W., Belliardo, J. J., and Wagstaffe, P. J., 1986, "Polycyclic Aromatic Hydrocarbons of Environmental and Occupational Importance", Fresenius. Z. Anal. Chem., Vol. 323, pp. 1-10.

Jacobs, M. W., Coates, J. A., Delphino, J. J., Bitton, G., Davis, W. M., and Garcia, K. L., 1993, "Comparison of Sediment Extract Microtox Toxicity with Semi-Volatile Organic Priority Pollutant Concentrations", Arch. Environ. Contam. Toxicol., Vol. 24, pp. 461-168.

Kagan, J., Kagan, E. D., Kagan, I. A., Kagan, P. A., and Quigley, 1985, "Phototoxicity of Non-carcinogenic PAHs in Aquatic Organisms", Chemosphere, Vol. 14, pp. 1829-1834.

Kaiser, K. L., and Devillers, J., 1994, " Ecotoxicity of Chemicals to *Photobacterium phosphoreum*", Handbooks of Ecotoxicological Data, (Devillers J. ed), London, Gordon and Breach, Vol. 2.

Kochevar, I. E., 1982, "Coal Tar Phototoxicity: Active Compounds and Action Spectra", Photochem. Photobiol., Vol. 36, pp. 65-69.

Krylov, S. N., Huang, X.-D., Zeiler, L. F., Dixon, D. G., and Greenberg, B. M., 1997, "Mechanistic QSAR Model for the Photoinduced Toxicity of Polycyclic Aromatic Hydrocarbons", I. Physical Model Based on Chemical Kinetics in a Two Compartment System, Environ. Toxicol. Chem., Vol. 16, pp. 2283-2295.

Mallakin, A., McConkey, B. J., Miao, G., McKibben, B., Snieckus, V., Dixon, D. G., and Greenberg, B. M., 1999, "Impacts of Structural Photomodification on the Toxicity of Environmental Contaminants: Anthracene Photooxidation Products", Ecotoxical. Environ. Saf., Vol. 43, pp. 204-212.

Oris, J. T., Hall, A. T., and Tylka, J. D., 1990, "Humic Acids Reduced the Photo-Induced Toxicity of Anthracene to Fish and Daphnia", Environ. Toxicol. Chem., Vol. 9, pp. 575-583.

Ren, L., Huang, X. -D., McConkey, B. J., Dixon, D. G., and Greenberg, B. M., 1994, "Photoinduced Toxicity of Three Polycyclic Aromatic Hydrocarbons (Fluoranthene, Pyrene, and Naphthalene) to the Duckweed *Lemna gibba* L. G-3", Ecotoxical. Environ. Saf., Vol. 28, pp. 160-171.

Steinberg, S. M., Poziomek, E. J., Engelmann, W. H., and Rogers, K. R., 1995, "A Review on Environmental Applications of Bioluminescence Measurements", *Chemosphere*, Vol. 30, No. 11, pp. 2155-2197.

Jerry M. Neff,[1] Theodor C. Sauer,[2] and Alan D. Hart[3]

Monitoring Polycyclic Aromatic Hydrocarbon (PAH) Bioavailability Near Offshore Produced Water Discharges

Reference: Neff, J. M., Sauer, T. C., and Hart, A. D. "**Monitoring Polycyclic Aromatic Hydrocarbon (PAH) Bioavailability Near Offshore Produced Water Discharge,**" *Environmental Toxicology and Risk Assessment: Science, Policy, and Standardization - Implications for Environmental Decisions: Tenth Volume, ASTM STP 1403*, B. M. Greenberg, R. N. Hull, M. H. Roberts, Jr., and R. W. Gensemer, Eds., American Society for Testing and Materials, West Conshohocken, PA, 2001.

Abstract: Produced water is the largest volume waste associated with production of oil and gas on offshore platforms. Produced water that meets effluent limitations for total oil and grease contains low concentrations of petroleum hydrocarbons, low molecular weight organic acids, and several metals. The U.S. EPA has expressed concern that some of these chemicals could be bioaccumulated to potentially toxic concentrations by marine organisms in the receiving waters of offshore produced water discharges. This paper presents the results of an intensive monitoring study to determine if marine animals bioaccumulate polycyclic aromatic hydrocarbons (PAHs) from produced water discharges to offshore waters of the Gulf of Mexico.

Two platform pairs, each consisting of a produced water-discharging platform and a nearby non-discharging reference platform were selected for monitoring in offshore waters (90 to 260 m depth) of the northern Gulf of Mexico. Produced water, ambient sea water, two species of bivalve mollusks, and several species of fish were collected from each platform pair. Forty PAH analytes, including parent and alkyl PAHs, were analyzed in all samples.

The two discharging platforms discharged an average of 1.75 million L/d and 1.13 million L/d of produced water containing 30 to 43 μg/L (ppb) and 24 to 51 μg/L of PAHs, respectively. More than 90 percent of the PAHs were naphthalene and alkylnaphthalenes. The two bivalves, jewel boxes and thorny oysters, collected from legs of the platforms, contained up to 800 ng/g dry wt (ppb) total PAHs in their soft tissues. Muscle tissues of fish collected from the platform pairs contained <1 to 120 ng/g dry wt total PAHs. The dominant PAHs in the bivalve tissues were alkylnaphthalenes, fluorenes, phenanthrenes, and dibenzothiophenes, all characteristic of a petroleum source. A few individual PAHs were present at a significantly higher concentration in tissues of thorny oysters, but not jewel boxes, from one of the produced water-discharging platforms than from the paired reference platform. The relative concentrations of different PAHs in

[1] Senior Research Leader, Battelle Ocean Sciences, 397 Washington St., Duxbury, MA 02332.
[2] Senior Management Consultant, ENTRIX, 232 Washington St., Duxbury, MA 02331.
[3] Senior Consultant, Continental Shelf Associates, 759 Parkway St., Jupiter, FL 33477.

oysters was different than that in the produced water. The evidence for bioaccumulation of PAHs from produced water by shellfish was considered weak and inconclusive, because bioaccumulation of petroleum-derived PAHs was demonstrated in only one instance, and the source(s) of the PAHs was unclear. Concentrations of individual PAHs in fish muscle were low. Higher concentrations of individual PAHs were detected with similar frequency in fish from the reference and discharging platforms. Thus, the fish were not bioaccumulating PAHs from the produced water discharges. Bivalves are more suitable than fish for monitoring bioaccumulation of petroleum hydrocarbons near offshore produced water discharges.

Keywords: polycyclic aromatic hydrocarbons, bioaccumulation, bivalve mollusks, fish, produced water

Introduction

During millions of years of geologic time, petroleum, natural gas, and water may accumulate in porous sediments (e.g., sands) trapped between layers of impermeable rock deep within the earth (Collins 1975). The water may be derived from ancient fresh or sea water (connate water) and often is as old as the fossil fuels in the reservoir. When the hydrocarbon reservoir is tapped by a well, the produced fluids may contain water. Also, in some oil fields, fresh or sea water may be injected into the reservoir through injection wells to displace oil into the production wells. Sometimes, this injection water channels through to the production well and is produced with the oil and gas. The water produced with oil and gas is called produced water, formation water, or oilfield brine (Neff et al. 1987, Black et al. 1994).

Produced water must be removed before the crude oil can be refined or the gas processed. During offshore oil and gas production operations, separation of the produced water from the oil and gas may take place on the production platform or the oil/gas/water mixture may be sent through a pipeline to a shore facility where the produced water is separated from the oil and gas. If not re-injected into another well, the produced water is treated to meet local regulatory limits for oil and grease before it is discharged to the ocean from the platform or from an ocean outfall from a shore-based treatment facility. Even with the most advanced separation equipment, the oil/water separation is not 100 percent efficient. Treated produced water that is discharged to the ocean often contains small amounts of hydrocarbons, other organic chemicals, dissolved salts, and metals

The current limit for total oil and grease (dispersed and dissolved oil, measured by gravimetric analysis) in treated produced water destined for ocean disposal in U.S. federal waters and state waters of Upper Cook Inlet, AK, is 42 mg/L (ppm) daily maximum and 29 mg/L monthly average (Otto and Arnold 1996, Veil 1997). Discharge of produced water to coastal estuarine and marine waters is no longer permitted in the United States.

Produced water represents the largest volume waste stream in production operations on most offshore platforms (Stephenson 1991). Current discharge permits for the U.S. Gulf of Mexico prohibit discharge of more than 25 000 bbl/d (4 million L/d) of produced water from a single platform. The total volume of produced water discharged to

US waters of the Gulf of Mexico in 1991 was approximately 549 million L/d (Rabalais et al. 1991).

The U.S. Environmental Protection Agency is concerned about the potential for bioaccumulation and toxicity of chemicals in produced water to marine organisms living in the vicinity of offshore production activities. In December 1993, EPA Region VI published a modified version of the final National Pollutant Discharge Elimination System (NPDES) General Permit (GMG290000) for the western Gulf of Mexico Outer Continental Shelf. The modified permit required that operators monitor bioaccumulation of selected chemicals at existing facilities that discharge more than 4 600 bbl/d (731 000 L/d) of produced water. The permit gave operators the option of doing a site-specific monitoring study according to an EPA-specified protocol or participating in an alternative joint industry monitoring program designed by industry and approved by EPA.

The site-specific monitoring study design included collection of at least one species each of mollusk, crustacean, and fish twice each year from the immediate vicinity of all platforms discharging more than 4 600 bbl/d of produced water and analysis of soft tissue samples from these marine animals for volatile organic chemicals (benzene, toluene, and ethylbenzene), semivolatile organic compounds (phenol, fluorene, benzo(a)pyrene, and bis(2-ethylhexyl)phthalate), metals (arsenic, cadmium, and mercury), and radionuclides (^{226}radium and ^{228}radium).

The Gulf of Mexico Offshore Operators Committee, representing most of the offshore oil and gas industry in the Gulf of Mexico, proposed an industry-wide bioaccumulation monitoring study that was approved by EPA. The study consisted of two components: a definitive component and a platform survey component. The definitive component involved intensive, statistically designed sampling to determine if marine animals at two produced water-discharging platforms were bioaccumulating produced water chemicals to concentrations higher than those in tissues of the same species from nearby non-discharging platforms. In the platform survey component of the monitoring program, marine animals were sampled and analyzed from the immediate vicinity of a large number of platforms spanning a wide range geographic locations, water depths, and proximity to the mouth of the Mississippi River. This paper summarizes the results of the definitive component monitoring of concentrations of polycyclic aromatic hydrocarbons (PAHs) in the tissues of marine animals near offshore production platforms.

Materials and Methods

Two platform pairs (discharging/non-discharging) were selected based on the results of a screening survey of five discharging and six non-discharging platforms in federal waters of the western and central Gulf of Mexico. The candidate sites were selected by evaluating a database of offshore production and produced water discharge information from the Minerals Management Service and EPA. In the screening survey, the proximity of each candidate platform to other offshore structures, the numbers and species of marine animals available for sampling, and concentrations of selected target chemicals in their tissues (used to determine the amount of tissue needed in each sample for analysis) were determined. Based on the results of this survey, two platform pairs were selected for the definitive field surveys (Table 1).

Table 1 – *Two platform pairs (produced water discharging and non-discharging) in the Gulf of Mexico were selected for monitoring bioaccumulation of PAHs by bivalve mollusks and fish*

Platform	Water Depth (m)	Produced Water (L/d)
East Breaks 165A (Discharge)	262	1,750,000
High Island 356A (No Discharge)	91	---
Green Canyon 19A (Discharge)	229	1,130,000
Eugene Island 361 A (No Discharge)	91	---

Two field surveys were performed to the two platform pairs, the first in May 1999 and the second between October and December 1995. An attempt was made to collect two species each of bivalve mollusks, crustaceans, and fish, as requested by EPA. It was not possible to collect sufficient biomass of crustaceans for analysis. Two species of bivalve mollusks and three species of fish were collected from each discharging and reference platform. Divers collected the bivalves from submerged platform structures in the depth interval between 2 and 22 m below the sea surface. Modeling had indicated that this was the depth interval of the produced water plume. Fish were collected from the upper water column within a 100 m radius of the platform by hook and line from the platform or by spear-fishing by divers. To the extent possible, the same species were collected from both the discharging and reference platform in a pair.

Marine animal samples were placed in pre-cleaned glass jars or aluminum foil and frozen for air shipment to the analytical laboratory. Produced water samples were collected in 2-L precleaned glass bottles from the two produced water discharging platforms. Ambient sea water samples were collected from produced water discharging and non-discharging (reference) platforms and placed in 2-L precleaned glass bottles. The water samples were fixed with 150 mL of ultrapure dichloromethane, chilled to ~4°C, and shipped by air to the analytical laboratory.

Analysis of water and tissue samples for PAHs was performed by Arthur D. Little, Inc., Cambridge, MA. Quality assurance comparison samples were analyzed by Battelle Ocean Sciences Laboratory, Duxbury, MA. The samples were extracted and analyzed for the PAHs listed in Table 2. Prior to extraction, samples were spiked with surrogate compounds, naphthalene-d_8, fluorene-d_{10}, phenanthrene-d_{10}, and benzo(a)pyrene-d_{12}. After extraction, seawater samples were analyzed directly by gas chromatography/mass spectrometry (GC/MS) for all target PAHs; produced water extracts were fractionated by high performance liquid chromatography (HPLC) and then analyzed by GC/MS for target PAHs. Tissue sample extracts were passed through a silica gel cleanup column, fractionated by HPLC, and split in half: one half was analyzed for phenols; the other half was cleaned up by passage through an alumina column and then analyzed by GC/MS for PAHs.

Two-liter water samples were extracted for PAHs by liquid-liquid extraction in separatory funnels. The water samples were acidified with clean 6N HCl and spiked with 1 mL of acetone containing between 0.4 and 10 μg of several PAH surrogate standards.

The samples then were extracted with three 120-mL volumes of ultrapure dichloromethane. The three solvent extracts were combined and dried with sodium sulfate. The extracts then were concentrated to approximately 1 ml in a Kuderna-Danish concentrator under a stream of purified nitrogen gas. The ambient sea water extracts were spiked with appropriate internal standards. The 1 ml produced water extracts were fractionated by HPLC.

Table 2 – *Polycyclic aromatic hydrocarbons (PAHs) analyzed in produced water, ambient sea water, and the tissues of marine animals near offshore production platforms in the Gulf of Mexico*

Naphthalene	C_3-Phenanthrenes/Anthracenes
C_1-Naphthalenes	C_4-Phenanthrenes/Anthracenes
C_2-Naphthalenes	Fluoranthene
C_3-Naphthalenes	Pyrene
C_4-Naphthalenes	C_1-Fluoranthenes/Pyrenes
Acenaphthene	C_2-Fluoranthrnes/Pyrenes
Acenaphthylene	Benz(a)anthracene
Biphenyl	Chrysene
Fluorene	C_1-Chrysenes
C_1-Fluorenes	C_2-Chrysenes
C_2-Fluorenes	C_3-Chrysenes
C_3-Fluorenes	C_4-Chrysenes
Dibenzothiophene	Benzo(b)fluoranthene
C_1-Dibenzothiophenes	Benzo(k)fluoranthene
C_2-Dibenzothiophenes	Benzo(a)pyrene
C_3-Dibenzothiophenes	Benzo(e)pyrene
Phenanthrene	Perylene
Anthracene	Indeno(1,2,3-cd)pyrene
C_1-Phenanthrenes/Anthracenes	Dibenz(a,h)anthracene
C_2-Phenanthrenes/Anthracenes	Benzo(ghi)perylene

The soft tissues of bivalves and muscle tissue (filet) of fish were analyzed. Tissues from several individuals of the same species from the same station and sampling time were combined into three composite samples. Two subsamples of each composite sample were taken for analysis. Each 25-g wet wt subsample was thawed, homogenized, and extracted for PAH analysis. Sodium sulfate was added to dehydrate the sample which then was spiked with 0.4 to 10 μg of selected PAH surrogate standards. The surrogate standards were mixed directly with the tissue/sodium sulfate mixture, which was then extracted with three 100-mL volumes of dichloromethane with maceration. The three extracts were combined and concentrated to approximately 1 mL with Kudurna-Danish concentrators under a stream of purified nitrogen gas.

Each produced water or tissue extract was applied to a cleanup column packed with sodium sulfate and 5% deactivated silica gel in a slurry of 9:1 dichloromethane:ethyl ether and eluted with 9:1 dichloromathane:ethyl ether. The eluate was collected and concentrated under nitrogen to the appropriate HPLC injection volume.

The extracts were fractionated by HPLC using a size-exclusion chromatography column (Envirosep Gel Permeation Column). The extract was injected onto the column and eluted with dichloromethane. The HPLC collection windows were calibrated with a solution containing phenol, 4,4'-dibromo-octafluorobiphenyl, bis(2-ethylhexyl)phthalate, benzo(ghi)perylene, and the primary sample interferences, lipid (corn oil) and sulfur, prior to the analysis of a sample sequence. The PAH fraction of the extract was collected by an automated fraction collector programmed to collect the specified fraction based on the HPLC calibration solution.

The final sample extract was concentrated to between 0.25 and 0.5 mL, spiked with recovery standards (acenaphthene-d_{10} and chrysene-d_{12} at 1 μg/mL), and analyzed for the target analytes by GC/MS in the selected ion monitoring (SIM) mode. The GC/MS was tuned and calibrated with a six-point PAH calibration spanning the linear range of the mass spectrometer prior to analysis of a sample set. The six-point calibration ranged from 10 to 5 000 ng/mL. The PAHs were quantified versus the surrogate compounds added to the samples prior to extraction. The analyte concentrations were corrected for instrumental response based on average response factors generated from the calibration. The recoveries of the surrogate compounds were determined versus the internal standards added to samples just prior to instrumental analysis.

Concentrations of individual and total PAHs in samples are reported in μg/L (parts per billion) for produced water and sea water, and ng/g dry wt (parts per billion) for tissue samples. Method detection limits (MDLs) for individual PAHs in water samples range from 1.0 to 11 ng/L (parts per trillion). MDLs for individual PAHs in tissue samples range from 1.3 to 16 ng/g dry wt (parts per billion).

The purpose of the statistical analysis was to determine whether statistically significant bioaccumulation of PAHs from produced water is occurring in edible tissues of invertebrates and fish near representative offshore platforms discharging more than 4 600 bbl/d of treated produced water. Choice of statistical tests was affected by the observation that concentrations of many PAH analytes were below the method detection limit in a large number of tissue samples. Concentrations of semivolatile organic chemicals (PAHs, phenol, and bis(2-ethylhexyl) phthalate) in soft tissues were below the method detection limit 87% of the time. The number of ND values was tabulated for each platform pair, taxon, and target chemical, in order to determine the appropriate statistical testing procedure (Table 3).

An analysis of variance (ANOVA) was used to test for differences between concentrations of individual PAHs in marine animal tissues from discharging and reference platforms if less than 15% of the analytical results for a particular analyte and taxon were ND. ANOVA included field survey as a blocking factor that reduced the error due to seasonal variability between the two field surveys and increased the sensitivity of the statistical tests. Comparisons between the discharging and reference platforms were made for individual field surveys with contrasts. When ANOVA tested for equality in means that was consistent over the two field surveys, contrasts tested for equality of mean concentrations between platform pairs within each field survey.

Table 3 – *Statistical analysis performed with PAH tissue residue data sets from platform pairs with different numbers of ND values*

Percent ND	No. Analyses	Analysis Recommended by EPA (1989)	Statistical Test
<15% ND	20	Replace NDs with ½ MDL and perform parametric test	Two-way analysis of variance with subsampling and contrasts to compare platforms within surveys
15%≤ND<50 %	38	Use NDs as ties (2 or more observations with the same value) and perform non-parametric analysis of variance	Friedman's Test with a correction for ties; Mann-Whitney Test to determine within-survey differences
50%≤ND<90 %	127	Test of proportions	Fisher's Exact Test
90%≤ND	332	No statistical analysis	No statistical analysis

When between 15 and 50% of the analytical results for an analyte and taxon were NDs, the data were transformed to ranks and the Friedman test (Conover 1980) was used to test for equality of concentrations between platform pairs. Field survey was used as a blocking factor. The form of the Friedman test that incorporates multiple observations was used, because there were three observations for each platform/field survey combination. The Mann-Whitney test (Conover 1980) was used to test for differences between the platform pairs for each field survey.

The statistical methods described above were inappropriate when the numbers of NDs ranged from 50 to 90%. These data were transformed to binary values, either ND or not ND, and Fisher's exact test (Conover, 1980) of proportions was used. Data from each field survey were tested separately. If more than 90% of the analytical results for a particular analyte and taxon were ND, no statistical test was performed because too few data were available to make a reliable comparison.

Results

The production platform in East Breaks Block 165A in 262 m of water discharged an average of 1.75 million liters/day of produced water at the time of the field surveys (Table 1). The other discharging platform, located in Green Island Block 19A in 229 m of water, discharged an average of 1.13 million liters/day of produced water. The produced water from Platform EB165A contained averages of 43 and 30 μg/L total PAHs at the time of the first and second definitive surveys, respectively (Table 4). PAH concentrations were more variable in produced water from Platform GC19A; mean concentrations were 51 μg/L at the time of the first survey and 24 μg/L at the time of the second survey. A low-volume, intermittent secondary produced water discharge from GC19A at the time of the second definitive field survey contained an average of 130 μg/L total PAHs. (Method detection limits for individual PAHs in produced water were in the range of 0.001 to 0.01 μg/L.)

Table 4 – *Mean concentrations of polycyclic aromatic hydrocarbons in produced water collected from the two discharging production platforms in the Gulf of Mexico during the two field surveys. Concentrations are μg/L (parts per billion).*

Polycyclic Aromatic Hydrocarbon	Platform EB165A		Platform GC19A	
	Survey 1	Survey 2	Survey 1	Survey 2
Naphthalene	15	10	14	5.5
C_1-Naphthalenes	12	7.1	11	4.4
C_2-Naphthalenes	6.4	5.0	8.1	5.3
C_3-Naphthalenes	3.0	2.7	4.7	3.0
C_4-Naphthalenes	1.9	1.1	2.8	1.7
Acenaphthyylene	0.17	ND	ND	0.37
Acenaphthene	0.018	ND	ND	0.076
Biphenyl	1.0	0.55	0.78	0.37
Fluorene	0.16	0.11	0.26	0.20
C_1-Fluorenes	0.22	0.17	0.40	0.10
C_2-Fluorenes	0.39	0.22	0.76	0.25
C_3-Fluorenes	0.51	0.33	0.95	0.35
Anthracene	0.020	0.030	0.021	0.048
Phenanthrene	0.15	0.12	0.34	0.16
C_1-Phenanthrenes/Anthracenes	0.25	0.27	0.65	0.29
C_2-Phenanthrenes/Anthracenes	0.27	0.30	0.82	0.29
C_3-Phenanthrenes/Anthracenes	0.26	0.53	0.68	0.13
C_4-Phenanthrenes/Anthracenes	0.28	0.54	0.58	0.21
Dibenzothiophene	0.087	0.072	0.35	0.18
C_1-Dibenzothiophenes	0.20	0.18	0.73	0.27
C_2-Dibenzothiophenes	0.28	0.43	1.2	0.49
C_3-Dibenzothiophenes	0.35	0.38	1.3	0.45
Fluoranthene	0.002	ND	0.010	0.008
Pyrene	0.010	0.018	0.024	0.010
C_1-Fluoranthenes/Pyrenes	ND	0.057	0.081	ND
C_2-Fluoranthenes/Pyrenes	ND	0.064	0.11	ND
Chrysene	ND	ND	0.011	ND
C_1-Chrysenes	ND	ND	0.034	ND
C_2-Chrysenes	ND	ND	0.061	ND
C_3-Chrysenes	ND	ND	0.077	ND
Benzo(e)pyrene	ND	0.002	ND	0.002
Benzo(a)pyrene	ND	ND	ND	0.002
Perylene	0.047	0.036	0.18	0.036
Benzo(ghi)perylene	ND	ND	ND	0.003
Total PAHs	42.97	30.31	51.01	24.20

The most abundant PAHs in produced water from both platforms were naphthalene and alkylnaphthalenes. Collectively, they represented 90% or more of the total PAHs detected in the produced water samples. Alkyl fluorenes, phenanthrenes, and dibenzothiophenes were present at less than one-tenth the concentrations of alkyl-naphthalenes. A few four- and five-ring PAHs were present at concentrations below 0.05 µg/L. All the PAHs were present in the produced waters at concentrations below their single-phase aqueous solubilities, suggesting that all or most were in solution in the produced water.

Concentrations of total PAHs in ambient sea water at the discharge and reference platforms at the time of the two definitive field surveys ranged from below the method detection limit to 2.24 µg/L. Small amounts of naphthalene and methylnaphthalenes (to 0.01 µg/L) were detected in a few laboratory and field blanks. The highest PAH concentration was in an ambient sea water sample from the reference platform, HI356A. The dominant PAHs in these samples were alkyl fluorenes, phenanthrenes, dibenzothiophenes, and chrysenes, indicating that they were from a petroleum origin, probably micro-tar balls.

Two species of bivalve mollusks, the jewel box *Chama macerophylla* and the American thorny oyster *Spondylus americanus* were found in sufficient numbers on the legs of both discharging and non-discharging platforms to be useful for monitoring (Table 5). Offshore oil and gas platforms often attract reef-associated fish that may take up long-term residence near underwater platform structures. The species of fish attracted to a platform depend primarily on the species composition of nearby natural reef assemblages. On the outer continental shelf of the Gulf of Mexico there are abundant hard rock reef outcrops (topographic features) and a few coral reefs, with indigenous populations of reef fish. The four platforms monitored in this investigations are in the vicinity of some of these topographic features and have resident populations of several species of reef fish. However, only two species, the yellow chub *Kyphosus incisor* and the creole fish *Paranthias furcifer* were present in sufficient numbers at all four platforms for monitoring (Table 5). Three other species, the rockhind *Epinephelus adscensionis*, the sergeant major *Abudefduf saxatilis*, and the gray triggerfish *Balistes cupriscus*, were present in sufficient numbers at one or both platform pairs on one field survey to serve the needs of monitoring.

Concentrations of individual PAHs in soft tissues of jewel boxes from the legs of discharging and non-discharging platforms ranged from below the method detection limit (most samples) to 64 ng/g dry wt (Table 6). Of the 40 target PAH analytes (Table 2), only 18 were present in at least one jewel box at a concentration above the method detection limit which ranged from 1.3 to 16 ng/g dry wt. There were no statistically significant differences in the concentration of any PAH in tissues of jewel boxes from the EB165/HI356 platform pair. However, C_2- and C_3-dibenzothiophenes were present at significantly higher concentrations in jewel boxes from discharging Platform GC19 than in those from the paired non-discharging Platform EI361. The differences in mean concentrations were small.

More PAHs were detected, and at higher mean concentrations, in soft tissues of American thorny oysters (Table 7). Concentrations of individual PAHs ranged from below the method detection limit to 180 ng/g dry wt. Among oysters from the EB165/HI356 platform pair, concentrations of C_4-naphthalenes and C_2-dibenzothiophenes were significantly higher in individuals from the reference platform (HI356);

the concentration of anthracene was slightly, but significantly higher in oysters from the discharging than from the reference platform. Among oysters from the GC19/EI361 platform pair, concentrations of C_3- and C_4-naphthalenes, C_1-, C_2-, C_3-, and C_4-phenanthrenes, C_1-. C_2-, and C_3-dibenzothiophenes, C_1-chrysenes, perylene, and benzo(ghi)perylene were present at significantly higher concentrations in tissues of oysters from the discharging than from the reference platform. All of these PAHs, except perylene and benzo(ghi)perylene, are characteristic of petroleum sources; therefore, the oysters probably were bioaccumulating PAHs from a petroleum source near the discharging platform. At the time of the second definitive survey, there was a low-volume secondary produced water discharge from Platform GC19. Although the volume of produced water discharged from the secondary discharge was smaller than that from the primary discharge, the concentration of total PAHs in it was higher (121-149 µg/L). The relative concentrations of PAHs in the PAH assemblage in the tissues of thorny oysters was different from that in produced water from either the primary or secondary source, suggesting that some of the PAHs in the oyster tissues were from another source than the produced water.

Table 5 – *Species of bivalve mollusks and fish collected at each platform pair during the spring and fall field surveys 1995*

Platform Pair	Sampling Survey	Species
EB 165A (D)/HI 356A (R)	Spring 1995	Jewel Box *Chama macerophylla*
		Thorny Oyster *Spondylus americanus*
		Yellow Chub *Kyphosus incisor*
		Creole Fish *Paranthias furcifer*
		Rockhind *Epinephelus adscensionis*
	Fall 1995	Jewel Box *Chama macerophylla*
		Thorny Oyster *Spondylus americanus*
		Yellow Chub *Kyphosus incisor*
		Creole Fish *Paranthias furcifer*
		Sergeant Major *Abudefduf saxatilis*
GC 19A (D)/EI 361 A (R)	Spring 1995	Jewel Box *Chama macerophylla*
		Thorny Oyster *Spondylus americanus*
		Yellow Chub *Kyphosus incisor*
		Creole Fish *Paranthias furcifer*
		Gray Triggerfish *Balistes capriscus*
	Fall 1995	Jewel Box Chama *macerophylla*
		Thorny Oyster *Spondylus americanus*
		Yellow Chub *Kyphosus incisor*
		Creole Fish *Paranthias furcifer*
		Gray Triggerfish *Balistes capriscus*

None of the fish monitored in this investigation contained greater than trace concentrations of a few PAHs in edible muscle tissues (Table 8). Yellow chub contained the largest number (4) and highest concentrations of individual PAHs in its muscle tissues. Both total C_1-naphthalenes and 1-methyl- and 2-methyl-naphthalene were measured. Concentrations of 2-methylnaphthalene were higher than concentrations of 1-methylnaphthalene. The concentration of 2-methyl naphthalene was slightly, but significantly higher in muscle of yellow chub from the two discharging platforms than in muscle of yellow chub from the paired reference platforms. Phenanthrene was present at a significantly higher concentration in muscle of yellow chub from discharging Platform GC19 than in muscle of fish from the paired reference Platform EI361. The concentration of C_2-naphthalenes was significantly higher in muscle of yellow chub from reference Platform EI361 than in yellow chub from discharging platform GC19. There were no other statistically significant differences in concentrations of individual PAHs in muscle tissues of any of the five species of fish. Concentrations of individual PAHs in muscle tissue of the five species of fish ranged from below the method detection limit (most samples) to 16 ng/g dry wt.

Table 6 – *Concentration ranges of PAHs in tissues of jewel boxes* Chama macerophylla *from produced water discharge (D)/reference (R) platform pairs in the northwestern Gulf of Mexico. PAHs are listed only if one or more values is above the method detection limit. Differences between pairs in bold type are statistically significant. Concentrations are ng/g dry wt (parts per billion).*

Polycyclic Aromatic Hydrocarbon	Platform Pair		Platform Pair	
	EB165 (D)	HI356 (R)	GC19 (D)	EI361 (R)
Naphthalene	<9	<9 – 16	<9	<9
C_1-Naphthalenes	5 – 12	4 – 30	6 – 18	<3 – 13
C_2-Naphthalenes	<5 – 31	<5 – 36	<5 – 34	<5 – 25
C_3-Naphthalenes	<5 – 42	<5 – 32	<5 – 37	<5 – 24
C_4-Naphthalenes	<5	<5 – 34	<5 – 54	<5
Biphenyl	<2 – 6	<2	<2 – 6	<2 – 5
C_1-Fluorenes	<4 – 28	<4 – 32	<4 – 23	<4 – 16
Phenanthrene	<4 – 6	<4 – 8	<4 – 9	<4
C_1-Phenanthrenes/Anthracenes	<6 – 15	<6 – 23	<6	<6 – 15
C_2-Phenanthrenes/Anthracenes	<16	<16 – 58	<16 – 44	<16 – 38
C_1-Dibenzothiophenes	<1	<1	<1 – 15	<1
C_2-Dibenzothiophenes	<1 – 28	<1 – 28	**<1 – 40**	**<1 – 19**
C_3-Dibenzothiophenes	<1 – 23	<1 – 22	**<1 – 64**	**<1 – 18**
Fluoranthene	<3	<3 – 4	<3	<3
Benz(a)anthracene	<2 – 58	<2	<2	<2
Benzo(e)pyrene	<2 – 25	<2 – 20	<2 – 41	<2 – 26
Benzo(a)pyrene	<3 – 8	<3 – 9	<3 – 21	<3 – 21
Perylene	<3 – 49	<3 – 34	<3 – 75	<3 – 41

Discussion

The composition of the PAH assemblage in produced water from the two offshore platforms monitored in this investigation is similar to that in produced water from other offshore platforms in the Gulf of Mexico, North Sea, Australia, and Indonesia (Terrens and Tait 1996, DOE 1997, Utvik 1999, Neff 2000). However, concentrations of total

PAHs in produced water from the two platforms are lower than those from most other platforms in U.S. waters and abroad. For example, mean total PAH concentrations (measured by the same methods as used in this investigation) in seven produced waters (including the two evaluated in this investigation) from the Gulf of Mexico range from 24 μg/L to 600 μg/L and concentrations in eight produced water samples from the North Sea and Indonesia range from 230 μg/L to 1 560 μg/L (Neff 2000).

Table 7 – *Concentration ranges of PAHs in tissues of thorny oysters* Spondylus americanus *from produced water discharge (D)/reference (R) platform pairs in the northwestern Gulf of Mexico. PAHs are listed only if one or more values is above the method detection limit. Differences between pairs in bold type are statistically significant. Concentrations are ng/g dry wt (parts per billion).*

Polycyclic Aromatic Hydrocarbon	**Platform Pair**		**Platform Pair**	
	EB165 (D)	**HI356 (R)**	**GC19 (D)**	**EI361 (R)**
Naphthalene	<9	<9	<9 – 17	<9
C_1-Naphthalenes	3 – 9	<3 – 10	3 – 11	<3 – 8
C_2-Naphthalenes	<5 – 28	<5 – 57	<5 – 24	<5 – 15
C_3-Naphthalenes	<5 – 32	<5 – 140	**<5 – 40**	**<5 – 9**
C_4-Naphthalenes	**<5**	**<5 – 170**	**<5 – 54**	**<5**
Biphenyl	<2	<2	<2 – 7	<2 – 19
C_1-Fluorenes	<4 – 24	<4 – 41	<4 – 23	<4 – 22
Anthracene	**<2 – 10**	**<2 – 9**	<2 – 10	<2 – 6
Phenanthrene	<5	<4 – 14	<4	<4
C_1-Phenanthrenes/Anthracenes	<6 – 19	<6 – 80	**<6 – 16**	**<6**
C_2-Phenanthrenes/Anthracenes	<16 – 44	<16 – 120	**<16 – 57**	**<16 – 40**
C_3-Phenanthrenes/Anthracenes	<16	<16	**<16 – 180**	**<16**
C_4-Phenanthrenes/Anthracenes	<16	<16	**<16 – 55**	**<16**
Dibenzothiophene	<1	<1 – 6	<1 – 2	<1
C_1-Dibenzothiophenes	<1	<1 – 36	**<1 – 16**	**<1**
C_2-Dibenzothiophenes	**<1 – 33**	**<1 – 70**	**25 – 60**	**<1 – 22**
C_3-Dibenzothiophenes	<1 – 26	<1 – 47	**41 – 100**	**<1 – 25**
Fluoranthene	<3	<3	<3 – 4	<3 – 5
Pyrene	<3	<3	<3	<3 – 11
C_1-Fluoranthenes/Pyrenes	<3	<3 – 17	<3	<3
C_2-Fluoranthenes/Pyrenes	<3	<3	<3 – 16	<3 – 6
Benz(a)anthracene	<2	<2 – 58	<2	<2 – 4
Chrysene	<2 – 4	<2	<2	<2
C_1-Chrysenes	<2 – 9	<2	**<2 – 12**	**<2 – 5**
C_2-Chrysenes	<2 – 11	<2	<2 – 27	<2
Benzo(e)pyrene	<2 – 6	<2 – 4	<2 – 11	<2 – 4
Benzo(a)pyrene	<3 – 9	<3 – 6	<3 – 12	<3 – 5
Perylene	<3	<3 – 5	**<3 – 35**	**<3**
Benzo(ghi)perylene	<3	<3	**<3 – 6**	**<3**

Table 8 – *Concentration ranges of selected PAHs in muscle tissues of five species of fish from produced water discharge (D)/reference (R) platform pairs in the northwestern Gulf of Mexico. PAHs are listed only if one or more values is above the method detection limit. Differences between pairs in bold type are statistically significant. Concentrations are ng/g dry wt (parts per billion).*

Polycyclic Aromatic Hydrocarbon	**Platform Pair**		**Platform Pair**	
	EB165 (D)	**HI356 (R)**	**GC19 (D)**	**EI361 (R)**
Yellow Chub *Kyphosus incisor*				
2-Methylnaphthalene	**3 – 5**	**3 – 4**	**<2 – 5**	**4 – 16**
1-Methylnaphthalene	<3	<3	<3 – 3	<3 – 8
C_1-Naphthalenes	3 – 5	<3 – 5	<3 – 7	4 – 8
C_2-Naphthalenes	<5 – 6	<5 – 17	**<5 – 7**	**5 – 16**
C_1-Fluorenes	<4 – 9	<4 – 21	<4 – 24	<4 – 12
Phenanthrene	<4	<4	**<4 – 4**	**<4**
Creole Fish *Paranthias furcifer*				
2-Methylnaphthalene	<2 – 4	<2 – 4	<2 – 4	<2 – 5
C_1-Naphthalenes	3 – 5	<3 – 4	<3 – 5	4 – 6
C_1-Fluorenes	<4	<4 – 10	<4 – 5	<4 – 13
Rockhind *Epinephelus adscensionis*			Gray Triggerfish *Balistes capriscus*	
2-Methylnaphthalene	<2 – 5	<2 – 5	<2 – 4	<2 – 4
C_1-Naphthalenes	<3 – 4	<3 – 6	<3 – 4	<3 – 4
C_1-Fluorenes	<4 – 9	<4 – 11	<4 – 5	<4 – 11
Sergent Major *Abudefduf saxatilis*				
2-Methylnaphthalene	<3 – 7	3 – 4	---	---
1-Methylnaphthalene	<3 – 5	<3	---	---
C_1-Naphthalenes	4 – 7	3 – 5	---	---

The concentration of PAHs in treated produced water discharges is dependent on the efficiency of oil-water separation. The oil-water treatment system on the platform removes primarily oil droplets from the produced water. If droplet removal is essentially complete, the only hydrocarbons remaining in the produced water are in solution or colloidal suspension and concentrations of PAHs, because of their low aqueous solubilities, are low. More than 90% of the PAHs in the produced water from the two platforms were naphthalene and alkylnaphthalenes, the most water-soluble PAHs. Concentrations of the nearly insoluble four- through six-ring PAHs were extremely low, suggesting that most of the PAHs in the produced water were in solution.

Marine animals near an ocean discharge of produced water may be exposed to a rapidly-diluting plume containing a wide variety of metals and organic chemicals characteristic of produced water (Johnsen et al. 1998). In order to bioaccumulate chemicals from the diluting plume, marine organisms must be exposed to elevated concentrations (compared to natural concentrations in clean ambient sea water) of chemicals for long enough (days or weeks) to permit significant bioaccumulation. Mobile animals, such as platform-associated fish and crustaceans, are unlikely to be exposed to the chemicals in the diluting produced water plume long enough and at high enough concentrations to allow for biologically significant bioaccumulation. Biofouling organisms on submerged platform structures, such as bivalve mollusks and barnacles, may be exposed intermittently to relatively undiluted produced water chemicals as the plume drifts away from the platform in different directions with local tidal and wind-driven currents.

Saline produced waters dilute rapidly upon discharge to well-mixed marine waters. Dispersion modeling studies of the fate of produced water differ in specific details but all predict a rapid initial dilution of discharges by 30- to 100-fold within the first few tens of meters of the outfall, followed by a slower rate of dilution at greater distances (Terrens and Tait 1993, Strømgren et al. 1995, Brandsma and Smith 1996). Terrens and Tait (1993) modeled the fate of produced water discharged to the Bass Strait off southeastern Australia. Under typical oceanographic conditions for the area, the produced water was diluted nearly 30-fold within 10 m of the discharge and by 1 800-fold 1 000 m down-current of the produced water discharge. Sommerville (1987) measured a 2 800-fold dilution of produced water 1 000 m down-current from a North Sea produced water discharge.

Brandsma and Smith (1996) modeled the fate of produced water discharged under typical Gulf of Mexico conditions. For a median produced water discharge rate of 115 m^3/d (722 bbl/d), a 500-fold dilution was predicted 10 m from the outfall and a 1 000-fold dilution was predicted 100 m from the outfall. In the present investigation, the 1.13 million L/d produced water discharge from Platform GC19A was predicted to dilute by a factor of 100-fold within a few meters of the outfall under stratified water column conditions. The larger volume (1.75 million L/d), more saline discharge from Platform EB165A was predicted to descend deeper following discharge and dilute nearly as rapidly as the produced water plume from Platform GC19A.

Despite the rapid dilution of produced water in ambient sea water, PAH concentrations in surface sea water near produced water discharges often are above background concentrations. In the present investigation, concentrations of total PAHs in ambient sea water at the discharge and reference sites at the time of the two field surveys ranged from below the method detection limit to 2.24 μg/L. The highest total PAH concentration and the only one above 0.1 μg/L was from the vicinity of the reference platform HI356A. The highest measured concentrations of total PAHs in ambient water from the two discharging platforms were 0.01 and 0.07 μg/L, close to background. The PAH assemblage in the water samples was dominated by alkyl PAHs, indicating that the PAHs were from a petroleum origin (Youngblood and Blumer 1975). The concentration of total PAH, estimated from concentrations in tissues of caged mussels and in semipermeable membrane devices, in surface waters of an area in the Norwegian Sector of the North Sea with a large number of production platforms was in the range of 0.005 to 0.07 μg/L (Johnsen et al. 1998).

Thorny oysters collected from the legs of offshore production platforms in this study contained up to 800 ng/g dry wt. total PAHs in their soft tissues. Most composite samples of bivalve soft tissues contained less than 100 ng/g total PAHs. These PAH concentrations generally were lower than those in bivalves collected by others from shallow coastal waters throughout the world (Table 9). Bivalve mollusks, primarily mussels and oysters collected and analyzed as part of the NOAA National Status and Trends Mussel Watch Program, from coastal and estuarine environments usually contained more than about 500 ng/g total PAHs. The "high" concentration (defined as the geometric mean concentration plus one standard deviation of the lognormal distribution of concentrations among sampling sites) of total PAHs in tissues of mussels and oysters from the Mussel Watch Program is 1 020 ng/g dry wt (O'Connor and Beliaeff, 1995).

Mussels *Mytilus edulis* that had been deployed in cages 10 m below the sea surface for one month 500 m down-current from two production platforms in the North Sea contained means of 1 540 ng/g and 2 910 ng/g dry wt total PAHs (Johnsen et al., 1998). Mean concentrations of total PAHs in mussels deployed 10 km down-current from the production platforms were 141 ng/g and 540 ng/g; PAH concentrations in mussels from more remote reference sites were in the range of 17.7 ng/g to 51 ng/g. The higher concentrations of PAHs in mussels deployed near North Sea platforms than in two species of bivalves collected from submerged platform structures in the Gulf of Mexico probably is due primarily to differences in monitoring program design. The mussels can be deployed directly down-current from the produced water discharge, assuring maximal exposure to the produced water plume, whereas, the extent of exposure of bivalves from submerged platform structures to the produced water plume is uncertain and variable. However, the latter exposure scenario is more realistic. The North Sea discharges monitored by Johnsen et al. (1998) are high-volume discharges. The produced water discharge from the Statfjord Field is the largest in the North Sea (30.9 million L/d in 1992: Ynnesdal and Furuholt 1994). About 12 million L/d of produced water is discharged from the Troll platform (Utvik 1999). PAH concentrations in the high-volume North Sea produced water discharges tend to be higher than those in the two produced water discharges monitored in the Gulf of Mexico. Produced water from 12 North Sea platforms monitoried by Utvik (1999) contain 300 μg/L to 1 800 μg/L total PAHs. As a result, mussels in the North Sea deployments were exposed to higher concentrations of produced water-derived PAHs than bivalves from platform structures in the Gulf of Mexico.

Table 9 – *Concentration ranges of total PAHs in the soft tissues of bivalve mollusks and muscle tissue of marine fish from throughout the world. Concentrations are ng/g dry wt (parts per billion). From Neff (2000)*

Taxon	Number of Sample Means	Range of Concentrations
Bivalve Mollusks	153	3 – 1,729,000
Fish	84	2 – 23,450

Jewel boxes and thorny oysters collected at paired discharge and reference sites EB165A(D)/HI356A(R) contained low concentrations of several PAHs. Alkyl homologues of naphthalene were present in most bivalve samples. C_2- and C_3-dibenzothiophenes, C_1-fluorenes, and C_1-phenanthrenes also were present at measurable concentrations in some bivalve samples. These PAHs all are typical of petroleum sources. Several bivalves from the EB165A/HI356A platform pair contained small amounts of predominantly pyrogenic PAHs, benzo(e)pyrene, benzo(a)pyrene, and perylene. Thorny oysters collected from the reference Platform HI356A on the second definitive survey contained elevated concentrations of several PAHs, probably of petroleum origin. However, there were only a few statistically significant differences in concentrations of individual PAHs in tissues of thorny oysters, but not jewel boxes, from the EB165A/HI356A platform pair. Two PAHs were present at higher concentrations in oysters from the reference platform and one was higher in oysters from the discharging platform. Therefore, there is no real evidence of bioaccumulation of PAHs from the produced water discharge at Platform EB165A.

PAH concentrations in tissues of jewel boxes and thorny oysters from the discharge/reference platform pair GC19A(D)/EI361A(R) were, in a few cases, higher than those in bivalves from the other platform pair. Some jewel boxes from this platform pair contained detectable concentrations of alkylnaphthalenes, biphenyl, C_1-fluorenes, C_1- and C_2-phenanthrenes, C_1-, C_2-, and C_3-dibenzothiophenes, all primarily petrogenic, and benzo(e)pyrene, benzo(a)pyrene, and perylene, all primarily pyrogenic. The only PAHs that were significantly more abundant in jewel boxes from the discharging than from the reference platform were C_2- and C_3-dibenzothiophenes, both petrogenic.

Thorny oysters from the GC19A/EI361A platform pair contained higher concentrations of several PAHs than did jewel boxes. The most abundant PAH in the thorny oyster tissues were alkylnaphthalenes, C_1-fluorenes, alkylphenanthrenes, alkyldibenzothiophenes, alkylchrysenes, all primarily petrogenic, and benzo(e)pyrene, benzo(a)pyrene, perylene, and benzo(ghi)perylene, all primarily pyrogenic. Several of the petrogenic PAHs were present at significantly higher concentrations in oysters from the discharging than from the reference platform at the time of the first definitive survey. The PAH profile in the tissues of most of the thorny oysters collected from the discharging platform GC19A during the first definitive survey resembles that of petroleum. The source of these PAHs in the thorny oyster tissues probably was produced water or a light refined petroleum product. Evidence of bioaccumulation of PAHs from produced water by thorny oysters was considered weak and inconclusive, because bioaccumulation of petroleum-derived PAHs was demonstrated in only one instance, and the source(s) of the PAHs was unclear. Bivalves from both the discharging and reference platforms contained similar concentrations of total PAHs and most individual PAHs.

The abundance of C_2- and C_3-dibenzothiophenes in the produced water from GC19 (Table 4) and in the tissues of jewel boxes (Table 6) and thorny oysters (Table 7) suggests that some of the PAHs in the bivalve soft tissues was derived from produced water. However, the abundance of C_3-phenanthrenes in oyster tissues but not in the produced water and the similarity in concentrations of total PAHs in bivalves from both discharging and reference platforms indicates that much of the body burden of PAHs was derived from other sources.

Sources of PAH assemblages in environmental samples sometimes can be identified by PAH fingerprinting (Page et al. 1995). The relative concentrations (ratios) of different PAHs remain relatively constant or change in a systematic manner in PAH assemblages as they are transported and weathered in the environment. Some petroleum components, such as steranes and triterpanes, are stable in the environment and characteristic of the petroleum source. They can be used to identify crude oils and some residual oils in environmental samples.

However, fingerprinting has limited applicability for identifying PAH assemblages from produced water in tissues of marine animals. Treated produced water contains primarily low molecular weight, slightly soluble hydrocarbons and does not contain quantifiable concentrations of the highly insoluble sterane and triterpane biomarkers. Bivalve mollusks have only a limited ability to metabolize and actively excrete accumulated PAHs (Stegeman, 1981). Nevertheless, they can bioaccumulate particulate, colloidal, and dissolved PAHs and the PAH assemblage in their tissues may not resemble that in the source material or in the water to which they are exposed (Neff and Burns 1996, Axelman et al. 1999). Fish have an active mixed function oxygenase system that rapidly metabolizes PAHs, changing the composition of the PAH assemblage in their tissues (Meador et al. 1995).

Two frequently-used PAH fingerprinting ratios are C_2-phenanthrenes/C_2-dibenzothiophenes (P2/D2) and C_3-phenanthrenes/C_3-dibenzothiophenes (P3/D3). In the present investigation, P2/D2 ranged from 0.51 to 0.71 in produced water from Platform GC19A and from 0.86 to 1.57 in soft tissues of thorny oysters from GC19A. P3/D3 ranged from 0.25 to 0.61 in produced water and from 0.59 to 2.67 in thorny oyster tissues. Thus, it is not possible to attribute the PAHs in tissues of thorny oysters from GC19A to produced water from the platform.

Muscle tissues of fish collected in this study contained <1 to 120 ng/g dry wt total PAHs. This concentration range is in the lower part of the range reported for muscle of fish from elsewhere in the world (Table 9). Although fish can bioaccumulate PAHs rapidly from solution, they are able to metabolize and excrete them rapidly, keeping concentrations in tissues low (Meador et al. 1995). Fishes tend to metabolize high molecular weight PAHs more rapidly than low molecular weight PAHs (Varanasi and Stein 1991), possibly accounting for the higher concentrations of low molecular weight PAHs sometimes encountered in fish tissues (Hellou et al. 1994, 1995).

The five species of fish sampled in this study contained only traces of a relatively few PAHs in their edible muscle tissue. Only five of the 40 target PAH analytes were detected in muscle of one or more of the fish species. All the detected PAHs were low molecular weight 2- or 3-ring PAHs. The only statistically significant differences were for alkylnpahthalenes and phenanthrene in muscle tissues of yellow chub. There were two cases each of higher concentrations in muscle of fish from the discharging and reference platforms. Thus, fish were not bioaccumulating PAHs from the produced water discharges.

This study has shown, as others have, that bivalve mollusks are preferable to fish for monitoring the bioavailability of petroleum hydrocarbons from wastewater effluents. The bivalves are immobile and have only a limited ability to metabolize and excrete accumulated PAHs. Different species may be able to bioaccumulate dissolved, colloidal, and particulate PAHs. Most fish are highly motile and are able to rapidly metabolize and excrete accumulated PAHs. However, it is useful to monitor edible tissues of fish from offshore platforms for contaminant residues to ensure that fish caught for human consumption do not contain potentially toxic concentrations of contaminants.

Acknowldegments

This work was supported by a contract from the Offshore Operators Committee to Continental Shelf Associates, Inc., Jupiter, FL. Analysis of PAHs in produced water, ambient sea water, and tissues of marine animals was performed by Arthur D. Little, Inc., Cambridge, MA. We would like to thank the members of the Bioaccumulation Working Group of the OOC for their helpful guidance in the design and performance of this investigation.

REFERENCES

Axelman, J., Naes, K., Näf, C., and Broman, D., 1999, "Accumulation of polycyclic aromatic hydrocarbons in semipermeable membrane devices and caged mussels (*Mytilus edulis* L.) in relation to water column phase distribution," *Environmental Toxicology and Chemistry*, Vol. 18, pp. 2454-2461.

Black, K.P., Brand, G.W., Grynberg, D.H., Gwyther, D., Hammond, L.S., Mourtikas, S., Richardson, B.J., and Wardrop, J.A. 1994. "Production facilities," *Environmental Implications of Offshore Oil and Gas Development in Australia - The Findings of an Independent Scientific Review,* J.M. Swan, J.M. Neff, and P.C. Young, Eds., Australian Petroleum Exploration Association, Canberra, Australia, pp. 209-407.

Brandsma, M.G. and Smith, J.P., 1996, "Dispersion modeling perspectives on the environmental fate of produced water discharges," *Produced Water 2: Environmental Issues and Mitigation Technologies,* M. Reed and S. Johnson, Eds., Plenum Press, New York, pp. 215-224.

Collins, A.G., 1975, *Geochemistry of Oilfield Waters,* Elsevier Scientific Publishers, New York. 496 pp.

Conover, W.J., 1980, *Practical Nonparametric Statistics,* 2nd Ed., John Wiley & Sons, Inc., New York.

Continental Shelf Associates, 1993, "Measurements of Naturally Occurring Radioactive Materials at Two Offshore Production Platforms in the Northern Gulf of Mexico," Final Report to the American Petroleum Institute, Washington, DC.

DOE (U.S. Dept. of Energy), 1997, "Radionuclides, Metals, and Hydrocarbons in Oil and Gas Operational Discharges and Environmental Samples Associated with Offshore Production Facilities on the Texas/Louisiana Continental Shelf with an Environmental Assessment of Metals and Hydrocarbons," Report to U.S. Dept. of Energy, Bartlesville, OK.

EPA (U.S. Environmental Protection Agency), 1989, "Statistical Analysis of Ground-Water Monitoring Data at RCRA Facilities. Interim Final Guidance," EPA/530/SW-89/026, EPA, Office of Solid Waste, Washington, DC.

Hellou, J., Mackay, D., and Fowler, B., 1995, "Bioconcentration of polycyclic aromatic compounds from sediments to muscle of finfish," *Environmental Science and Technology*, Vol. 29, pp. 2555-2560.

Hellou, J., Upshall, C., Payne, J.F., and Hodson, P.V., 1994, "Polycyclic aromatic compounds in cod (*Gadus morhua*) from the northwest Atlantic and St. Lawrence Estuary," Science of the Total Environment, Vol. 145, pp. 71-79.

Johnsen, S., Røe, T.I., and Durell, G., 1998, "Dilution and bioavailability of produced water compounds in the northern North Sea. A combined modeling and field study," SPE 46269. The 1998 SPE International Conference on Health, Safety and Environment in Oil and Gas Exploration and Production. Society of Petroleum Engineers, Richardson, TX. 11 pp.

Meador, J.P., Stein, J.E., Reichert, W.L., and Varanasi, U., 1995, "Bioaccumulation of polycyclic aromatic hydrocarbons by marine organisms," *Reviews in Environmental Contamination and Toxicology*, Vol. 143, pp. 79-165.

Neff, J.M., 2000, "Bioaccumulation in Marine Organisms: Effects of Contaminants from Oil Well Produced Water," Elsevier Science Publishers, London (in press).

Neff, J.M. and Burns, W.A., 1996, "Estimation of polycyclic aromatic hydrocarbon concentrations in the water column based on tissue residues in mussels and salmon: an equilibrium partitioning approach," *Environmental Toxicology and Chemistry*, Vol. 15, pp. 220-2254.

Neff, J.M., Rabalais, N.N., and Boesch, D.F., 1987, "Offshore oil and gas development activities potentially causing long-term environmental effects," *Long-Term Environmental Effects of Offshore Oil and Gas Development,* D.F. Boesch and N.N. Rabalais, Eds., Elsevier Applied Science Publishers, London, pp. 149-174.

O'Connor, T.P. and Beliaeff, B., 1995, "Recent Trends in Coastal Environmental Quality: Results from the Mussel Watch Project," National Oceanic and Atmospheric Administration, National Ocean Service, Office of Ocean Resources, Conservation and Assessment, Coastal Monitoring and Bioeffects Assessment Division, Silver Springs, MD. 40 pp.

Otto, G.H. and Arnold, K.E., 1996, "U.S. produced water discharge regulations have tough limits," Oil and Gas Journal, Vol. 94, pp. 54-61.

Page, D.S., Boehm, P.D., Douglas, G.S., and Bence, A.E., 1995, "Identification of hydrocarbon sources in benthic sediments of Prince William Sound and the Gulf of Alaska following the *Exxon Valdez* oil spill," *Exxon Valdez Oil Spill: Fate and Effects in Alaskan Waters. ASTM STP 1219,* P.G. Wells, J.N. Butler, and J.S.

Hughes, Eds., American Society for Testing and Materials, West Conshohocken, PA, pp. 41-83

Rabalais, N.N., McKee, B.A., Reed, D.J., and Means, J.C., 1991, "Fate and effects of nearshore discharges of OCS produced waters. Vol. 1: Executive Summary. Vol. 2: Technical Report. Vol. 3. Appendices," OCS Studies MMS 91-004, MMS 91-005, and MMS 91-006. U.S. Dept. of the Interior, Minerals Management Service, Gulf of Mexico OCS Regional Office, New Orleans, LA.

Somerville, H.J., 1987, "Environmental aspects of offshore operations," *Microbiological Problems in the Offshore Oil Industry, International Conference, Aberdeen, Scotland.* John Wiley & Sons, London, pp.105-124

Stegeman, J.J., 1985, "Benzo(a)pyrene oxidation and microsomal enzyme activity in the mussel (*Mytilus edulis*) and other bivalve mollusc species from the western N. Atlantic," *Marine Biology*, Vol. 89, pp. 21-30.

Stephenson, M.T., 1991, "Components of produced water: a compilation of results from several industry studies," SPE 23313. Proceedings of the First International Conference on Health, Safety and Environment. The Hague, Netherlands. Society of Petroleum Engineers, Inc., Richardson, TX, pp. 25-38

Strømgren, T., Sørstrøm, S.E., Schou, L., Kaarstad, I., Aunaas, T., Brakstad, O.G., and Johansen, Ø., 1995, "Acute toxic effects of produced water in relation to chemical composition and dispersion," *Marine Environmental Research*, Vol. 40, pp.147-169.

Terrens, G.W. and Tait, R.D., 1993, "Effects on the marine environment of produced formation water discharges from Esso/BHPP's Bass Strait Platforms," Esso Australia Ltd., Melbourne, Australia. 25 pp.

Terrens, G.W. and Tait, R.D., 1996, "Monitoring ocean concentrations of aromatic hydrocarbons from produced formation water discharges to Bass Strait, Australia," SPE 36033. Proceedings of the International Conference on Health, Safety & Environment. Society of Petroleum Engineers, Richardson, TX, pp. 739-747.

Utvik, T.I.R., 1999, "Chemical characterization of produced water from four offshore oil production platforms in the North Sea," *Chemosphere*, Vol. 39, pp. 2593-2606.

Varanasi, U. and Stein, J.E., 1991, "Disposition of xenobiotic chemicals and metabolites in marine organisms," Environmental Health Perspectives, Vol. 90, pp. 93-100.

Veil, J.A., 1997, "NPDES permits have increased emphasis on control of toxic pollutants," *Oil and Gas Journal*, Vol. 95, pp. 46-52.

Youngblood, W.W. and Blumer, M., 1975, "Polycyclic aromatic hydrocarbons in the environment: homologous series in soils and recent marine sediments," *Geochimica et Cosmochimica Acta*, Vol. 39, pp. 1303-1314.

Lara C. Diener,[1] D. George Dixon,[2] Bruce M. Greenberg,[2] and Patricia M. Schulte [2]

Differential Display Polymerase Chain Reaction and Gene Expression in Copper-Exposed *Daphnia magna*

Reference: Diener, L. C., Dixon, D. G., Greenberg, B. M., and Schulte, P. M., **"Differential Display Polymerase Chain Reaction and Gene Expression in Copper-Exposed *Daphnia magna*,"** *Environmental Toxicology and Risk Assessment: Science, Policy, and Standardization- Implications for Environmental Decisions: Tenth Volume ASTM STP1403*, B. M. Greenberg, R. N. Hall, M. H. Roberts, Jr., and R. W. Gensemer, Eds., American Society for Testing and Materials, West Conshohocken, PA, 2001.

Abstract: Contamination of aquatic systems by metals and polycyclic aromatic hydrocarbons (PAHs) is a prevalent environmental problem. These contaminants are known to impact populations, organismal health, and survival negatively. Most of the organism and ecosystem level changes are a consequence of underlying molecular and subcellular damage. Therefore, molecular bioindicators are likely to be a sensitive tool for environmental assessment. We have demonstrated that both copper and phenanthrenequinone (PHEQ) alter protein expression in *Daphnia magna*. To investigate altered gene expression in *Daphnia magna* exposed to copper, PHEQ, and other contaminants, a technique based on the differential display polymerase chain reaction (ddPCR) is being developed for *D. magna*. This technique promises numerous applications as it permits a survey of the genes being expressed in any given organism. Furthermore, ddPCR allows one to monitor the changes in gene expression that result from any toxicant exposure. This paper reviews the applications of ddPCR and describes our development of ddPCR as a bioindicator of gene expression in *D. magna* in response to toxicant exposure. This is the first step in the development of a novel gene fingerprinting technique that can be applied to any compound and organism of interest.

Keywords: mRNA, molecular bioindicators, PCR, metal, aquatic, invertebrate, toxicity

Introduction

Contamination of aquatic systems by metals and polycyclic aromatic hydrocarbons (PAHs) is a prevalent environmental problem. These contaminants are known to impact organism health and survival negatively. Damage is often the result of molecular and biochemical changes, although acclimation can also be observed. Changes in gene expression are of particular importance because they can be among the first effects of

---

[1]Graduate student and [2]Professor, respectively, Department of Biology, University of Waterloo, Waterloo, Ontario, N2L 3G1, Canada.

toxicant exposure (Hightower 1998). Molecular bioindicators that can be used to monitor changes in gene expression therefore provide early warning signals of toxicant exposure and adverse biological effects. Molecular bioindicators such as the metallothioneins (MTs), heat shock proteins (HSPs), superoxide dismutase (SOD), and cytochrome P450, play a useful role in monitoring and assessing impacted sites. Some applications, advantages, and disadvantages of using MTs, HSPs, SOD, and cytochrome P450 as bioindicators in mammals, fish, insects, and crustaceans have been widely reviewed (Huggett et al. 1992). However, each of these indicators provides information regarding the physiological or biochemical effects of only one class of compounds. For example, metallothionein induction suggests metal exposure, while cytochrome P450 expression indicates exposure to PAHs or dioxins. Thus, a bioindicator that could provide information about multiple detoxification processes would be valuable both in screening for multiple chemicals and by clarifying mechanisms of toxicant action.

We are currently developing a molecular technique, differential display polymerase chain reaction (ddPCR), as a molecular bioindicator of gene expression in response to chemical exposure. ddPCR is a novel technique that permits a survey of the population of genes, among the thousands of genes in a given organism. It only reports the genes being expressed at a given time. Thus, using ddPCR a systematic comparison of mRNA expression between cell types, stages of development, or in tissues exposed to altered conditions such as hypoxia, temperature changes, or toxicants, is possible. Since its development by Liang and Pardee (1992), ddPCR has been exploited extensively for research on cancer, diabetes, heart disease, and drug treatment (Liang et al. 1992, Utans et al. 1994, Nishio et al. 1994, Wang et al. 1999). However, this technique has rarely been applied in the field of environmental toxicology.

The freshwater microcrustaceans, *Daphnia magna*, are widely utilized as a representative of other freshwater species in standard toxicity testing. *D. magna's* small size, ease of culturing, and short reproductive cycle facilitates its use in the laboratory. Furthermore, it is possible to link whole organism endpoints such as growth and reproduction to changes in gene expression using this organism. Although ddPCR has been applied to many mammalian test organisms, it has not yet been applied to *D. magna*.

ddPCR was developed as an alternative method of identifying and isolating differentially expressed genes. It has numerous advantages over techniques such as construction of subtracted cDNA libraries, or differential screening of genomic or cDNA libraries (Matz and Lukyanov 1998, Rockett et al. 1999). While a tremendous amount of time was required for analysis of differentially expressed genes in the past, ddPCR permits rapid screening. A ddPCR analysis (RNA isolation, PCR amplification, and polyacrylamide gel electrophoresis) can be generated within a single day. DNA bands from these gels can be cloned and then sequenced within a week. This dramatically decreases the time needed for identification of genes, particularly because the time required for construction of cDNA libraries is eliminated. Less RNA is required for ddPCR analysis as only 0.02 μg of RNA is needed for each reaction. Both increases and decreases in levels of mRNA can be monitored simultaneously. The combination of arbitrary primers and PCR allows identification of even rare mRNA sequences that have previously been difficult to obtain. Variations of the original protocol have resulted in improved reproducibility between PCR runs and decreased occurrence of false positives (Graf et al. 1997, Diachenko et al. 1996, Miele et al. 1998, Mathieu-Daude et al. 1996).

ddPCR is based on two common molecular tools: PCR and electrophoresis. Using these tools in combination with selected arbitrary primers, differentially expressed genes can be rapidly identified. RNA is first extracted from control and treated organisms, then reverse transcribed to generate the 1st strand of the cDNAs. cDNA is subsequently PCR amplified using a pair of arbitrary primers. The arbitrary primers are an essential feature of ddPCR (Liang and Pardee 1992). These primers anneal to a variety of cDNA fragments, yielding PCR products of varying lengths. Thus, a large subset of genes is amplified. If different pairs of arbitrary primers are used, different subsets of genes will be amplified. The PCR products can be radioactively labeled and separated by size using denaturing polyacrylamide gel electrophoresis. The visualized products are 'displayed' as bands on the gel. The distinct pattern of bands, or gene profile, for control and treated organisms can be directly compared. Differences in band intensity suggest inhibition or induction of a gene in response to the treatment. Similarly, the appearance or disappearance of a band indicates a gene has been turned on or off.

The objective of this study is to generate gene profiles for *D. magna* using ddPCR. The resulting profile of expressed genes provides a clearer picture of the organism's response to a given treatment. The effects of toxicant exposure on multiple genes can be monitored simultaneously. The gene profile can be used as a species-specific 'fingerprint' of toxicant exposure, thus representing a potentially powerful bioindicator. This bioindicator has great potential for investigations of contaminant mixtures as well as providing an idea of organismal response at the gene level to toxicants. Further, it requires no prior knowledge about the mechanisms of toxicant action. Genes that respond to a toxicant can be identified by sequencing the differentially expressed bands, and subsequently comparing the sequences obtained to those in genome project databanks.

Development of ddPCR as a Bioindicator

ddPCR analysis begins with the extraction of either mRNA or total RNA (Liang and Pardee 1992). We have evaluated several commonly available RNA extraction methods for use on *D. magna*, including the RNeasy Mini Kit (Qiagen Inc., Mississauga, Ontario) and Tripure kit (Roche Diagnostics, Laval, Quebec). The RNeasy kit utilizes a column that selectively binds RNA and the Tripure method involves a rapid guanidinium isothiocyanate-phenol-chloroform extraction. We found the Tripure isolation method resulted in high quality, undegraded total RNA from *D. magna* (Fig. 1), while the RNeasy method was more variable. The appearance of two ribosomal RNA bands indicates minimal degradation of the RNA and the underlying smear contains mRNA fragments. Only a single *D. magna* is necessary to obtain sufficient RNA for multiple ddPCR assays. We chose to pool ten *D. magna* in order to provide ample amounts of RNA and to control for animal to animal variability in response to a test chemical. In preliminary experiments we found that there was no significant change in the profile generated in pools ranging from 5-20 animals (data not shown). Following extraction, total RNA was first reverse transcribed to generate cDNA and then the cDNA was PCR amplified. Reverse transcription followed standard protocols. RNA (1 μg) was incubated for 1 hour at approximately 37°C with 20 U MMLV-reverse transcriptase, 25 U RNasin (MBI Fermentas Inc.), 1 μL dNTPs (25 mM) and 1 μL of each primer (25 μM primers).

A key feature of this ddPCR analysis, however, is the use of arbitrary primers. These arbitrary primers anneal and extend from complementary sites contained within the RNA, yielding a subset of cDNA fragments of various sizes. The cDNA is then PCR amplified using the same pair of arbitrary primers. We selected six 18-mer arbitrary primers out of a variety available from Stratagene Corp. Different primer pair combinations were tested. For every RNA-arbitrary primer combination a control was included that did not contain RNA. Certain primer pairs resulted in amplification from negative controls (containing no added *D. magna* cDNA). This suggests that some primer sets may anneal to bacterial genomic DNA contaminants present in certain preparations of *Taq* DNA polymerase. Thus, various primer pairs were tested and pairs that successfully yielded cDNA without bands in the negative control were applied to subsequent ddPCR analysis.

For PCR amplification, 5 μL of the cDNA template (diluted 1:10) was used in 25 μL reactions containing the two arbitrary primers (1 μL each) and Ready-To-Go PCR Beads (Amersham Pharmacia Biotech Inc., Baie d'Urfe, Quebec). The PCR conditions were as follows: one cycle at low-stringency 1 min @ 94°C, 5 min @ 36°C, 5 min @ 72°C and 39 cycles at high stringency 1 min @ 94°C, 2 min @ 50°C and 2 min @ 72°C.

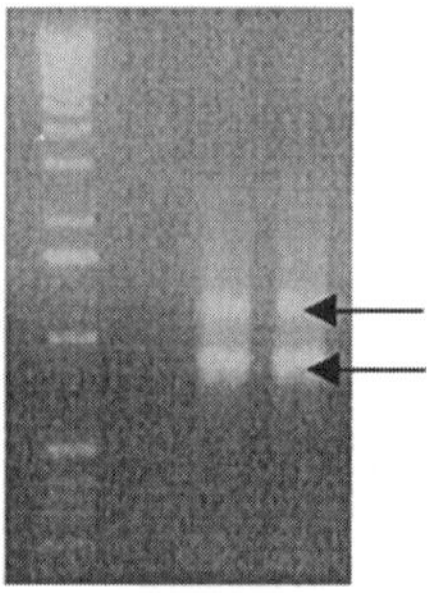

Figure 1-*Total RNA extracted from D. magna using Tripure. The arrows indicate the undegraded ribosomal RNAs.*

PCR was performed under mineral oil in a Perkin-Elmer thermocycler. The PCR products were subsequently purified in order to remove excess primer that might interfere with subsequent fluorescent labeling. Both Microcon (Amicon, Bedford, MA) and Qiagen PCR purification kits successfully removed excess primers.

Techniques for visualizing PCR products on electrophoresis gels using radioactive labeling are well established (Liang and Pardee 1992). However, disadvantages associated with the use of radioactivity include high disposal costs, safety hazards, and a requirement of substantial time for film or phosphorscreen exposure for detection. To address these issues we have developed a method that exploits the many novel fluorescent tags. Purified PCR products were incubated with a fluorescently labeled adapter primer, dNTPs, Klenow buffer and Klenow polymerase at 37°C for one hour. The adapter primer, labeled with Cy 5.0 (AGCT Inc.) contains a region that is complementary to a conserved region in all 6 arbitrary primers. This technique generates fluorescently tagged complementary strands (strategy illustrated in Fig. 2). The fluorescently tagged PCR products were then mixed 1:1 with a formamide loading buffer and separated on a 6% acrylamide-7 M urea denaturing sequencing gel prepared in 10x TBE buffer run at 1700 V, 55 W for 2 hours. PCR products were visualized using the red fluorescence mode on a Storm Imaging System (Molecular Dynamics Corp).

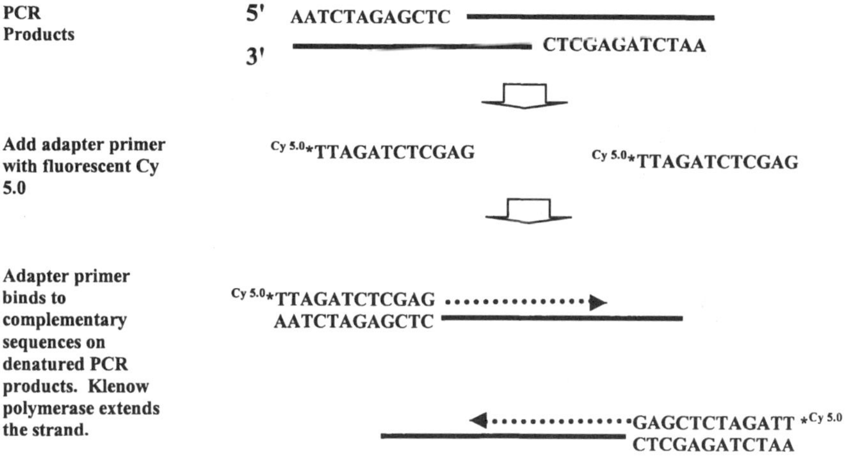

Figure 2-*PCR products are fluorescently tagged using an adapter primer that is labeled with Cy 5.0. PCR products are denatured and adapter primer is added. Fluorescently tagged complementary strands are generated.*

Results

In pilot experiments, ddPCR was first applied to the teleost fish, *Fundulus heteroclitus,* as this organism is frequently used in gene expression studies in our laboratory. Gene profiles for untreated fish were generated using arbitrary primer pairs as described above. Different primer pairs yielded distinct gene profiles as anticipated. Two different fingerprints generated by different primer pairs using *F. heteroclitus* RNA are shown (Fig. 3A). These fingerprints were accurately reproduced in separate PCR reactions as shown by similar profiles in lanes 1-4 and lanes 5-8.

Next, ddPCR was applied to *D. magna*. Different primer sets were tested and found to generate distinct gene profiles. *D. magna* profiles were accurately reproduced in triplicate ddPCR reactions using RNA extracted from different pools of 10 *D. magna* (Fig. 3B).

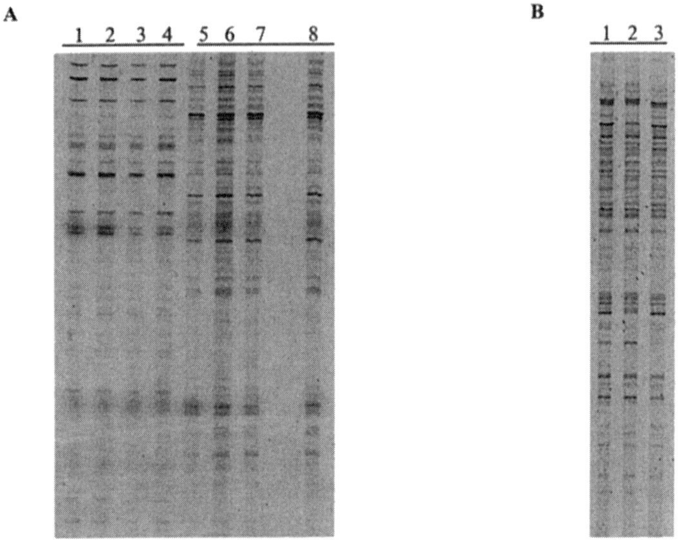

Figure 3-A: *PCR amplified cDNA from Fundulus heteroclitus separated using polyacrylamide gel electrophoresis. PCR products in lanes 1-4 were amplified using a different pair of primers than the PCR products seen in lanes 5-8. The different subset of cDNA fragments amplified by the different set of primers is evident.* B: *The cDNAs from three different pools of 10 D. magna were PCR amplified in separate reactions and yielded reproducible gene profiles.*

Following the production and validation of gene profiles for untreated organisms, profiles were generated for copper-treated *D. magna*. Organisms were exposed to 0.4 μM $CuSO_4$ for 24 hours and analyzed using ddPCR. Gene profiles can be compared between controls and copper-treated *D. magna* (Fig. 4). Bands that were different in only one lane were considered artefacts and were not used for subsequent analysis. Those bands that were consistent within a treatment, but which differed from controls were analyzed using peak height and/or area using densitometric software (ImageQuant, Molecular Dynamics Corp.). It is evident that copper exposure resulted in up-regulation of genes in *D. magna*. Up-regulated genes are represented by arrows on the left. Subsequent work will include identification of these differentially expressed genes by cloning and sequencing, as well as development of dose-response relationships between copper and gene expression in these organisms.

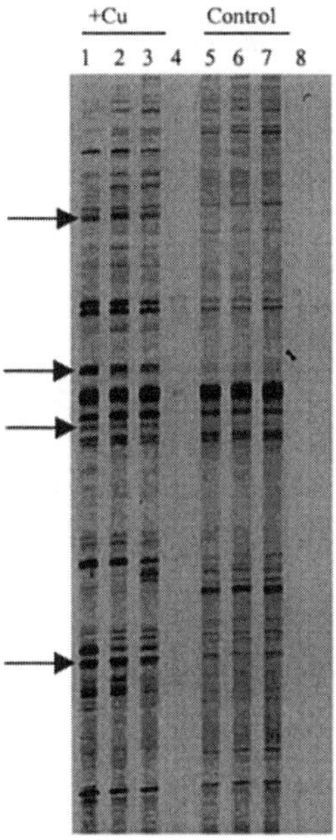

Figure 4-*PCR products for copper-exposed D. magna (lanes 1-3) and control organisms (lanes 5-7) separated using a polyacrylamide sequencing gel. Reverse transcription control (no RNA template) and PCR control (no cDNA template) are in lanes 4 and 8.*

Applications of ddPCR as a Bioindicator

A primary role of bioindicators is to provide early warning signals of exposure and adverse effects to toxicants. Although molecular bioindicators cannot replace the use of whole organism endpoints for risk assessment, monitoring changes at the mRNA level can provide a sensitive indication of exposure and adverse effects to toxicants. A bioindicator that could monitor many genes simultaneously would represent a useful ecotoxicological tool. Using ddPCR, gene induction profiles can be generated for organisms exposed to any given chemical. These fingerprints have great potential as bioindicators of exposure. Moreover, they further our understanding of the mechanisms of toxicant action by identifying the genes that are affected by toxicants. This technique has only recently been exploited in the field of environmental toxicology.

Using ddPCR, toxicant specific fingerprints have been generated for different species exposed to a range of toxicants. Several studies have used ddPCR to investigate the effects of various organic compounds on gene expression. For example, ddPCR was used to discover a novel gene that is regulated by the environmental contaminant 2,3,7,8-tetrachlorodibenzo-p-dioxin (TCDD) in mouse cells. This gene encodes ecto-ATPase and its induction requires both the aromatic hydrocarbon receptor (AhR) and the AhR nuclear translocator (Gao et al., 1998). In a similar manner, ddPCR was employed to detect altered gene expression in the soft-shell clam, *Mya arenaria*, exposed to [super(3)H]tetrachlorodibenzo-p-dioxin (Rhodes et al. 1997). Exposure to this compound results in tumor induction. Differentially expressed genes in *M. arenaria* tumors were identified that may have roles in signal transduction pathways (Van Beneden et al. 1996).

A variety of conventional methods have been used to show that exposure to metals also results in the induction of numerous genes, including those coding for MT, HSPs, and the antioxidant defense proteins, SOD, catalase and peroxidase (Lam et al. 1998, Murata et al. 1999, Sanders et al. 1994, Starcevic and Zielinkski 1997, Dalton et al. 1999, Jacob et al. 1999). ddPCR can be used to survey the genes induced by metal-exposure. Liao and Freeman (1998) surveyed the genes induced by cadmium exposure in the nematode, *Caenorhabditis elegans,* using ddPCR. Forty-nine cDNAs were identified, including those encoding metallothionien-1, HSP70, collagens, ribosomal RNAs, as well as numerous novel genes. Genes that are solely induced by a specific metal compound have also been identified using ddPCR. The Cap43 gene is involved in signaling pathways and is uniquely induced by exposure to nickel in human and rodent cell lines (Zhou et al. 1998). Similarly, genes involved in lead resistance have been identified using ddPCR (Rossman 1997).

Alterations in gene expression due to exposure to endocrine modulators have also been detected using ddPCR. While increased levels of vitellogenin mRNA are reported to be specific and reliable evidence of estrogenic contamination in the environment (Mellanen et al. 1999, Flouriot et al. 1996), other genes affected by 17-β-estradiol were identified in sheepshead minoows using ddPCR (Denslow et al. 1999). Certain phthalate compounds are also reported to have weak estrogenic activity in vitro (Jobling et al. 1995, Zacharewski et al. 1998), as well as being hepatocarcinogenic in rodents (Anderson et al. 1999). ddPCR has been used to investigate the effects of diethylhexyl phthalate (DEHP) on gene expression in rodent livers. Genes encoding the glucose-regulated protein (GRP58), and several acute-phase proteins were affected by DEHP exposure (Anderson et al. 1999, Muhlenkamp and Gill 1998). These applications of ddPCR have helped to elucidate the gene induction pathways that underlie disruption of endocrine systems.

Thus, ddPCR has been successfully used to identify genes altered by exposure to environmental contaminants in a variety of species. This, however, is the first reported application of ddPCR to *D. magna*. Having optimized ddPCR for *D. magna*, gene expression fingerprints can now be easily generated. The copper-specific gene profile did indicate altered gene expression when compared to control gene profiles. The specific genes that were altered by copper treatment can now be identified, enhancing our understanding of this organism's response to copper exposure. This represents a powerful tool for investigating the sublethal effects of any contaminant, such as metals, PAHs or polychlorinated biphenyls. Further, effective monitoring of the biological effects of cumulative mixtures may now be feasible as multiple gene expression changes can be detected. *D. magna's* rapid generation time facilitates measurements of whole organism endpoints such as inhibited growth or reproductive success. This is only the first step in the development of a gene fingerprinting tool that will provide a rapid and sensitive means of predicting whether a contaminant will have adverse effects. As with any biochemical or molecular bioindicator, field validation will be essential as organisms cultured in the laboratory are maintained under controlled conditions and often demonstrate limited genetic diversity. Future analysis will include an examination of *D. magna* sampled from the field in order to assess the variability in gene expression due to factors such as life stage and individual fitness. Ultimately, the changes in gene expression can then be linked to whole organism endpoints such as reproduction and growth. As understanding of gene function continues to grow, techniques such as ddPCR will only become increasingly useful in assessing the risk of contaminants in the environment.

References

Anderson, S. P., Cattley, R. C., and Corton, J. C., 1999, "Hepatic Expression of Acute-Phase Protein Genes During Carcinogenesis Induced by Peroxisome Proliferators," *Molecular Carcinogenesis,* Vol. 26, No. 4, pp. 226-238.

Dalton, T. P., Shertzer, H. G., and Puga, A., 1999, " Regulation of Gene Expression by Reactive Oxygen," *Annual Review in Pharmacology and Toxicology*, Vol. 39, pp. 67-101.

Denslow, N. D., Bowman, C. J., Robinson, G., Lee, H. S., Ferguson, R. J., Hemmer, M. J., and Folmar, L. C., 1999, "Biomarkers of Endocrine Disruption at the mRNA Level," *Environmental Toxicology and Risk Assessment, Vol. 8, STP 1364*, D. S. Henshel, M. C. Black, and M. C. Harrass, Eds., American Society for Testing and Materials, West Conshohocken, PA, pp. 24-35.

Diachenko, L. B., Ledesma, J., Chenchik, A. A., and Siebert, P. D., 1996, "Combining the Technique of RNA Fingerprinting and Differential Display to Obtain Differentially Expressed mRNA," *Biochemical and Biophysical Research Communications,* Vol. 219, pp. 824-828.

Flouriot, G., Pakdel, F., and Valotaire, Y., 1996, "Transcriptional and Post-Transcriptional Regulation of Rainbow Trout Estrogen Receptors and Vitellogenin Gene Expression," *Molecular and Cellular Endocrinology*, Vol. 124, pp. 173-83.

Gao, L., Dong, L., and Whitlock, Jr., J. P., 1998, "A Novel Response to Dioxin: Induction of Ecto-ATPase Gene Expression," *Journal of Biological Chemistry,* Vol. 273, No. 25, pp. 15358-15365.

Graf, D., Fisher, A. G., and Merkenschlager, M., 1997, "Rational Primer Design Greatly Improves Differential Display-PCR (DD-PCR)," *Nucleic Acids Research*, Vol. 25, No. 11, pp. 2239-2240.

Hightower, L., 1998, "The Promise of Molecular Biomarkers for Environmental Monitoring," *Biological Chemistry*, Vol. 379, pp. 1213-1215.

Huggett, R. J., Kimerle, R. A., Mehrle Jr., P. M., and Bergment, H. L., 1992, *Biomarkers: Biochemical, Physiological, and Histological Markers of Anthropogenic Stress*, Lewis Publishers, Boca Raton, Florida.

Jacob, S. T., Ghoshal, K., and Sheridan, J. F., 1999, "Induction of Mt by Stress and its Molecular Mechanisms," *Gene Expression*, Vol. 7, No. 4-6, pp. 301-310.

Jobling, S., Reynolds, T., White, R., Parker, M. G., and Sumpter, J. P., 1995, "A Variety of Environmentally Persistent Chemicals, Including Some Pthalate Plasticizers, are Weakly Estrogenic," *Environmental Health Perspectives*, Vol. 103, No. 6, pp. 582-587.

Liang, P. and Pardee, A. B., 1992, "Differential Display of Eukaryotic Messenger RNA by Means of the Polymerase Chain Reaction," *Science*, Vol. 257, No. 5072, pp. 967-971.

Liang, P., Averboukh, L., Keyomarsi, K., Sager, R., and Pardee, A. B., 1992, "Differential Display and Cloning of Messenger RNAs from Human Breast Cancer Versus Mammary Epithelial Cells," *Cancer Research*, Vol. 54, pp. 6966-6968.

Liao, V. H. and Freeman, J. H., 1998, "Cadmium-Regulated Genes from the Nematode *Caenorhabditis elegans*: Identification and Cloning of New Cadmium-Responsive Genes by Differential Display," *Journal of Biological Chemistry*, Vol. 273, No. 48, pp. 31962-31970.

Mathieu-Daude, F., Cheng, R., Welsh, J., and McClelland, M., 1996, "Screening of Differentially Amplified cDNA Products from RNA Arbitrarily Primed PCR Fingerprints Using Single Strand Conformation Polymorphisms (SSCP) Gels," *Nucleic Acids Research*, Vol. 24, No. 8, pp. 1504-1507.

Matz, M. V. and Lukyanov, S. A., 1998, "Different Strategies of Differential Display: Areas of Application," *Nucleic Acids Research*, Vol. 26, No. 24, pp. 5537-5543.

Mellanen, P., Soimasuo, M., Holmbom, B., Oikari, A., and Santii, R., 1999, "Expression of the Vitellogenin Gene in the Liver of Juvenile Whitefish (*Coregonus lavaretus*) Exposed to Effluents from Pulp and Paper Mills," *Ecotoxicology and Environmental Safety*, Vol. 43, No. 2, pp. 133-137.

Miele, G., MacRae, L., McBride, D., Manson, J., and Clinton, M., 1998, "Elimination of False Positives Generated Through PCR Re-Amplification of Differential Display cDNA," *BioTechniques*, Vol. 25, pp. 138-144.

Muhlenkamp, C. R., and Gill, S. S., 1998, "A Glucose-Regulated Protein, GRP58, is Down-Regulated in C57B6 Mouse Liver After Diethylhexyl Pthalate Exposure," *Toxicology and Applied Pharmacology*, Vol. 148, No. 1, pp. 101-108.

Murata, M., Gong, P., Suzuki, K., and Koizumi, S., 1999, "Differential Metal Response and Regulation of Human Heavy Metal-Inducible Genes," *Journal of Cell Physiology*, Vol. 180, pp. 105-113.

Nishio, Y., Aiello, L. P., and King, G. L., 1994, "Glucose Induced Genes in Bovine Aortic Smooth Muscle Cells Identified by mRNA Differential Display," *FASEB Journal*, Vol. 8, pp. 103-106.

Rhodes, L. D., Gardner, G. R., and Van Beneden, R. J., 1997, "Short-Term Tissue Distribution, Depuration and Possible Gene Expression Effects of [super(3)H]TCDD Exposure in Soft-Shell Clams (*Mya arenaria*)," *Environmental Toxicology and Chemistry*, Vol. 16, No. 9, pp. 1888-1894.

Rockett, J. C., Esdaile, D. J., and Gibson, G. G., 1999, "Differential Gene Expression in Drug Metabolism and Toxicology: Practicalities, Problems and Potential," *Xenobiotica*, Vol. 29, No. 7, pp. 655-691.

Rossman, T. G., 1997, "Lead Induced Gene Activation," Crisp Data Base National Institute of Health, Agency Project ID: 1R01ES08453-01.

Sanders, B. M., Martin, L. S., Howe, R., Nelson, W. G., Hegre, E. S., and Phelps, D. K., 1994, "Tissue-Specific Differences in Accumulation of Stress Proteins in *Mytilus edulis* Exposed to a Range of Copper Concentrations," *Toxicology and Applied Pharmacology*, Vol. 125, pp. 206-213.

Starcevic, S. L., and Zielinkski, B. S., 1997, "Neuroprotective Effects of Glutathione on Rainbow Trout Olfactory Receptor Neurons During Exposure to Copper Sulphate," *Comparative Biochemistry and Physiology*, Vol. 117C, pp. 211-219.

Utans, U., Liang, P., Wyner, L. R., Karnovsky, M. J., and Russell, M., 1994, "Chronic Cardiac Rejection: Identification of Five Upregulated Genes in Transplanted Hearts by Differential mRNA Display," *Proceedings of the National Academy of Science, USA*, Vol. 91, pp. 6463-6467.

Van Beneden, R. J., Rhodes, L. R., Brown, D. J., and Gardner, G. R., 1996, "Investigation of Molecular Mechanisms of Tumorigenesis in Bivalve Gonadal Tumors," *Journal of Shellfish Research*, Vol. 15, No. 2, p. 520.

Wang, J., Brown, C., and Trevor-Young, L., 1999, "Differential Display PCR Reveals Novel Targets for Mood-Stabilizing Drug Valproate Including the Molecular Chaperone GRP78," *Molecular Pharmacology*, Vol. 55, pp. 521-527.

Zhou, D., Salnikow, K., and Costa, M., 1998, "Cap43, a Novel Gene Specifically Induced by Ni Super(2+) Compounds," *Cancer Research,* Vol. 58, No. 10, pp. 2182-2189.

Zacharewski, T. R., Meek, M. D., Clemons, J. H., Wu, Z. F., Fielden, M. R., and Matthews, J. B., 1998, "Examination of the in Vitro and in Vivo Estrogenic Activities of Eight Commercial Phthalate Esters," *Toxicological Sciences*, Vol. 46, No. 2, pp. 282-293.

L. E. J. Lee,[1] T. Mann,[1] K. Pagniello,[1] I. Mikaelian,[2] and Y. de Lafontaine[3]

Examination of EROD Activity and Fibronectin Levels in Lake Whitefish as Biomarkers of Neoplasia

---

Reference: Lee, L. E. J., Mann, T., Pagniello, K., Mikaelian, I. and de Lafontaine, Y., "**Examination of EROD Activity and Fibronectin Levels in Lake Whitefish as Biomarkers of Neoplasia,**" *Environmental Toxicology and Risk Assessment: Science, Policy, and Standardization – Implications for Environmental Decisions: Tenth Volume, ASTM STP 1403*, B. M. Greenberg, R. N. Hull, M. H. Roberts, Jr., and R. W. Gensemer, Eds., American Society for Testing and Materials, West Conshohocken, PA, 2001.

Abstract: The study of tumors in fish has been hampered by the lack of suitable bioindicators especially because the ultimate diagnosis is not achieved until the fish are dead or killed. The present study was undertaken to develop simple, reliable and minimally invasive procedures to detect neoplasms in lake whitefish (*Coregonus clupeaformis*) and investigate their applicability as fish tumor biomarkers. Ethoxyresorufin-o-deethylase (EROD) assays have been widely used as an indicator of the activity of cytochrome P450-1A1, an isozyme located in a variety of tissues and in measurable amounts in the liver of many vertebrates. A fluorometric protocol using very small sized samples such as those from biopsies was used to measure EROD activity. Although no direct correlation could be made between EROD activity and liver tumor occurrence, EROD activity was significantly higher in livers with high melanomacrophage aggregates ($P<0.001$). Fibronectin (Fn) is a plasma and cellular protein that can be conveniently measured from biological fluids and has been used as tumor biomonitor in humans. Changes in Fn within serum and tissue samples of whitefish were monitored. Mean Fn levels in serum samples ($n=65$) was 2.03% of total serum proteins. Among the serologically evaluated fish, three had hepatic neoplasia as diagnosed by histological means. Fn levels in two of these were reduced at 1.89 and 1.22% of total serum proteins, however, no statistical correlations could be made with such small sample size, and further analysis is in progress.

Keywords: bioindicators, EROD, CytP450, fibronectin, neoplasia, lake whitefish

---

[1]Associate Professor and Honours Thesis Students, respectively, Department of Biology, Wilfrid Laurier University, Waterloo, Ontario, Canada N2L 3C5.

[2]Pathologist and Research Scientist, Canadian Cooperative Wildlife Health Centre, St. Hyacynthe, Quebec, Canada J2S 7C6.

[3]Research Scientist, Environmental Biology Section, Environment Canada, Montreal, Quebec, Canada H2Y 2E7.

Introduction

Lake whitefish, *Coregonus clupeaformis* are commercially valuable fish widely distributed throughout North America (Coad et al. 1995). They are abundant in the Great Lakes and the St. Lawrence River and its tributaries (Scott and Crossman 1973; Coad et al. 1995). Lake whitefish are among the top predators of the food chain amid the natural inhabitants of the St. Lawrence River. They are a benthivorous species and have a long life span (>30 years), thus water and sediment contaminants may bioaccumulate to critical levels affecting their health. Mikaelian et al. (1998) reported a high incidence of abnormalities in lake whitefish collected from the St. Lawrence near Quebec City, Canada in 1995, with a prevalence of hepatic tumors at 5% of the specimens sampled. No tumors were observed in other species caught at the same site which included channel catfish (*Ictalurus nebulosus*), longnose suckers (*Catostomus catostomus*) and white suckers (*Catostomus commersoni*). This high incidence of tumors in whitefish prompted further studies and the present report constitutes part of a long term project to develop a health monitoring program for various fish species, specifically to predict the incidence of neoplasia.

Environmental contamination by anthropogenic compounds is widespread and is associated with several ecotoxicological implications, including the occurrence of neoplasia in fish (Williams et al. 1998). Although, information about the relationship between contamination and biological response is complex, several conventional methods that measure the levels of contamination and the state of environmental health have been developed. Measuring concentrations of chemicals within organisms does not necessarily indicate the biological significance and biologically harmful concentrations may be below the levels of analytical detection. Even more, the concentration of pollutants in tissue has limited value because it is not well understood how tissue concentration relates to the toxic effect of a substance. Conventional toxicity tests which estimate LC_{50} and LD_{50}s do not account for bioaccumulation through the food chain or chemical speciation in the environment. Thus, traditional tests may not reflect true ecological systems. Biomarkers, on the other hand, although still being characterized (Travis 1993), reflect the "cumulative, synergistic, or antagonistic effect of a complex mixture of anthropogenic contaminants on biological systems" (Bucheli and Fent 1995) and several biomarkers have been developed to link contamination and biological response (Huggett et al. 1992; Timbrell 1998).

In humans and various other mammalian systems, biomarkers have been developed that could facilitate and speed up the detection of abnormalities and tumors with minimal discomfort in the organisms involved (Ghosh and Ghosh 1987; Kaiser 1989). Few efforts have been made in fish to develop simple biomarkers, and health diagnosis including cancer occurrence, are only made following death of the organisms and ulterior microscopical analysis of affected tissues. This is despite the fact that in fish, as in other vertebrates, carcinogen exposure through aquatic pollutants has been linked to incidence of cancers in recent years (Harshbarger and Clark 1990; Bunton 1996). The present study was undertaken to investigate possible fish health biomarkers using lake whitefish as a model system.

Cytochrome P450 as a Biomarker

There is overwhelming evidence that certain types of anthropogenic compounds such as planar aromatic hydrocarbons (PAHs) and organochlorine compounds like polychlorinated biphenyls (PCBs), certain pesticides and dioxins influence abnormal physiological and pathological effects such as immunological disturbances, effects on reproduction and development, and even neoplasms (Goksoyr and Husoy 1998). Many of these chemicals have also been shown to induce specific isozymes of cytochrome P450 (eg. CYP1A) (Bucheli and Fent 1995). Exposure to some of these toxicants leads to stimulation of the *CYP1A* gene and increased levels of the P450 isozymes. A common method to measure the catalytic activity of CYP1A is by quantification of ethoxyresorufin O-deethylase (EROD) activity (Stegeman et al. 1992). EROD activity is relatively simple to measure, which makes it advantageous as a biomarker. It has been suggested that the induction of P450 as measured by EROD, provides a sensitive biological response and may serve as an early warning system indicating the presence of organic pollutants (Bucheli and Fent 1995; Stegeman et al. 1992). Many laboratory and field experiments have shown a direct correlation between amount of contaminants and EROD activity. This response has been the basis for a sensitive biomonitoring tool of ecosystem health for a number of years (Williams et al. 1998), and many studies have documented a correlation between CYP1A induction, pollutant levels and tumor incidence, especially in benthivorous species. Thus this study investigated whether histologic lesions in whitefish could be correlated to enhanced EROD activity.

Fibronectin as a Biomarker

Fibronectin (Fn) is a large glycoprotein present in many tissues and body fluids (Mosher 1989). This protein exists in soluble and insoluble forms and has a multitude of biological functions. These include cell adhesion, morphology, migration, proliferation and differentiation, as well as phagocytosis, blood clotting, wound healing and metastasis (Hynes and Yamada 1982; Mosher 1989). Fn has been shown to be present throughout the animal kingdom from sea sponges to mammals (Akiyama and Johnson 1983), but studies of Fn in fish have been comparatively few. The presence or function of Fn in lake whitefish has not been previously reported.

Fn levels and distribution have been shown to change with disease in higher vertebrates (Proctor 1987; Carsons 1989) and Fn has been touted as a potential tumor marker for humans (Ylatupa et al. 1995). Aside from external tumors that are readily visible, the occurrence of internal tumors in fish are only diagnosed following necropsy and microscopic examination of the organs involved. Ulterior identification of tumors involves specialized histological and histochemical analysis (Boorman et al. 1997).

In the present study, the normal distribution of Fn in feral whitefish collected from the St. Lawrence River in 1996 is investigated using biochemical and immunological methods and relationships between EROD and Fn level changes to biological parameters of fish are assessed.

Materials and Methods

Sampling

Lake whitefish, *Coregonus clupeaformis* were collected from the St. Lawrence River at Saint Nicolas (46°43'N, 71°19'W), 15 km upstream from Quebec City, Canada, using fixed tidal traps in the fall of 1996. Fish were anesthetized with tricaine methanosulfonate (MS222) and physical parameters were recorded with special notation for gross morphological abnormalities. Blood samples were collected by heart puncture, plasma and serum samples were prepared by centrifugation and quickly frozen in liquid nitrogen after which they were stored at -80°C. Similarly, liver tissue samples were quickly frozen in liquid nitrogen and subsequently stored frozen at -80°C. Of over 500 fish collected, 65 samples were analyzed for serum Fn content, 60 for EROD assays and 21 for liver Fn distribution from cryostat sections. Samples of all major organs were fixed in formalin and routinely prepared for histopathology. Age was determined upon microscopic examination of one section of the otoliths.

EROD Assays

Liver microsomal fractions were prepared from 200 to 500 mg tissue samples following a modified protocol described in Clemons et al. (1996) for microsomal preparation from fish cells. The microsomal fractions were then evaluated for ethoxy-rerufin-O-deethylase activity (EROD). The conversion of 7-ethoxyresurufin to the fluorescent molecule resorufin was detected using an automated microplate fluorescence reader (Cytofluor) following a modification of the protocol described by Lee et al. (1993) and further refined in Clemons et al. (1996) for EROD activity in fish liver cells.

Immunoscreening

Dot blotting in nitrocellulose membranes (Bio Rad, Richmond, CA) was used for preliminary testing of immunoreactive antisera. Two microlitres of each antigen was applied to the membranes cut in strips and allowed to dry. Antigens included lake whitefish serum samples, bovine Fn (Sigma, St. Louis, MO) and rainbow trout plasma. The antigen blotted strips were then washed three times with 0.01% Tween-20 in phosphate buffered saline (PBS) (Sigma) and were blocked with a 3% non fat dry milk in PBS overnight. Each membrane was then transferred to a diluted antisera at 1:100, 1:500 and 1:1000 in PBS for 1 to 6 h depending on the dilution in a sealed 10 mL vial. Primary antiserum controls included normal rabbit serum (NRS), normal goat serum (NGS), and pre-immune rabbit serum. Various anti-Fns tested included commercially purchased anti-human Fn generated in rabbits from Sigma, Calbiochem (San Diego, CA) and UBI (Lake Placid, NY), anti-bovine Fn from rabbit (Calbiochem) and anti-human Fn developed in goat (Sigma). Two anti-fish Fn were also tested: anti-trout Fn (Miller et al. 2000) and anti-salmon Fn. The latter was prepared from plasma of Pacific salmon

(*Oncorhynchus tschawitscha*) (courtesy of Stephen Rafferty, Nanaimo Biological Station, BC) following a protocol similar to that reported for anti-trout Fn. Subsequent to the incubation with the various antisera, the membranes were washed three times with 0.01% Tween-20 in PBS, and two additional washes that included soaking the membranes in the wash for 5 min each. All the membranes were then transferred to an appropriate peroxidase-labeled secondary antibody diluted 1:1000 with PBS and incubated for 3 h. Membranes were extensively washed and developed using Bio Rad Immuno Blot Assay kit as indicated by manufacturer.

Purification of Whitefish Plasma Fibronectin

Whitefish Fn was purified by gelatin affinity chromatography from whitefish plasma following a similar procedure to that described for rainbow trout Fn (Lee and Bols 1991). The isolated whitefish plasma Fn was lyophilized using a Speedvac concentrator (Savant, Hicksville, NY) and stored at -20°C. Purity was tested by gel electrophoresis and immunoblotting.

Gel Electrophoresis and Fn Quantification

Sample polypeptides were separated in 5, 7.5 or 10% SDS-PAGE and run on Mini-Protean II electrophoretic systems (Bio Rad). Purified Lake whitefish Fn and serum samples were mixed with sample buffer (0.5M Tris, glycerol, SDS, beta-mercaptoethanol and bromophenol blue) and equivalent protein (in 10 μL volume) was loaded into the gel wells. A prestained molecular weight standard (Bio-Rad, Kaleidoscope Prestained Standards) was run along with the serum samples for molecular weight calibration. The standard contained myosin, beta-galactosidase, bovine serum albumin, carbonic anhydrase, soybean trypsin inhibitor, lysozyme and aprotinin (molecular weights ranging from 7,000-200,000 daltons). Protein bands were visualized after 30 min staining with 0.1% Coomassie Blue (Bio Rad) in 40% methanol and 10% acetic acid and destaining overnight in a solution containing 5% methanol and 10% acetic acid. For quantification, the gels were scanned using a computing densitometer (Molecular Dynamics, Sunnyvale, CA). Protein bands were then analyzed using ImageQuant software (Molecular Dynamics) and the percent Fn was determined relative to the total protein content per lane.

Western Blotting

Proteins separated by SDS-PAGE were transferred into nitrocellulose for approximately one hour at 10-20 V using a semi-dry electrophoretic transfer unit (Bio Rad). Immunodetection for Fn was performed as described for the immunoscreening protocol using various anti-Fn antisera. The remaining proteins in the transferred gels were stained with Coomassie blue to test for efficiency of transfer.

Protein Assay

Lake whitefish serum samples were diluted 1:40 with sterile distilled water for protein quantitation. Bovine serum albumin (BSA) standards (Pierce, Rockford, IL) were prepared from 25 to 2000 μg/mL. Ten μL of each sample, standards and a water blank were added in duplicates to a 96 well plate (Nunc, Roskilde, Denmark). A bicinchoninic acid (BCA) protein assay kit (Pierce) was used for the color reaction. Absorbance at 550 nm was read using a microplate reader (Bio-Rad). The total protein content for each sample was determined from the standard curve after correcting for the dilution factor.

Immunocytochemical Detection of Fn in Liver Sections of Lake Whitefish

Frozen liver sections were cut at a thickness of 8 to 10 μm with a cryostat (Ames LabTek Microtome Cryostat, Elkhart, IN) at -20°C. A Histostain SP kit (Zymed, CA) was used for immunochemical staining. Essentially, the slides were incubated first with a serum blocking solution for 10 min at room temperature in a humidified chamber. Following removal of the blocking solution, the slides were exposed to a 1:1000 dilution in PBS of the various antisera or control NRS or an irrelevant sera, anti-chum salmon vitellogenin (gift from Dr. Sullivan, NCSU). Following 60 min incubation in a humidified chamber, slides were washed twice with 0.05% Tween-PBS (T-PBS) and exposed to a biotinilated secondary antibody from the kit for 10 min. After further washes with T-PBS, sections were incubated for 10 min with peroxidase labelled streptavidin. After another two washes with T-PBS, slides were exposed to the chromogen substrate (3-amino-ethylcarbazole) for 10 min at room temperature. Sections were then washed and counterstained with hematoxylin for 3-5 min. After final rinses with deionized water, the slides were mounted with a glycerol vinyl alcohol mounting media and observed by light microscopy. Each immunostained liver was subjectively rated for intensity of immunostaining by the following criteria: (-) no visible staining, (+) minimal staining/light pink, (++) moderate staining/dark pink to red, (+++) intense staining/brigth to dark red.

Statistical Analysis

InStat, v. 2.01 (GraphPad, San Diego, CA) was used for statistical analysis. An initial assumption for linear correlations was made to compare relationships between physiological parameters and EROD activity or Fn content. Analysis of variance (ANOVA) tests at the 95% confidence level were used and P values equal or less than 0.05 were considered significant. ANOVA tests were done on those relationships where the linear regression gave an $R^2 > 0.1$. When a graph's linearity was in doubt, a runs test was performed (InStat). This involved counting the number of points above and below the line as well as the number of runs. If the data deviates substantially from linearity, the number of runs will be small. A P value less than 0.05 for this test indicates significance and therefore a departure from linearity.

Results

EROD and Whitefish Biotic Parameters

Whitefish biotic parameters such as weight, length, age, gonado-somatic index (GSI) (gonadal weight /body weight), liver-somatic index (LSI) (liver weight/body weight) and results from histological analysis (data to be reported elsewhere) were compared to EROD activity values obtained for 60 fish and Fn values obtained for 65 fish. The 65 fish sampled varied in age and size. The age ranged from 5-17 years and the average length and body weight were 473.26 mm and 770.37 grams. No significant correlations were obtained for most of the evaluated parameters, however, significant inverse correlations were noted for EROD values compared to LSI ($P<0.01$) (Fig. 1) for both sexes and GSI for females ($P<0.001$) (Fig. 2). EROD values were also positively correlated to incidence of melano-macrophage aggregates in the liver ($P<0.001$) (Fig. 3).

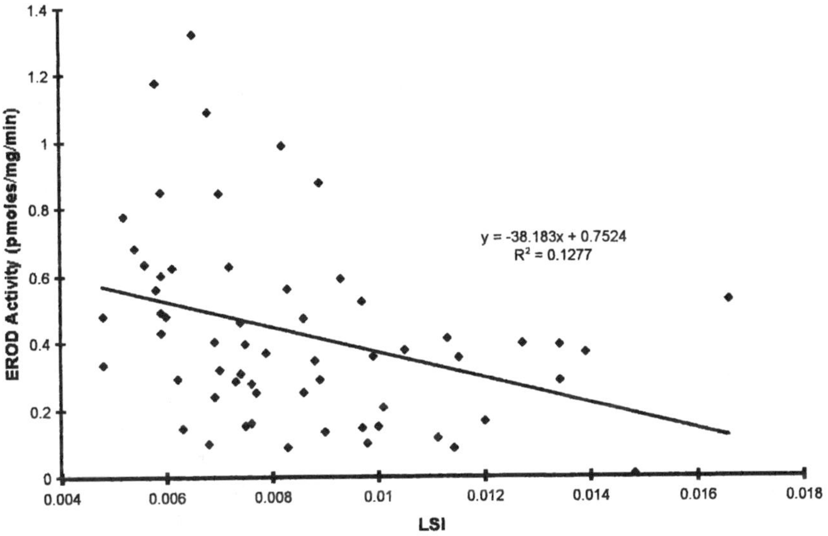

Figure 1 *Relationship between Liver Somatic Index and Hepatic EROD Activity in Lake Whitefish. A comparison between the LSI (Liver Somatic Index) of both sexes and hepatic EROD activity in whitefish (n=60) suggests an inverse linear correlation with an* R^2 *value of 0.1277. An ANOVA gives a P value of 0.0051 indicating the relationship is very significant and the slope is different from zero. A runs test was used to verify the relationship is linear. The P value for this test was 0.0938 which is not quite significant so the relationship can be considered linear.*

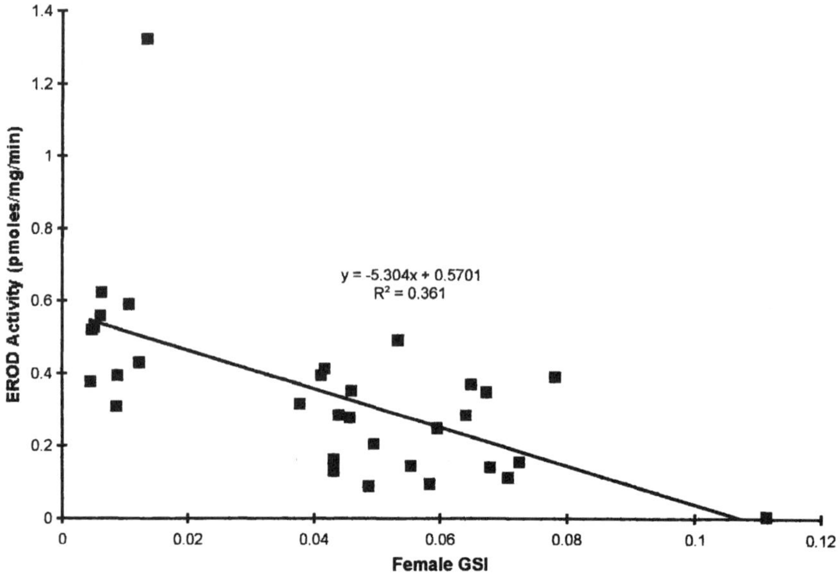

Figure 2 *Relationship Between Female Gonadosomatic Index and Hepatic EROD Activity in Lake Whitefish. There is an inverse linear correlation between female gonadosomatic index (n = 32) and hepatic EROD activity. The R^2 value is 0.3610 and the P value is 0.0003 suggesting that the slope is extremely significant and is not zero. A runs test with a P value of 0.6525 indicates that the relationship is linear.*

Fibronectin Detection in Lake Whitefish

In order to identify antisera with affinity for lake whitefish Fn, various commercial anti mammalian Fn and two anti-fish Fn were tested by dot blotting. Immunoreactions were detected and described by the intensity of the color observed after developing for the peroxidase label. The NRS, NGS, and the pre immune sera from rabbits injected with fish Fn did not give any immunological reaction with any samples tested. Anti-human Fn UBI (A), Sigma (B) and anti-bovine Fn from Calbiochem (C) reacted with bovine Fn (bFn). The only commercial anti-human Fn that had a reaction with Fn in whitefish serum samples and trout plasma was from Sigma (B). The anti-human Fn generated in goat (Sigma) and anti human Fn (Calbiochem) did not recognize any of the Fns in the serum samples or standards. Anti-cellular trout Fn (E51) recognizes trout and whitefish serum Fn but the immunoreaction is weak compared to anti plasma salmon Fn (E52). E52 and B generated the strongest immunoreactions among all antisera tested and were used for subsequent detections.

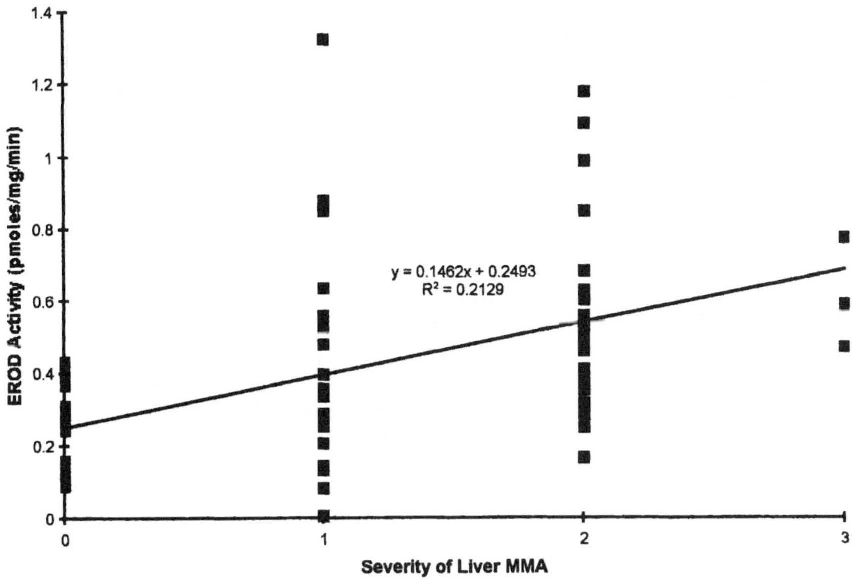

Figure 3 *Correlation Between Hepatic EROD Activity and the Severity of Liver Melano-macrophage Aggregates. Hepatic EROD activity is positively correlated to the severity of liver melano-macrophage aggregates (MMA) in males and females combined. The occurrence of MMA was rated on a scale of 0 to 3 with a value of 0 indicating MMA is rarely present in histological sections, and increasing to 3 where liver MMA accounted for more than 20% of the liver section. The R^2 value for this positive linear correlation is 0.2129 while the P value is 0.0002 which makes the relationship extremely significant. A runs test gave a P value of 0.0752 which is not quite significant, indicating linearity.*

Purification and Characterization of Whitefish Fn

Lake whitefish Fn was isolated from plasma by gelatin affinity chromatography (Fig. 4a). The amount of Fn in the eluate plasma (lane B) is noticeably less than that of the plasma (lane A). The Fn bands (lanes D and E) are positioned at a slightly higher molecular weight than the 200 kD (MW) standard. Lake whitefish Fn appears slightly heavier in molecular weight than the commercial bovine Fn (Sigma) standard (not shown) of 220 kD.

The purification only isolated one of the subunits of Fn indicated by one distinct band. Fn appears as two subunits in SDS-PAGE represented by the doublet banding pattern at approximately 220 kD (Fig. 4b). This was confirmed by western blots with anti-Fn antibodies (data not shown). The remaining lanes illustrate the occurrence of Fn in various serum samples of lake whitefish. Levels of each subunit varied among the sampled fish.

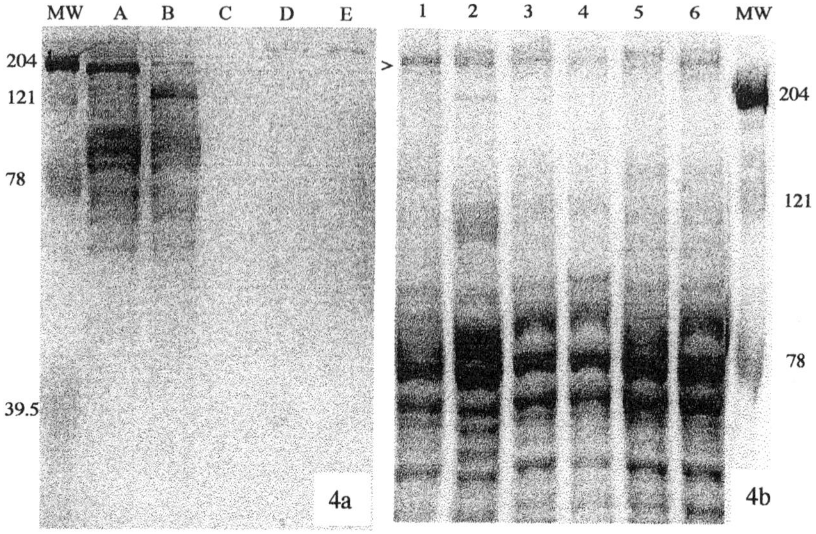

Figure 4 *Purification and Characterization of Lake Whitefish Fn.* (4a) *10% SDS-PAGE depicting whitefish plasma profile and gelatin-affinity column eluates. MW indicates lane with molecular weight standards indicated by numbers on the left. LaneA. Lake whitefish plasma profile. Lane B. Plasma eluted through affinity column, note reduction in band intensity around 220 kD. Lane C. Wash through affinity column, note absence of proteins. Lanes D, E. Primary and secondary eluates containing the Fn fractions from affinity column, note absence of proteins other than band at 220 kD.* (4b) *7.5% SDS-PAGE serum profiles from six lake whitefish. Fn which appear as doublets around 220 kD is indicated by (>). Note that levels of individual subunits vary among sampled fish.*

Quantification of Lake Whitefish Serum Fn Levels

There were variations in the levels of Fn and total protein content in the serum of the whitefish sampled. Most of the fish sampled had Fn serum levels ranging from 0-3 % of total serum proteins, with most individuals concentrated in the 1-3 % range (Fig. 5). Mean Fn levels in serum samples (n=65) was 2.03% of total serum proteins. The observed Fn levels range from as low as 0.040 to 7.050 %. The total protein content in the serum of the fish sampled ranged from 9.49mg/mL to 76.53mg/mL with most fish having levels between 30-50mg/mL. The mean total serum protein content of the fish sampled was 39.50mg/mL. The percent Fn of each individual fish was not correlated to their total serum protein content.

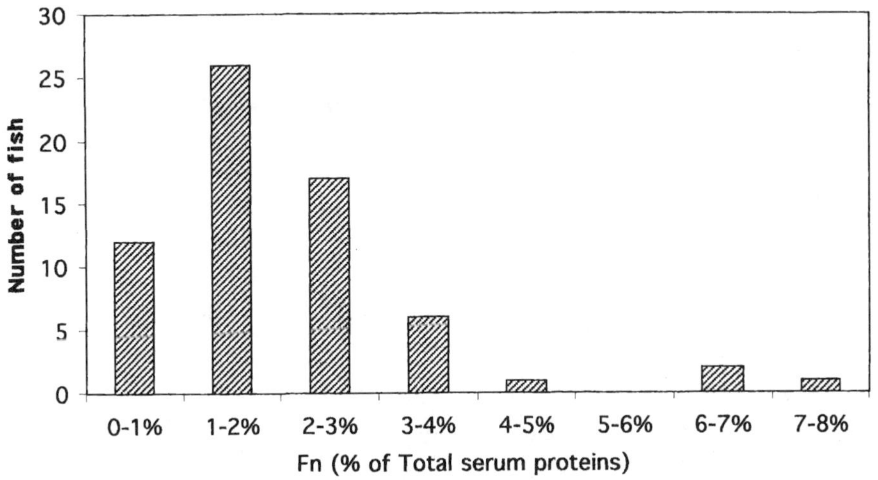

Figure 5 *Distribution of Fn Levels Among Sampled Lake Whitefish. Serum Fn levels expressed as % of total serum proteins obtained by densitometric quantification is plotted in one percent increment groups.*

Correlations of Fn Levels and Distribution to Whitefish Biotic Parameters

There was no relation between the age, length or body weight and the serum Fn levels of the fish sampled. No correlation could be drawn between EROD and Fn levels among the examined 42 fish that overlapped for both measurements. This lack of relationship was also noted for the other parameters investigated including gonado-somatic and liver-somatic indices. However, the immunostaining of Fn in livers with tumors showed a clustered occurrence in those with decreased Fn staining (Table 1). Fn staining was generally decreased in liver areas with tumors. This correlated with decreased serum Fn levels observed in two of three fish with tumors evaluated for Fn levels which were 1.89 and 1.22% of total serum proteins. Fn distribution in livers was mainly restricted to the liver stroma with strong positive staining for Fn using anti-human Fn (B) and anti-salmon Fn (E52). Fn appeared red among the collagenous fibers of the extracellular matrix surrounding bile ducts and blood vessels (not shown). Fn could also be seen in scattered punctate form around hepatocytes and fibroblasts within the hepatic lobules. Among the 21 liver samples examined histologically for Fn distribution, not all stained for Fn and the intensity of staining also varied, even though the irrelevant anti-vitellogenin was generally positive for female livers.

Table 1 *Occurrence of liver neoplasms and correlation to intensity of Fn staining. A subsample of 21 livers of which 7 had been diagnosed to have liver tumors (data to be presented elsewhere) were processed for Fn immunostaining. Samples containing tumors clustered among those with low Fn staining.*

Whitefish Sample No.	Sex	Liver tumors	Intensity of staining with anti-hFn
124	M	-	-
130	M	-	-
214	F	-	-
221	F	Cholangiocarcinoma	-
466	F	Hepatocellular carcinoma	-
96	M	-	+
40	M	Cholangioma	+
69	M	Cholangiocarcinoma	+
3	M	Cholangiocarcinoma	+
82	M	Cholangiocarcinoma	+
107	F	-	+
113	M	Hepatocellular carcinoma	+
212	F	-	+
90	F	-	++
407	M	-	++
112	F	-	++
204	M	-	++
56	M	-	+++
115	M	-	+++
118	M	-	+++
129	F	-	+++

Discussion

Species differences in response to xenobiotics has been reported (reviewed by Lewis et al. 1998). It is possible that some species of fish are more sensitive to xenobiotic chemicals than others, which could make them better biomonitors of contamination. Lake whitefish could be sensitive biomonitors as they show differential tissue accumulation to pollutants. Mikaelian et al. (1997) reported that several contaminants, such as polychlorinated biphenyls, occurred in higher concentrations in lake whitefish compared to other species, such as channel catfish, white suckers and walleye, collected in 1995 from the same site on the St. Lawrence River. As well, laboratory exposure to TCDD in juvenile whitefish and trout showed whitefish to have greater assimilation efficiency of the toxicant and be more sensitive than trout in terms of EROD response which could be induced faster and at lower toxicant levels (Fisk et al. 1997). This may be more so because of the bottom-dwelling behavior of whitefish that may predispose them to higher levels of persistent pollutants which tend to accumulate in sediments.

Xenoestrogens have been shown to modulate enzymes of cytochrome P450 and suggestions have been made for their potential use as bioindicators of carcinogenesis (reviewed by Williams et al. 1998). Most studies have been performed with the trout as a model system, and comparatively fewer studies have been reported with whitefish despite their economical importance. The present study suggests the use of EROD activity as bioindicator for abnormalities in whitefish. An inverse correlation between EROD activity and liver somatic index was seen as well as with female gonadosomatic index. Whyte et al. (1998) found a similar correlation between hepatic EROD activity and liver mass in Lake trout. Munkittrick et al. (1994) showed a decrease in gonadal size for white suckers in the presence of higher concentrations of contaminants. This may correlate to the present study since an increase in contaminants usually causes an increase in EROD activity which would then be associated with a decrease in gonadal size.

An increase in pigmented macrophage aggregates with exposure to contaminants has been observed (Couillard and Hodson 1996) and suggestions have been made as to the usefulness of monitoring the occurrence of these pigment aggregates or melanomacrophages as biomarkers of immune function, and thus of contaminant exposure (Blazer et al. 1997). Couillard and Hodson (1996) have suggested the presence of macrophage aggregates can be a particularly useful indicator of bleached-kraft mill effluent (BKME) exposure. EROD activity has also been a useful marker of exposure to BKME (Kloepper-Sams and Benton 1994; Kloepper-Sams et al. 1994; Soimasuo et al. 1998). Thus the present observation of increasing EROD to severity of MMA correlates well with these findings. Couillard and Hodson (1996) have proposed a mechanism linking CYP1A induction to pigmented macrophage aggregate proliferation. They suggest that the induction of CYP1A can cause oxidant damage to cellular membranes by generating superoxide ions or generating electrophiles. This can result in an increased rate of cell death or lipid peroxidation of the cellular membranes to yield lipofuscin. Lipofuscin can then accumulate within the MMA and lead to the proliferation of MMAs.

Couillard and Hodson (1996) also suggest that enhanced density of pigmented macrophage aggregates may be associated with a higher frequency of neoplasms. This may be because CYP1A induction in the liver can cause bioactivation of carcinogens that lead to altered hepatocytes (preneoplastic lesions), adenomas and eventually hepatocellular carcinomas. Their study found that both EROD activity and proliferation of MMAs were associated with exposure to higher concentrations of BKME in mirror carp and there was no correlation to preneoplastic lesions (Couillard and Hodson 1996).

The presence of hepatic EROD activity is not in itself indicative of contamination. As mentioned earlier, cytochrome P450 is responsible for the metabolism of several natural hormones, including estradiol (Bucheli and Fent 1995). This means it is important to understand the seasonal changes in EROD activity before interpreting the data (Levine et al. 1995). Other environmental variables such as pH, temperature, and nutrition can play a role in the induction of cytochrome P450 in different species of fish (Andersson and Nilsson 1989; Jimenez et al. 1988) and should be taken into consideration.

Immunological Detection and Role of Fn in Whitefish

The availability of suitable antibodies and tissue preparation, limit the qualitative detection of antigens in immunohistochemical procedures. This study indicates that a fibronectin-like material in whitefish serum and liver tissues cross reacted against anti-salmon Fn, as well as with anti-human Fn. This cross reactivity illustrates the similarity of Fn from various species and thus its conservation through evolution (Akiyama and Johnson 1983) and agrees with similar findings of Fn cross rectivity such as that reported by Wright (1986) for lamprey and hagfish Fn with anti-human Fn. Antibodies to whitefish Fn should be prepared and tested to confirm these results, even though animal Fns are known to share immunological determinants and cross react with heterologous Fn antisera (Gomez-Lechon and Castell 1985).

Fn was isolated by gelatin affinity chromatography and shows similar characteristics to mammalian Fn, although the affinity to gelatin may differ among the subunits. Lake whitefish serum Fn is composed of two similar molecular weight subunits, approximately 220 kD which is typical of plasma Fn from many species under the reducing conditions of SDS-PAGE. However, following affinity chromatography only a singlet could be seen rather than the doublet seen in whole sera as was visualized by SDS-PAGE and Western blotting. As various forms of Fn have been reported to occur in higher vertebrates (Hynes and Yamada 1982), and at least two forms of plasma Fn were reported in carp (Uchida et al. 1992), it is advisable that a study be performed in detecting the various types of Fn that might occur in whitefish.

Levels of Fn in serum samples were quantified by densitometric scanning of electrophoretically separated proteins. Fn levels varied in the sera of the fish sampled ranging from as low as 0.040 to 7.050% of total serum proteins, with a mean of 2.03% which is in agreement with reported Fn concentrations for other vertebrates (Gomez-Lechon and Castell 1985). No definite correlations could be made between changes in Fn levels and total protein content, gender, age, size, gonado-somatic index or other physiological state, although, serum samples from two of three fish with hepatic tumors evaluated for serologic Fn levels, showed decreased Fn levels compared to average values. However, the evaluated sample size was too small and further fish are currently being evaluated. The above findings contrast to human studies in which changes in Fn levels had been shown to modulate with sex, age and some physiological states (Proctor 1987; Carsons 1989). There are no reported correlations of Fn levels documented in fish to support any of these findings and further studies are needed.

Changes in circulating Fn levels may be location specific and may not be represented by fluctuations in serum Fn. Analysis of Fn distribution in 21 livers by immuno-cytochemistry shows a clustered occurrence of liver neoplasms in those with decreased Fn staining intensity. This agrees with neoplasm studies in humans were decreased Fn had been observed (Carsons 1989), which may allow cells to detach and metastasize, as Fn's main role is that of cell adhesion (Hynes and Yamada 1982). This observation is of value for the development of Fn as a tumor biomarker in fish and further studies are underway.

Conclusions

Changes in EROD activity in Lake whitefish, *C. clupeaformis*, correlated with some biotic parameters that could also be indicators of contaminant exposure, namely LSI and GSI in females. Additionally, increased MMA correlated with increased EROD activity which further validates the usefulness of EROD as was described for many other vertebrates. However, further sample analysis is required to correlate changes in EROD activity and health abnormalities including neoplasms. Another bioindicator could be Fn, and for the first time, Fn was detected in Lake whitefish serum by immunoreactivity against various Fn anti-sera and purified by affinity chromatography. The characteristics of this molecule correspond to those reported for other vertebrate's Fn.
Preliminary results indicate variable levels of Fn in the serum samples analyzed but mean levels correspond to those reported for other vertebrates. Although no direct correlation was found between changes in Fn levels and occurence of tumors, the low staining intensity of tissues with hepatic tumors as seen in immunostained sections suggests a possible role of Fn as a biomarker of tumors in fish.

Acknowledgments

This project was funded in part by an operating grant from the Natural Sciences and Engineering Research Council of Canada to LEJL. We thank the Science and Technology Endowment Program (STEP) funded by science students from WLU for partial support with TM's work. Special thanks to Dr. NC Bols (Biology, U. of Waterloo) for use of the Cytofluor.

References

Akiyama, S. K. and Johnson, M. D., 1983, "Fibronectin in Evolution: Presence in Invertebrates and Isolation from *Microciona prolifera*," *Comparative Biochemistry and Physiology*, Vol. 76B, pp. 687-694.

Andersson, T. and Nilsson, E. 1989, "Characterization of Cytochrome P-450-Dependent Activities in Hagfish, Dogfish, Perch and Spectacle Caiman," *Comparative Biochemistry and Physiology*, Vol. 94B, pp. 99-105.

Blazer, V. S., Fournie, J. W. and Weeks-Perkins, B. A., 1997, "Macrophage aggregates: biomarker for immune function in fishes," *Environmental Toxicology and Risk Assessment: Modeling and Risk Assessment: Sixth Volume, ASTM STP 1317*. F. J. Dwyer, T. R. Doane, and M. L. Hinman, Eds. American Society for Testing and Materials, West Conshohocken, PA.

Boorman, G. A., Botts, S., Bunton, T. E., Fournie, J. W., Harshbarger, J. C., Hawkins, W. E., Hinton, D. E., Jokinen, M. P., Okihiro, M. S. and Wolfe, M. J., 1997, "Diagnostic Criteria for Degenerative, Inflammatory, Proliferative Nonneoplasyic and Neoplastic Liver Lesions in Medaka (*Oryzias latipes*): Consensus of a National Toxicology Program Pathology Working Group," *Toxicology Pathology*, Vol. 25, pp. 202-210.

Bucheli, T. D. and Fent, K., 1995, "Induction of Cytochrome P450 as a Biomarker for Environmental Contamination in Aquatic Ecosystems," *Critical Reviews in Environmental Science and Technology*, Vol. 25, No. 3, pp. 201-268.

Bunton, T. E., 1996, "Experimental Chemical Carcinogenesis in Fish," *Toxicologic Pathology*, Vol. 24, pp. 603-618.

Carsons, S. E., 1989, "Fibronectin in Health and Disease," CRC Press, Boca Raton, FL.

Clemons, J. H., Lee, L. E. J., Myers, C. R., Dixon, D. G. and Bols, N. C., 1996, "Cytochrome P450 1A1 Induction by Polychlorinated Biphenyls (PCBs) in Liver Cell Lines from Rat and Trout and the Derivation of Toxic Equivalency Factors," *Canadian Journal of Fisheries and Aquatic Sciences*, Vol. 53, pp. 1177-1185

Coad, B. W., Wasczuk, H. and Labignon, I., 1995, "Encyclopedia of Canadian Fishes," *Canadian Museum of Nature*, Singapore, pp. 386-388.

Couillard, C. M. and Hodson, P. V., 1996, "Pigmented Macrophage Aggregates: A Toxic Response in Fish Exposed to Bleached-Kraft Mill Effluent?," *Environmental Toxicology and Chemistry*, Vol. 15, pp. 1844-1854.

Fisk, A. T., Yarechewski, A. L., Metner, D. A., Evans, R. E., Lockhart, W. L. and Muir, D. C., 1997, "Accumulation, Depuration and Hepatic Mixed-Function Oxidase Enzyme Induction in Juvenile Rainbow Trout and Lake Whitefish Exposed to Dietary 2,3,7,8-Tetrachlorodibenzo-*p*-dioxin," *Aquatic Toxicology*, Vol. 37, pp. 201-220.

Ghosh, B. C. and Ghosh, L., 1987, "Tumor Markers and Tumor Associated Antigens," McGraw-Hill Book Co. NY.

Goksoyr, A. and Husoy, A. M., 1998, "Immunochemical Approaches to Studies of CYP1A Localization and Induction by Xenobiotics in Fish," *EXS*, Vol. 86, pp. 165-202.

Gomez-Lechon, M. J. and Castell, J. V., 1985, "Enzyme-Linked Immunosorbent Assay to Quantify Fibronectin," *Analytical Biochemistry*, Vol. 145, pp. 1-8.

Harshbarger, J. C. and Clark, J. B., 1990, "Epizootiology of Neoplasms in Bony Fish of North America," *Science of the Total Environment*, Vol. 94, pp. 1-32.

Huggett, R.J., Kimerle, R.A., Mehrle, P.M., and Bergman, H.L, 1992, "Biochemical, Physiological, and Histological Markers of Anthropogenic Stress," Society of Environmental Toxicology and Chemistry (SETAC) Inc., Lewis Publishers, Boca Raton, FL.

Hynes, R. O. and Yamada, K. M., 1982, "Fibronectins: Multifunctional Modular Glycoproteins," *Journal of Cell Biology*, Vol. 95, pp. 369-77.

Jimenez, B. D., Burtis, L. S., Ezell, G. H., Egan, B. Z., Lee, N. E., Beauchamp, J. J. and McCarthy, J. F., 1988, "The Mixed Function Oxidase System of Bluegill Sunfish, *Lepomis macrochirus*: Correlation of Activities in Experimental and Wild Fish?," *Environmental Toxicology and Chemistry*, Vol. 7, pp. 623-634.

Kaiser H. E., 1989, "Comparative Aspects of Tumor Development," Kluwer Academic Publishers, Netherlands.

Kloepper-Sams, P. J. and Benton, E., 1994, "Exposure of Fish to Biologically Treated Bleached-Kraft Effluent. 2. Induction of Hepatic Cytochrome P4501A in Mountain

Whitefish (*Prosopium williamsoni*) and Other Species," *Environmental Toxicology and Chemistry,* Vol. 13, pp. 1483-1496.

Kloepper-Sams, P. J., Swanson, S. M., Marchant, T., Schryer, R. and Owens, J. W., 1994, "Exposure of Fish to Biologically Treated Bleached-Kraft Effluent. 1. Biochemical, Physiological and Pathological Assessment of Rocky Mountain Whitefish (*Prosopium williamsoni*) and Longnose Sucker (*Catostomus catostomus*)," *Environmental Toxicology and Chemistry,* Vol. 13, pp. 1469-1482.

Lee, L. E. J. and Bols, N. C., 1991, "Identification of Fibronectin in Rainbow Trout and Influence of Cortisol on Fibronectin Accumulation by Rainbow Trout Cell Cultures," *Journal of Aquatic Animal Health,* Vol. 3, pp. 31-40.

Lee, L. E. J., Clemons, J. H., Bechtel, D. G., Caldwell, S. J., Han, K. B., Pasitschniak-Arts, M., Mosser, D. D. and Bols, N. C., 1993, "Development and Characterization of a Rainbow Trout Liver Cell Line Expressing Cytochrome P450-dependent Monooxygenase Activity," *Cell Biology and Toxicology,* Vol. 9, pp. 279-294.

Levine, S. L., Oris, J. T. and Wissing, T. E., 1995, "Influence of Environmental Factors on the Physiological Condition and Hepatic Ethoxyresorufin O-Deethylase (EROD) Activity of Gizzard Shad (*Dorosoma cepedianum*)," *Environmental Toxicology and Chemistry,* Vol. 14, pp. 123-128.

Lewis, D. F., Ioannides, C., Parke, D. V., 1998, "Cytochromes P450 and Species Differences in Xenobiotic Metabolism and Activation of Carcinogen," *Environmental Health Perspectives,* Vol. 106, pp. 633-641.

Mikaelian, I., Ménard, C., de Lafontaine, Y., Tellier, P., Harshbarger, J.C. and Martineau, D., 1997, "Liver Neoplasms and Contaminants in Lake Whitefish (*Coregonus clupeaformis*) from the Saint Lawrence River, Québec, Canada," *Twenty-Second Annual Eastern Fish Health Workshop.*

Mikaelian, I., de Lafontaine, Y., Ménard, C., Tellier, P., Harshbarger, J.C., and Martineau, D., 1998, "Neoplastic and Nonneoplastic Hepatic Changes in Lake Whitefish (*Coregonus clupeaformis*) from the St. Lawrence River, Quebec, Canada," *Environmental Health Perspectives,* Vol. 106, No. 4, pp. 179-183.

Miller, M. G., Kapron, C. M., Metcalfe, C. D., and Lee, L. E. J., 2000, "Down-regulation of Fibronectin in Rainbow Trout Gonadal Cells Exposed to Retinoic Acid," *Aquatic Toxicology* Vol. 48, pp. 119-126.

Mosher, D. F., 1989, "Fibronectin," Academic Press, San Diego, CA.

Munkittrick, K. R., Van der Kraak, G. J., McMaster, M. E., Portt, C. B., Van den Heuvel, M. R., and Servos, M. R., 1994, "Survey of receiving-water environmental impacts associated with discharges from pulp mills. 2. Gonad size, liver size, hepatic EROD activity and plasma sex steroid levels in white sucker," *Environmental Toxicology and Chemistry,* Vol. 13, No. 7, pp. 1089-1101.

Proctor, R. A., 1987, "Fibronectin and the Pathogenesis of Infections," *Reviews of Infectious Diseases* Vol. 9, pp. S317-S430.

Scott, W. and Crossman, E. , 1973, "Freshwater fishes of Canada," *Fisheries Research Board of Canada*, Ottawa.

Soimasuo, M. R., Karels, A. E., Leppänen, H., Santti, R. and Oikari, A.O., 1998, "Biomarker Responses in Whitefish (*Coregonus lavaretus* L. s.l.) Experimentally Exposed in a Large Lake Receiving Effluents from Pulp and Paper Industry," *Archives of Environmental Contaminant Toxicology,* Vol. 34, pp. 69-80.

Stegeman, J.J., Brouwer, M., Di Giulio, R.T., Förlin, L., Fowler, B.A., Sanders, B.M., and Van Veld, P.A., 1992, "Molecular Responses to Environmental Contamination: Enzyme and Protein Systems as Indicators of Chemical Exposure and Effect," R. J. Huggett, R. A. Kimerle, P. M. Mehrle, and H. L. Bergman, Eds. *Biochemical, Physiological, and Histological Markers of Anthropogenic Stress*, Society of Environmental Toxicology and Chemistry (SETAC) Inc., Lewis Publishers, Boca Raton, FL, pp. 235-335.

Timbrell, J. A., 1998, "Biomarkers in Toxicology," *Toxicology*, Vol. 129, pp. 1-12.

Travis, C. C., 1993, "Use of Biomarkers in Assessing Health and Environmental Impacts of Chemical Pollutants," *NATO ASI Series Vol. 250,* Plenum Press, NY.

Uchida, N., Watanabe, M., Kakiuchi, M., Anzai, H. and Nishide, E., 1992, "Isolation and Characterization of a Novel Fibronectin from the Plasma of Carp," *Nippon Suisan Gakkaishi,* Vol. 58, pp. 1107-1113.

Whyte, J. J., van den Heuvel, M. R., Clemons, J. H., Huestis, S. Y., Servos, M. R., Dixon, D. G., and Bols, N. C., 1998, "Mammalian and Teleost Cell Line Bioassay and Chemically Derived 2,3,7,8-TetraChloroDibenzo-*p*-Dioxin Equivalent Concentrations in Lake Trout (*Salvelinus namaycush*) from Lake Superior and Lake Ontario, North America," *Environmental Toxicology and Chemistry,* Vol. 17, pp. 2214-2226.

Williams, D. E., Lech, J. J. and Buhler, D. R., 1998, "Xenobiotics and Xenoestrogens in Fish: Modulation of Cytochrome P450 and Carcinogenesis," *Mutation Research*, Vol. 399, pp. 179-192

Wright, G. M., 1986, "Immunocytochemical Study of Fibronectin in the Sea Lamprey, *Petromyzon marinus*, and the Atlantic Hagfish, *Myxine glutinosa,*" *Cell and Tissue Research,* Vol. 244, pp. 549-555.

Ylatupa, S., Haglund, C., Mertaniemi, P., Vahtera, E. and Partanen, P., 1995, "Cellular Fibronectin in Serum and Plasma: A Potential New Tumor Marker?," *British Journal of Cancer*, Vol. 71, pp. 578-582.

Mark A. Lampi,[1] Xiao-Dong Huang,[2] Yousef S. El-Alawi,[1] Brendan J. McConkey,[1] D. George Dixon,[3] and Bruce M. Greenberg[†3]

Occurrence and Toxicity of Photomodified Polycyclic Aromatic Hydrocarbon Mixtures Present in Contaminated Sediments

---

Reference: Lampi, M. A., Huang, X.-D., El-Alawi, Y. S., McConkey, B. J., Dixon, D. G., and Greenberg, B. M., **"Occurrence and Toxicity of Photomodified Polycyclic Aromatic Hydrocarbon Mixtures Present in Contaminated Sediments,"** *Environmental Toxicology and Risk Assessment: Science, Policy, and Standardization — Implications for Environmental Decisions: Tenth Volume, ASTM STP 1403*, B. M. Greenberg, R. N. Hull, M. H. Roberts, Jr., and R. W. Gensemer, Eds., American Society for Testing and Materials, West Conshohocken, PA, 2001.

Abstract: Exposure of PAHs to solar radiation results in the generation of oxygenated products. Many of these oxyPAHs are more toxic and/or carcinogenic than the parent compounds. Environmental photomodification of PAHs could result in formation of toxic compounds not anticipated by regulatory agencies. We have confirmed the presence of oxyPAHs at toxic levels in sediment samples taken from a known contaminated site. Contaminated sediment samples were taken from Hamilton Harbour (Hamilton, Ontario). A reference site from the harbour, known to be free of contaminants was also analyzed. High performance liquid chromatography (HPLC) was used to fractionate, and analyze individual compounds present. Fractions were tested for toxicity using both short-term, and long-term assays on the bacterium *Vibrio fischeri*. OxyPAHs were found in sediments at concentrations comparable to intact PAHs. Testing confirmed toxicity in fractions containing oxyPAHs on the order of intact PAH-containing fractions. It is concluded that environmental photomodification of PAHs contributes to the presence of toxic compounds that are not properly addressed by current regulations in the U.S. and Canada.

Keywords: environmental photomodification, sediment, polycyclic aromatic hydrocarbons, *Vibrio fischeri*

Introduction

Polycyclic aromatic hydrocarbons (PAHs) are ubiquitous environmental contaminants, with well documented toxic, mutagenic, and carcinogenic properties.

---

[1] Graduate Students, [2]Research Associate, [3]Professors, Department of Biology, University of Waterloo, Waterloo, Ont., N2L 3G1.

[†] Corresponding author email: greenber@sciborg.uwaterloo.ca.

These compounds are produced by natural sources including forest and grass fires, volcanoes, and seepage of oil into the environment (Neff 1985, Eisler 1987). However, the majority of PAHs are released into the environment through a wide variety of anthropogenic activities, including petroleum spills, electric power generation, refuse incineration, home heating, internal combustion engines, and the production of coke, carbon black, coal tar and asphalt (Nikolaou et al. 1984, Neff 1985, Eisler 1987). As a result of the large fraction of PAHs produced by human activities, these contaminants are found in most industrialized regions.

The structure of PAHs includes conjugated π-bonding orbitals, resulting in the absorption of light in the UV/far blue region of the spectrum that is present in solar radiation (Larson and Berenbaum 1988, Newsted and Giesy 1987, Nikolaou et al. 1984, Huang et al. 1993, Mallakin et al. 1999). Absorption of light energy can alter the toxicity of the compound through two different mechanisms: photosensitization, and photomodification (Krylov et al. 1997). Photosensitization generally leads to the production of singlet oxygen, which is capable of damaging biological molecules (Foote 1987, Girotti 1983). Photomodification of PAHs is defined here as photooxidation and photolysis, and generally results in the formation of new compounds with increased polarity. They still possess some hydrophobicity, and thus the ability to accumulate in biological membranes (Huang et al. 1993, Ren et al. 1996, McConkey et al. 1997, Krylov et al. 1997). This process is rapid under environmentally relevant levels of actinic radiation (Katz et al. 1979, Huang et al. 1993, McConkey et al. 1997, Mallakin et al. 2000), from which it may be hypothesized that the contribution of modified PAHs to the environmental load is significant.

The presence of modified PAHs in the environment is now recognized, and a thorough assessment of loads of these contaminants is currently underway. Hazard assessment of these compounds is also ongoing, and recently some groups have reported that modified PAHs (including oxy- and nitro- derivatives) are widely distributed throughout the environment (Legzdins et al. 1995, Enya et al. 1997, Kosian et al. 1998). Legzdins et al. (1995) fractionated air samples collected from Hamilton, Ontario, a highly industrialized city, and found the samples contained many forms of modified PAHs . Included were anthraquinone (ATQ), benzanthrone (BAT), benzo[a]anthraquinone (BAQ), 9-nitroanthracene, and 2-nitrofluoranthene, all in comparable concentrations with intact PAHs. Enya et al. (1997)found the modified PAHs 3-nitrobenzanthrone, 3,9-dinitrobenzanthrone, and 1,8-dinitropyrene in diesel engine exhaust and air samples collected in Tokyo. All were produced by the combustion of diesel fuel, photooxidation, or a combination of both of the above processes. Kosian et al. (1998)reported that a number of modified PAHs, including BAT, and 1-hydroxyATQ were present in sediment pore water samples collected from a contaminated stream in close proximity to an oil refinery.

Photomodification can significantly alter the bioactivity of a compound, and many of the photooxidation products of PAHs (oxyPAHs) exhibit greater toxicity than the parent compounds. Oris and Giesy (1985) demonstrated that the LT50 decreased when juvenile sunfish were exposed to ultraviolet light, and anthracene (ANT) simultaneously. Newsted and Giesy (1987) showed that a number of PAHs, including ANT were phototoxic to the cladoceran, *Daphnia magna*. However, these studies attributed the observed phototoxicity to the photosensitization mechanism described above.

Evidence exists that modified PAHs are equally, or more toxic, mutagenic and/or carcinogenic than the parent compounds (Gibson et al. 1978, Legzdins et al. 1995, McConkey et al. 1997, Enya et al. 1997). It is well-established that PAHs become more toxic and mutagenic following cytochrome P450-catalyzed oxidation (Sims et al. 1974, Huberman et al. 1976, Yang et al. 1977). It is not surprising then, that PAHs modified by alternative means (e.g. photomodification) are more hazardous as well. In fact, the highest score ever reported in an Ames test was produced by the modified PAH 3-nitrobenzanthrone (Enya et al. 1997). Enya et al. (1997) also found 1,8-dinitropyrene to be a powerful mutagen. Further, oxy- and nitro-PAH-containing fractions have been found to be exhibit greater direct mutagenicity than fractions containing intact PAHs (Legzdins et al. 1995). Fractions of samples of sediment pore water collected from a contaminated stream were found to be phototoxic, despite a lack of intact PAHs (Kosian et al. 1997). These fractions did contain modified PAHs, although other compounds were present that may have contributed to toxicity. In another study, the toxicity of 14 of 16 PAHs increased upon photomodification (Krylov et al. 1997). It is important to note that modified PAHs require neither biological activation, nor UV radiation to exhibit toxicity and mutagenicity (Gibson et al. 1978, Legzdins et al. 1995, McConkey et al. 1997, Enya et al. 1997). However, toxicity and mutagenicity may be increased in the presence of UV radiation (Oris and Giesy 1985, Newsted and Giesy 1987, Huang et al. 1993, Ankley et al. 1994).

It is hypothesized that environmental photomodification of PAHs, will contribute significantly to the environmental load of toxic contaminants. Further, this class of compounds is currently overlooked by current regulations in the U.S. and Canada, and might pose a risk of unknown magnitude if undetected amounts of toxic compounds are indeed present. Therefore we have attempted to identify and quantify photomodified PAHs in contaminated environments, particularly aquatic environments. In this paper, the fractionation of contaminated sediments will be described, as will toxicity assays performed on specific sediment fractions.

Case Study: Hazards of Modified PAHs in Sediments from Hamilton Harbour

Sediment samples were taken 5 metres from shore at a depth of 1.5 metres in a docking port near Randle Reef in Hamilton Harbour (Hamilton, Ontario), and a reference site near the entrance to Coote's Paradise in Hamilton Harbour. A ponar was used to make surface sediment grabs of approximately 1 kg. This docking port is known to be contaminated with PAHs from the industry surrounding the harbour. The above samples were extracted using a modification of U.S. EPA method 3550B for ultrasonic extraction of sediments (U.S. EPA 1998). Briefly, 4 g of dry sediment was suspended in 10 mL of hexane:acetone (1:1, v/v), and ultrasonicated for 20 minutes. Particulate matter was removed by centrifugation and the extract was dried down to 2 mL with a gentle stream of N_2. The extracts were fractionated using a normal phase high performance liquid chromatography (HPLC) method developed for this study. A Whatman 5 μm Partisil PAC RAC column (Whatman, Clifton, NJ, 9.4 mm i.d. × 10 cm length) was used. Samples were eluted at a flow rate of 2 mL/min., with a step gradient of hexane:tetrahydrofuran (THF) (95:5, v/v, Solvent A) and methanol:THF (80:20, v/v,

Solvent B). The gradient used was as follows (elapsed time): initial, 100% Solvent A; 5-10 min, 90% Solvent A; 10-25 min., 50% Solvent A; 25-30 min., 100% Solvent B. This method was designed to elute compounds with increasing polarity as retention time increased, thus allowing isolation of more polar compounds like modified PAHs, in later fractions. Six fractions were collected for toxicity testing, and further analysis by reverse phase HPLC. The following retention time intervals were used to collect fractions: 2-4 min., fraction 1; 4-7 min., fraction 2; 7-12 min., fraction 3; 12-17 min., fraction 4; 17-22 min., fraction 5; 22-30 min., fraction 6. Chromatograms of the contaminated site, and the reference site are included (Fig. 1).

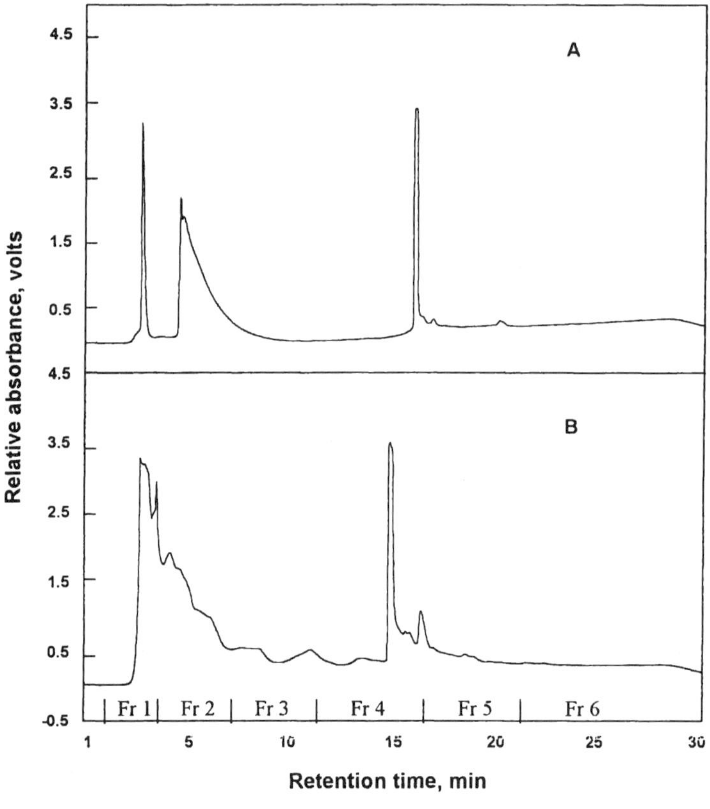

Figure 1--Normal phase HPLC chromatogram. A. Reference sediment. B. Contaminated Hamilton Harbour sediment. HPLC conditions as described in text.

Reverse phase HPLC has been used to tentatively identify some individual components of the fractions. Samples of fractions were eluted through a 5 µm Supelco Supelcosil LC-18 analytical column (Sigma-Aldrich Canada Ltd., Oakville, Ont., 4.6 mm i.d. × 25 cm length). A gradient beginning with 50:50 acetonitrile:water (v/v), and ramping to 100% acetonitrile over 40 min. was used, at a flow rate of 1.5 mL/min. A photodiode array detector scanning over 210 nm to 400 nm, was used to create absorbance spectra of individual components eluting off of the column. Spectra, and retention times were then compared with existing compounds in a library previously created, enabling identification of the components. The compounds identified are listed in Table 1.

Table 1--Components of fractions from contaminated Hamilton Harbour sediment. +- arbitrary concentration unit based on relative absorbance of reverse phase HPLC. +- relative absorbance from 0-1; ++- rel. abs. from 1-2; +++- rel. abs. greater than 2. Abbreviations are as follows: ANT-anthracene, FLA-fluoranthene, PHE-phenanthrene, PYR-pyrene, BAA-benzo[a]anthracene, TRL-triphenylene, CHR-chrysene, BBF/BKF-benzo[b or k}fluoranthene, BAP-benzo[a]pyrene, ATQ-anthraquinone, HATQ-2-hydroxyanthraquinone, HPHEQ-hydroxyphenanthrenequinone.

	Fraction 1	Fraction 2	Fraction 3	Fraction 4	Fraction 5	Fraction 6
ANT	+++	++	+	+	+	
FLA		+	+			
PHE		+				
PYR	+	++	+			
BAA		+	+			
TRL		+	+			
CHR		+	+			
BBF/BKF		+	+	+		
BAP		+				
ATQ				+	+	+
HATQ				+	+	+
HPHEQ					+	++

Whole sediment extracts, and fractions 1 to 6 from Hamilton Harbour, and the reference site were tested for toxicity using a bacterial bioluminescence assay previously developed (McConkey et al., 1997). Toxicity was tested with the luminescent marine bacterium *Vibrio fischeri* using inhibition of luminescence as the endpoint. Assays were performed in the dark, and under simulated solar radiation (SSR), and inhibition of luminescence was determined after 18 hours. Inhibition of bacterial growth is another factor that can be used as an endpoint in this assay. Data are presented in Table 2, as percent inhibition of luminescence of a control, with concentrations given as mg equivalents of extracted sediment per litre (mg EQS/L). This unit signifies the amount of extracted sediment that would be present in a litre of test media, and the concentration used corresponds to almost 250 ppm of extract or fraction. In this assay, the most toxic fraction was fraction 6, which was more toxic even than the whole extract.

Discussion

Based on this initial work, we have found modified PAHs in contaminated sediment samples at toxic levels. Reverse phase HPLC analysis has revealed modified PAHs in the polar sediment fractions. Intact PAHs were found in fractions 1 through 5, with the majority in fractions 1 to 3, the least polar fractions. Initial analysis shows the

Table 2--Percent inhibition of luminescence in V. fischeri after exposure to different fractions of Hamilton Harbour sediment. Long-term assay, in which inhibition of luminescence was measured after 18 h of exposure to fractions. Fraction concentration was 234.38 mg EQS/L. Data are means of six replicates ± 95 % confidence intervals. *SSR - simulated solar radiation; mg EQS/L - mg equivalents of extracted sediment per litre.*

Test Material	SSR	Dark
Whole Extract	91.0 ± 1.78	55.5 ± 1.33
Fraction 1	90.6 ± 1.50	35.4 ± 1.77
Fraction 2	3.31 ± 1.00	3.53 ± 0.83
Fraction 3	4.56 ± 1.00	3.22 ± 1.00
Fraction 4	35.9 ± 1.56	3.72 ± 1.22
Fraction 5	89.4 ± 1.4	57.8 ± 1.6
Fraction 6	94.9 ± 1.64	93.1 ± 2.00

presence of a large amount of anthracene, and a small amount of pyrene in fraction 1, which was expected to contain intact PAHs only. A wide variety of priority PAHs were identified in fractions 2 to 4 (Table 1). Increasingly polar compounds were expected to have longer retention times. Indeed fractions 4 to 6 contained several modified PAHs, as well as several putative oxyPAHs that we have not yet identified. Fraction 6 is the most polar of the fractions, and modified PAHs were found. Initial analysis does in fact show that fraction 6 contained hydroxyphenanthrenequinone, anthraquinone and 2-hydroxyanthraquinone. This initial data is consistent with other studies regarding the presence of modified PAHs in the environment (Legzdins et al. 1995, Enya et al. 1997, Kosian et al. 1998). Interestingly, there seem to be several modified PAHs present in the polar fractions, that we were not able to identify based on absorbance spectra, and retention time. Characterization of the identity of these compounds through alternative techniques such as GC/MS or LC/MS will facilitate greater insight into the toxicity of the polar fractions.

Whole sediment extracts and fractions 1 to 6 from Hamilton Harbour were tested for toxicity using *V. fischeri*. Results for the six fractions tested are quite striking. The highest inhibition of luminescence in all samples tested was produced by fraction 6 in SSR, and was higher even than the whole extract. An explanation for this might be the amelioration of toxicity in the whole extract by the presence of humic matter, which is known to decrease PAH toxicity (Gensemer et al. 1998). Although quantification of these compounds was not completed at the time of the preparation of this manuscript, it is evident from toxicity data that modified PAHs present in fractions from contaminated sediments contribute to overall toxicity of the sediments. Fractions containing compounds of higher polarity than intact PAHs, which are assumed to be modified PAHs were as, or more toxic than fractions expected to contain only intact PAHs. Phototoxicity was observed in long-term assays completed in SSR for all fractions. This is consistent with other reports on the toxicity of PAHs exposed to UV radiation (Oris and Giesy 1985, Kagan et al. 1985, Newsted and Giesy 1987, Ankley et al. 1994, Huang et al. 1993). However, many of these studies attribute toxicity to the photosensitized production of singlet oxygen, and preclude the toxic effects of photomodified PAHs.

To assess the direct toxicity of a compound, and eliminate any effects that might be caused by photosensitization, dark controls of the toxicity assays were also completed. The dark controls exhibited a similar response pattern to the SSR data, although the percent inhibition was lesser in the dark. Inhibition of luminescence by the polar fractions 5 and 6 completed in the dark was greater, or on the same order as that of the whole extract, or the non-polar fraction 1. This supports existing evidence that modified PAHs need neither biological activation, nor UV radiation to exhibit direct toxicity (Huang et al. 1993, Huang et al. 1995, Ren et al. 1996, McConkey et al. 1997, Mallakin et al. 1999).

It is important that the compounds that make up the profile of modified PAHs in the environment are identified and quantified. The elucidation of the individual compounds present in environmental samples will enable further determination of possible synergistic effects that may be observed in these complex mixtures. Mixtures of photomodified PAH anthracene have been found to inhibit photosynthesis (Huang et al. 1997). There is evidence that the modified PAH 1,2-dihydroxyanthraquinone (1,2-dhATQ), a product of the photomodification of anthracene (Mallakin et al. 2000), has an inhibitory site at the cytochrome b/c complex of the mitochondrial electron transport chain (Tripuranthakam et al. 1999). Also, inhibition in the chloroplast at the cytochrome b6/f complex has been observed, and synergism was found when 1,2-dhATQ was mixed with copper (Babu et al. 2000). As many oxyPAHs operate via different mechanisms, knowledge of components of relevant mixtures would be integral in evaluation of environmental risk.

Existing data, and that presented, indicates that the presence of modified PAHs in the environment should be studied more thoroughly. Further elucidation of the nature of the mixtures present, and the toxicity of these mixtures is required to understand the possible ramifications that may come about. Detailed evidence regarding the presence of a heretofore unmonitored class of toxic, mutagenic and/or carcinogenic compounds in the environment would be of great value. The data are needed to reassess regulations, and to understand the consequences of future environmental disasters like petroleum spills. The data will also help evaluate the risks associated with human, and environmental exposure from these compounds.

References

Ankley, G. T., Collyard, S. A., Monson, P. D., and Kosian, P. A., 1994, "Influence of Ultraviolet Light on the Toxicity of Sediments Contaminated with Polycyclic Aromatic Hydrocarbons," *Environmental Toxicology and Chemistry*, Vol. 13, pp. 1791-1796.

Babu, T. S., Marder, J. B., Tripuranthakam, S., Dixon, D. G., and Greenberg, B. M., 2000, "Synergistic Effects of a Photooxidized Polycyclic Aromatic Hydrocarbon and Copper on Photosynthesis and Plant Growth: Evidence that In Vivo Formation of Reactive Oxygen Species is a Mechanism of Copper Toxicity," submitted to Environmental Toxicology and Chemistry.

Eisler, R, 1987, *Polycyclic Aromatic Hydrocarbon Hazards to Fish, Wildlife, and Invertebrates: A Synoptic Review*, U.S. Fish and Wildlife Service Biological Report 85(1.11), U.S. Fish and Wildlife Service, Patuxent Wildlife Research

Center, Laurel, MD.

Enya, T., Suzuki, H., Watanabe, T., Hirayama, T., and Hisamtsu, Y., 1997, "3-Nitrobenzanthrone, a Powerful Bacterial Mutagen and Suspected Human Carcinogen Found in Diesel Exhaust and Airborne Particulates," *Environmental Science and Technology*, Vol. 31, pp. 2772-2776.

Foote, C S., 1987, "Type I and Type II Mechanisms of Photodynamic Action." In Heitz, J. R., and Downum, K. R., eds., *Light-Activated Pesticides,* American Chemical Society, Washington DC, pp. 22-38.

Gensemer, R. W., Dixon, D. G., and Greenberg, B. M., 1998, "Amelioration of the Photo-Induced Toxicity of Polycyclic Aromatic Hydrocarbons by a Commercial Humic Acid," *Ecotoxicology and Environmental Safety*, Vol. 39, pp. 57-64.

Gibson, T. L., Smart, V. B., and Smith, L. L., 1978, "Non-Enzymic Activation of Polycyclic Aromatic Hydrocarbons as Mutagens," *Mutation Research*, Vol. 49, pp. 153-161.

Girotti, A. W., 1983, "Mechanisms of Photosensitization," *Photochemistry and Photobiology,* Vol. 38, pp. 745-751.

Huang, X.-D., Dixon, D. G., and Greenberg, B. M., 1993, "Impacts of UV Radiation and Photomodification on the Toxicity of PAHs to the Higher Plant *Lemna gibba* (Duckweed)," *Environmental Toxicology and Chemistry,* Vol. 12, pp. 1067-1077.

Huang, X.-D., Dixon, D.G., and Greenberg, B.M., 1995, "Increased Polycyclic Aromatic Hydrocarbon Toxicity Following Their Photomodification in Natural Sunlight: Impacts on the Duckweed *Lemna gibba* L. G-3," *Ecotoxicology and Environmental Safety*, Vol. 32, pp. 194-200.

Huang, X.-D., McConkey, B. J, Babu, T. S., and Greenberg, B. M., 1997, "Mechanisms of Photoinduced Toxicity of Photomodified Anthracene to Plants: Inhibition of Photosynthesis in the Aquatic Higher Plant *Lemna gibba* (Duckweed)," *Environmental Toxicology and Chemistry*, Vol. 16, pp. 1707-1715.

Huberman, E., Sachs, L., Yang, S. K., and Gelboin, H. V., 1976, "Identification of Mutagenic Metabolites of Benzo[a]pyrene in Mammalian Cells," *Proceedings of the National Academy of Science, USA*, Vol. 73, pp. 607-612.

Kagan, J., Kagan, E. D., Kagan, I. A., Kagan, P. A., Quigley, S., 1985, "Phototoxicity of Non-Carcinogenic PAHs in Aquatic Organisms," *Chemosphere*, Vol. 14, pp. 1829-1834.

Katz, M., Chan, C., Tosine, H., and Sakuma, T., 1979, "Relative Rates of Photochemical and Biological Oxidation In Vitro of Polynuclear Aromatic Hydrocarbons," In

Jones, P. W., and Leber, P., eds., *Polynuclear Aromatic Hydrocarbon,* Ann Arbor Science, Ann Arbor, MI, pp. 171-189.

Kosian, P. A., Makeynen, E. A., Monson, P. D., Mount, D. R., Spacie, A., Mekenyan, O. G., and Ankley, G. T., 1998, "Application of Toxicity-Based Fractionation Techniques and Structure-Activity Relationship Models for the Identification of Phototoxic Polycyclic Aromatic Hydrocarbons in Sediment Pore Water," *Environmental Toxicology and Chemistry,* Vol. 17, pp. 1021-1033.

Krylov, S. N., Huang, X.-D., Zeiler, L. F., Dixon, D. G., and Greenberg, B. M., 1997, "Mechanistic Quantitative Structure-Activity Relationship Model for Photoinduced Toxicity of Polycyclic Aromatic Hydrocarbons: I. Physical Model Based on Chemical Kinetics in a Two-Compartment System," *Environmental Toxicology and Chemistry*, Vol. 16, pp. 2283-2295.

Larson, R. A., and Berenbaum, M. R., 1988, "Environmental Phototoxicity," *Environmental Science and Technology,* Vol. 22, pp. 354-360.

Legzdins, A. E., McCarry, B. E., Marvin, C. H., and Bryant, D. W., 1995, "Methodology for Bioassay-Directed Fractionation Studies of Air Particulae Material and Other Complex Environmental Matrices," *International Journal of Environmental Analytical Chemistry,* Vol. 60, pp. 79-94.

Mallakin, A., McConkey, B. J., Miao, G., McKibben, B., Snieckus, V., Dixon, D. G., and Greenberg, B. M., 1999, "Impacts of Structural Photomodification on the Toxicity of Environmental Contaminants: Anthracene Photooxidation Products," *Ecotoxicology and Environmental Safety*, Vol. 43, pp. 204-212.

Mallakin, A., Dixon, D. G., and Greenberg B. M., 2000, "Pathway of Anthracene Modification Under Simulated Solar Radiation," *Chemosphere,* Vol. 40, pp. 1435-1441.

McConkey, B. J, Duxbury, C. L., Dixon, D. G., and Greenberg, B. M., 1997, "Toxicity of a PAH Photooxidation Product to the Bacteria *Photobacterium phosphoreum* and the Duckweed *Lemna gibba*: Effects of Phenanthrene and its Primary Photoproduct, Phenanthrenequinone," *Environmental Toxicology and Chemistry,* Vol. 16, pp. 892-899.

Neff, J. M., 1985, "Polycyclic Aromatic Hydrocarbons." In Rand, G M. and Petrocelli, S. R., eds., *Fundamentals of Aquatic Toxicology,* Hemisphere Publishing Corporation, Toronto, Ont., pp. 416-454.

Newsted, J. L., and Giesy, J. P., 1987, "Predictive Models for Photoinduced Acute Toxicity of Polycyclic Aromatic Hydrocarbons to *Daphnia magna*, Strauss (Cladocera, Crustacea)," *Environmental Toxicology and Chemistry,* Vol. 6, pp. 445-461.

Nikolaou, K, Masclet, P., and Mouvier, G., 1984, "Sources and Chemical Reactivity of Polynuclear Aromatic Hydrocarbons in the Atmosphere-A Critical Review," *Science of the Total Environment*, Vol. 32, pp. 103-132.

Oris, J. T., and Giesy, J. P., 1985, "The Photoenhanced Toxicity of Anthracene to Juvenile Sunfish (*Lepomis* spp.)," *Aquatic Toxicology*, Vol. 6, pp. 133-146.

Ren, L., Zeiler, L. F., Dixon, D. G., and Greenberg, B. M., 1996, "Photoinduced Effects of Polycylic Aromatic Hydrocarbons on *Brassica napus* (canola) During Germination and Early Seedling Development," *Ecotoxicology and Environmental Safety*, Vol. 33, pp. 73-80.

Sims, P., Grover, L. L., Swaisland, A., Pal, K., and Hewer, A., 1974, "Metabolic Activation of Benzo[a]pyrene Proceeds by a Diol-Epoxide," *Nature*, Vol. 252, pp. 326-328.

Tripuranthakam, S., Duxbury, C. L., Babu, T. S., and Greenberg, B. M., 1999, "Development of a Mitochondrial Respiratory Electron Transport Bioindicator for Assessment of Aromatic Hydrocarbon Toxicity," *Environmental Toxicology and Risk Assessment: Standardization of Biomarkers for Endocrine Disruption and Environmental Assessment: Eighth Volume, ASTM STP 1364*, D.S. Henshel, M.C. Black, and M.C. Harrass, Eds., American Society for Testing and Materials, West Conshohocken, PA, 1999.

U.S. EPA, 1998, "Method 3550B – Ultrasonic Extraction", *SW-846, Test Methods for Evaluating Solid Waste, Physical/Chemical Methods, Fifth Revision*, United States Environmental Protection Agency, Office of Solid Waste, Washington, DC.

Yang, S. K., McCourt, D. W., Leutz, J. C., and Gelboin, H. V., 1977, "Benzo[a]pyrene Diol Epoxides: Mechanism of Enzymatic Formation and Optically Active Intermediates," *Science*, Vol. 196, pp. 1199-1201.

CURRENT ISSUES IN SOIL TOXICITY AND REMEDIATION

Windy A. Boyd,[1] Virginia A. Stringer,[1] and Phillip L. Williams[1]

Metal LC50s of a Soil Nematode Compared to Published Earthworm Data

Reference: Boyd, W. A., Stringer, V. A., and Williams, P. L., **"Metal LC50s of a Soil Nematode Compared to Published Earthworm Data,"** *Environmental Toxicology and Risk Assessment: Science, Policy, and Standardization – Implications for Environmental Decisions: Tenth Volume, ASTM STP 1403*, B. M. Greenberg, R. N. Hull, M. H. Roberts, Jr., and R. W. Gensemer, Eds., American Society for Testing and Materials, West Conshohocken, PA, 2001.

Abstract: A comparison of the acute LC50s for five metals between the standard test organism *Eisenia fetida* and the soil nematode *Caenorhabditis elegans* was made. Although the test with *C. elegans* is shorter (24 h vs. 2 wks) and uses less soil or testing medium (2.33 g vs. 200 g dry weight) than that for *E. fetida*, LC50s were comparable for the earthworm and nematode. The current study further investigated similarities by extending the exposure time to 48 h. Comparisons were made to 24-h *C. elegans* data, published *E. fetida* data, and U.S. Environmental Protection Agency (EPA) allowable concentrations. The nitrate salts of Pb, Ni, Cd, Zn, and Cu were used to generate LC50s. Two naturally occurring soils in Georgia were chosen to compare different soil properties on the metals' toxicity. Tifton soil was sampled from the southern region of Georgia and is characterized by relatively high sand and low clay and soil organic matter (SOM) contents. Cecil soil, in contrast, is found in the Piedmont region of Georgia and is characterized by relatively high amounts of clay and SOM. As anticipated, extending the exposure time to 48 h significantly increased the toxicity (i.e. decreased the LC50s) of the metals compared to published 24-h *C. elegans* data. Physical-chemical properties of soils are known to affect the binding of polyvalent metals and thus the bioavailability and toxicity of these metals. Increasing clay and SOM contents allow for an increased capacity to bind metals. For this reason, LC50s were higher in Cecil than in Tifton soil. Because tests using *C. elegans* are rapid, reliable, and generate data comparable to that of the earthworm, we suggest further studies that may lead to the standardization of the nematode for use as a soil toxicity-testing organism.

Keywords: *Caenorhabditis elegans*, *Eisenia fetida*, soil, metals, toxicity

In selecting an appropriate test species with which to assess toxicity of soils, both

[1]Graduate Students and Associate Professor, respectively, Department of Environmental Health Science, The University of Georgia, Athens, GA 30602-2102.

idealistic and realistic criteria must be considered (Lökke and van Gestel 1998). Ideally, a species should be ecologically and geographically relevant to the soil ecosystem, able to tolerate different soil conditions (pH, moisture content, etc.), and representative of multiple routes of exposure. Realistically, however, criteria for species selection often include consideration of the cost and duration of the test, ease of obtaining and culturing the test species, knowledge and understanding of the basic biology of the test species, and regulatory acceptance of the test. No single test species can meet all of the above criteria. However, nematodes appear to satisfy most of them.

Nematodes make up a major proportion of the soil biota. They help to maintain soil ecosystem stasis by contributing to the degradation of organic matter in soil and to the cycling of nutrients (Freeman et al. 1998). *C. elegans* is a non-parasitic nematode that lives in the interstitial water of soils, feeding on bacteria and other microbes. Since the 1970s, the advantages of using *C. elegans* for genetic studies have been known (Brenner 1974). The characterization of both the neural circuitry and cell lineage is more complete in *C. elegans* than in any other animal (Williams and Dusenbery 1988). The *C. elegans* Sequencing Consortium (1998) has now sequenced nearly the entire genome.

C. elegans is readily available from a national repository and can be cultured quickly and easily on agar plates (Williams and Dusenbery 1988) or in liquid medium (Williams and Dusenbery 1990) using *Escherichia coli*, another well-characterized organism, as a food source. Because the physiology and genetic makeup of *C. elegans* is well understood, the ability to quantify the lethality of toxicants can be supplemented by the possibility of determining the mechanisms associated with the toxic responses (Cressman and Williams 1997). *C. elegans* is currently being used as a model test organism.

Laboratory testing with *C. elegans* has included assessment of metal toxicity (Tatara et al. 1997), as well as recommendations for specific metals as reference toxicants in aquatic media (Cressman and Williams 1997). Besides metal studies, the nematode has also been used to estimate the lethality of such compounds as sodium pentachlorophenate (PCP) (Donkin and Williams 1995; Cressman and Williams 1997) and the breakdown products of glucosinolates (Donkin et al. 1995).

C. elegans is ideally suited to assess toxicity associated with porewater exposures because it resides in water within the soil matrix. Soil sorption (i.e., the capacity of soil particles to bind chemical substances) may alter the bioavailability of contaminants in soils and soil porewaters and influence the results of soil toxicity tests. As a result, the use of the nematode toxicity test has increased over the last ten years (Donkin and Dusenbery 1993, 1994; Donkin 1997; Freeman et al. 1999; Peredney and Williams 2000). Given the many advantages of *C. elegans* and the need for acceptable soil bioassays, a standardized method for soil toxicity testing with the nematode would be very useful.

Currently, the earthworm *E. fetida* is one of the few internationally standardized soil test organisms. Our proposal is not to replace the earthworm but to strengthen the validity of soil toxicity testing with multi-species comparisons. Although the earthworm test is widely accepted, in some situations, a nematode test might prove more applicable. The proposed nematode test consists of a 24-48 hour exposure time in 2.33 g dry weight (d.w.) of soil. The standardized earthworm test, however, has a 14-day exposure time in 200-400 g d.w. of soil (ASTM Standard Guide for Conducting Laboratory Soil Toxicity or Bioaccumulation Tests With the Lumbricid Earthworm *Eisenia fetida* E1676). In situations where time and/or soil quantities are limited, the nematode test would provide an attractive alternative. Other considerations may include species sensitivity to contaminants and previous studies have indicated that the sensitivities of *C. elegans* and *E. fetida* are comparable.

The objectives of this study were to assess the effects of exposure time and soil type on the toxicity of five metals (Cd, Cu, Ni, Pb, and Zn) to *C. elegans*. These metals were chosen based on the availability of earthworm data and 24-h data using *C. elegans*. Further assessment of the applicability of the soil nematode test as a standardized testing protocol was also examined.

Materials and Methods

The wild type N2 strain of *C. elegans* was obtained from the *Caenorhabditis* Genetic Center (Minneapolis, MN) and used in all tests. Cultures were maintained as previously described to yield age-synchronized adult worms (Cressman and Williams 1997). Reference toxicant tests with Cu were performed to verify the health of the worms (Freeman et al. 1998). Adult worms (3 days old) were rinsed from culture plates and transferred to exposure dishes at three days old. After a 48-h exposure period, the supernatants of test solutions were measured for pH (Orion Model 720 pH meter and Ross combination electrode). The pH of each sample was between 4.5 and 5.0, well within the acceptable range of approximately 3-12 for *C. elegans* (Khanna et al. 1997).

Soil Toxicity Testing

A modification of the soil test procedure previously described was used (Donkin and Dusenbery 1993, Freeman et al. 1999, and Peredney and Williams 2000). Thirty-five mm petri dishes were loaded with 2.33 g d.w. Cecil or Tifton soil and spiked with 1.5 mL of testing medium containing the appropriate concentration of nitrate metal salt. Metal concentrations were determined from range finding tests. Nematodes were exposed to nitrate salts of Cd (0, 10, 30, 50, and 70 mg/L for Tifton and 0, 50, 100, 150, and 200 mg/L for Cecil), Cu (0, 10, 20, 30, and 40 mg/L for Tifton and 0, 150, 250, 350, and 450 mg/L for Cecil), Ni (0, 20, 40, 60, and 80 mg/L for Tifton and 0, 50, 100, 150, and 200 mg/L for Cecil), Pb (0, 35, 70, 105, and 140 mg/L for Tifton and 0, 250, 500, 750, and 1000 mg/L for Cecil), and Zn (0, 75, 112.5, 150, and 187.5 mg/L for Tifton and 0, 200, 300, 400, and 500 mg/L for Cecil). For each metal tested, five dishes were spiked, a control and four increasing metal concentrations diluted in K-medium (Williams and Dusenbery 1990). Each test was replicated three times. After spiking, the test soils were allowed to equilibrate at 20°C for 7 days. Although 24-h exposures required no addition of bacteria as a source of food for the nematodes (Freeman et al. 1999 and Peredney and Williams 2000), it was necessary to add food for 48-h exposures to assure control survival. Fifty millilitres of an L-broth solution with *Escherichia coli* (OP50 strain) was centrifuged at 750 *g* for 10 minutes. The supernatant was removed and the pellet was re-suspended in 10 mL of K-medium for a 5:1 (L-broth to K-medium) concentration (Donkin and Williams 1995).

After the soil was allowed to equilibrate for 7 days, 1.5 mL of 5:1 L-broth was added to each test dish to re-wet the soils and provide food. Ten worms per dish were then transferred with a platinum wire to the soil surface (Freeman et al. 1999). Test units were incubated at 20°C for 48 h (±1 h). After exposure, the soil and worms were rinsed from the petri dishes into 50-mL centrifuge tubes with Ludox® (Dupont, East Chicago, IN), a colloidal silica suspension. Each tube was mixed with a vortex at low speed for ~ 20 s to ensure thorough mixing of the soil suspension. After centrifuging for 2 min, tubes were set aside for ~ 15 min to allow time for the worms to float to the top of the solution.

The solution was then poured into 100-mm glass petri dishes and viewed under a light microscope. Worms were removed from the solution with a platinum wire, placed in a separate petri dish containing K-medium, and examined under a microscope. If the worm did not respond to gentle probing with the platinum wire, it was scored as dead. Live worms were either obviously swimming or moving after probing. In accordance with previous testing in our lab, unrecovered worms were scored as dead, control survival was greater than or equal to 90% and percent recovery of all treatment groups exceeded 80% (Freeman et al. 1999).

Initial metal spiking solutions were collected into 20-mL polyethylene vials, acidified with 250 μL of concentrated HNO_3, and stored at 4°C. Actual measured concentrations were verified to be within 10% of the nominal concentrations with atomic absorption spectrometry. LC50s from each replicate were generated using log-transformed data in Toxstat® 3.4 (WEST Inc. and Gulley 1994). The LC50s were reported as the mean value of three replicates. Standard deviations (SD) and coefficients of variation (CV) were also calculated from LC50s.

A three-way analysis of variance (ANOVA) was used to test for interactive effects of metal, soil type, and exposure time. All data passed the normal assumptions of ANOVA (normality, homeoscedasticity, and independence). Because there was a significant interaction among all three factors, two-way ANOVA was then performed to test for interactive effects between soil type and exposure time within each metal. Paired comparisons were performed with a Student's t-Test. A p-value less than 0.5 indicated a significant difference in all statistical tests. All statistical operations were performed using SAS (SAS 1989).

Results

Average 48-h LC50s and CVs are presented in Table 1. All CVs for the 24-h test were <10% (Peredney and Williams 2000). In the current test, CVs were higher for two reasons: 1) two operators were performing the tests and 2) the average LC50s were lower.

Table 1 – *Average 48-h LC50s and coefficients of variation (CV) for* C. elegans *exposed to metals in two field-collected soils.*

Metal	CECIL Avg LC50 (mg/kg)	CECIL Avg LC50 (μM)	CV (%)	TIFTON Avg LC50 (mg/kg)	TIFTON Avg LC50 (μM)	CV (%)
Cd	80	1106	12	18	255	22
Cu	193	4716	8	16	383	17
Ni	71	1868	17	34	891	7
Pb	487	3650	3	43	322	8
Zn	219	5211	15	76	1810	10

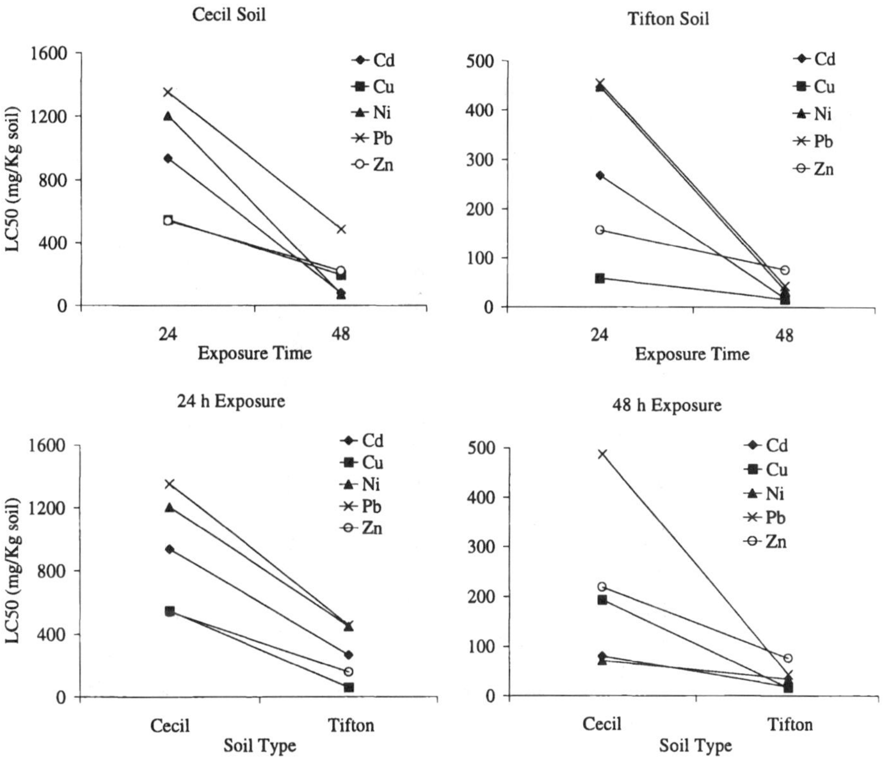

Figure 1 -- *Interactive effects of soil type and exposure time on the LC50s of five metals (Points joined for illustration only- not to imply a continnum).*

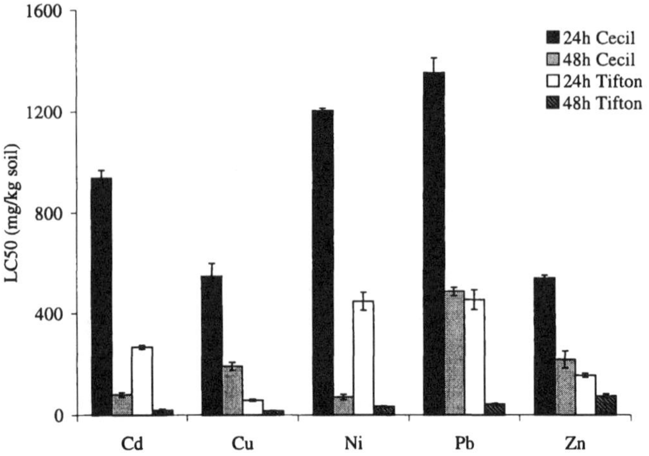

Figure 2-- *Average LC50s (mg metal/kg soil d.w.) for 24 and 48-h exposures of* C. elegans *to five metals in two field-collected soils.*

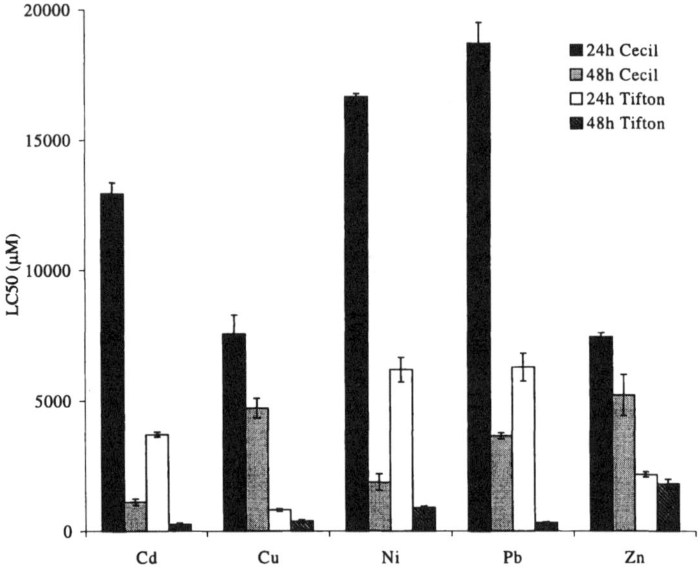

Figure 3-- *Average LC50s (μmole metal / L K-medium) for 24 and 48-h exposures of* C. elegans *to five metals in two field-collected soils.*

Significant interactive effects were found between soil type, exposure time, and metal using three-way ANOVA for LC50s expressed in terms of mg/kg of soil or µmol/L (Figure 1). Two-way ANOVAs also found significant interactions between soil type and exposure time within each metal. The Student's t-Test detected significant differences in means between soil type and exposure time for each metal. Average LC50s and standard deviations are presented in Figures 2 and 3. Increased exposure time resulted in increased toxicity or decreased LC50s. At both exposure times, higher LC50s were observed in Cecil soil than in Tifton soil for all metals.

Table 2 compares LC50s in soil tests with those in K-medium without soil present (24-h soil data from Peredney and Williams 2000; aquatic data compiled from Williams and Dusenbery 1990a, Cressman and Williams 1997, and Tatara et al. 1997 and 1998). In general, LC50s in Cecil soil were higher than in Tifton and Tifton LC50s were higher than aquatic values. The only exception for the 48-h data was Ni. The 48-h LC50 in K-medium only was higher than Cecil and Tifton values. This pattern was true for the 24-h data as well. In fact, all of the metals except Pb appeared to be more toxic in Tifton soil than in liquid medium at 24 h. In all exposure media, toxicity always increased with longer exposure time.

Table 2 – *Average 24- and 48-h LC50s in Tifton and Cecil soil and in K-medium (no soil present).*

Metal	Tifton 24-h LC50 (mg/L)	Tifton 48-h LC50 (mg/L)	Cecil 24-h LC50 (mg/L)	Cecil 48-h LC50 (mg/L)	Aquatic 24-h LC50 (mg/L)	Aquatic 48-h LC50 (mg/L)
Cd	416	29	1454	124	1307	10
Cu	90	25	851	300	109	1
Ni	696	52	1870	110	4039	185
Pb	707	67	2102	754	54	0.81
Zn	244	118	838	313	425	2

Discussion

Nematodes feed on bacteria and other microbes within the interstitial waters of the soil matrix, playing a substantial role in such processes as the nitrogen cycle, mineralization, decomposition, and nutrient mobilization (Wood et al. 1988). After exposure to toxicants in the soil, the ability of soil organisms to perform necessary functions may be impaired, leading to deleterious effects at the ecosystem level (Donkin 1997). Although the ecological significance of *C. elegans* has not been fully explored, the response of *C. elegans* to Cd is comparable to that of other nematode species (Kammenga et al. 1994). In addition, approximately 60% of *C. elegans* genome is shared by all nematodes (Blaxter 1998). A wealth of information exists on the biology, physiology, and genetics of *C. elegans* and stocks are easily cultured and maintained in the laboratory. These characteristics support the use of *C. elegans* in soil bioassays.

All metals appeared to be more toxic to *C. elegans* at an exposure time of 48 h in Tifton soil than to the earthworm *E. fetida* exposed for 14 days in ASTM soil (Table 3). When compared to the EPA's allowable limit for metals in land-applied sewage sludge, the ability of these limits to protect indigenous soil nematodes is questionable. While EC (European Commission) limits for soils are typically more stringent than U.S. limits, they are still higher in some cases.

Table 3- *LC50s and regulatory limits for metals in soils.*

Metal	*C. elegans* 48 h LC50 mg/kg (Tifton soil)	*E. fetida* 14 d LC50 mg/kg (ASTM soil)	US EPA 40 CFR 503 mg/kg (Max. yearly loading)	EC Limit Values mg/kg
Cd	19	1843	20	1-3
Cu	16	641	750	50-140
Ni	33	757	210	30-75
Pb	43	5947	150	50-300
Zn	76	661	1400	150-300

Acceptability criteria for 24-h soil testing have been established in our lab (Peredney and Williams 2000). The 24-h test required a percent recovery of live and dead worms >80% and control mortality <10%. Although the percent recovery of worms for the 48-h test was lower than that for the 24-h test (87% vs. >99%), each individual test had control survival ≥ 90%. A lower percent recovery with increased exposure time can be explained by the observation that most unrecovered worms were at the highest concentrations. If the worms died early in the exposure, decomposition processes would make the worms unidentifiable and, therefore, unrecoverable. For this reason, a lower percent recovery would be appropriate.

While the 48-h test produced lower LC50s than the 24-h test, the question remains: which exposure period produces results that reflect the actual toxicity of the soils? Our 24-h data were more comparable to those for the earthworm. Earthworm data are currently used to predict soil toxicity. If the earthworm test data accurately reflect metal toxicity then the 24-h test with nematodes should also be acceptable. Because nematodes perform such crucial roles in soil ecosystem processes, the 48-h test would more realistically reflect soil toxicity.

Besides lethality, additional endpoints of toxicity may also provide sensitive indications of sub-lethal toxic effects. Commonly-used sub-lethal endpoints used with invertebrates include reproduction, behavior, growth, and feeding and these have been previously explored with *C. elegans* in aquatic media (Anderson et al. 2001, Boyd et al. 2000, and Dhawan et al. 1999). Applications of these endpoints in soil toxicity tests require further study.

Toxic effects vary with soil conditions, species, and the specific contaminant and, thus, must be investigated on a site-specific basis. We feel that the nematode soil bioassay would prove useful as a supplement to existing standardized soil bioassays. The soil bioassay used in this study uses less soil (2.33 g) than the current standardized earthworm test (200g). In a situation where limited quantities of soil are available, the nematode soil bioassay would be an alternative to the earthworm test. Because a variety of species are involved with nutrient cycling and soil decomposition processes, single species tests may be an inadequate means of assessing toxicity of contaminants (Parmelee et al. 1997).

The bioavailability of metals in soil is dependent upon many factors. One of the most significant processes determining the fraction of chemical available in solution is sorption. Sorption is an electrostatic attraction between the positively charged metal cations in solution and negatively charged groups on SOM and clay particles. This phenomenon is dependent upon the physicochemical properties of the soil as well as environmental conditions. The pH of the soil is a most critical determining factor in soil sorption and soil speciation. Low pH values result in protonation of SOM functional groups and, therefore, in decreased sorption of cations.

The sorption of a particular metal is also dependent upon its chemical properties. Although the sorption selectivity is highly variable, in general, Cu, Pb, and Zn are sorbed more strongly than Cd and Ni (Sparks 1995). This could account for large differences between the 48-h LC50s for Cu and Pb (~ 12 and 11 times, respectively) between soil types (Figures 2 and 3). Toxic responses are a result of dose (or exposure concentration) and exposure time. Increased exposure time was shown to increase toxicity of all metals within a soil type. However, 24-h LC50s for Cu, Pb, and Zn in Tifton soil were either less than or equal to 48-h LC50s in Cecil soil. If these metals are strongly sorbed by SOM and Cecil contains significantly higher SOM than Tifton, it is reasonable to assume that the nematodes must have been receiving a lower dose of these metals over the exposure period.

These observations stress the importance of soil type on the resultant toxicity of metals. In standardized soil bioassays, an artificial medium typically replaces a natural soil as the testing medium. Organic carbon content gives a relative measure of the SOM content. ASTM artificial medium contains approximately 5% organic carbon compared to 2.5 and 0.7% in Cecil and Tifton soils, respectively. If metals were less toxic in Cecil soil than in Tifton soil, these same metals would appear to be even less toxic in ASTM artificial medium. This effect would be greatest for the most strongly sorbed metals described above and may partially explain the differences seen between the earthworm and nematode LC50s (Table 3). These results indicate the need for site-specific determinations of toxicity and assessment of toxicity in natural soils. A synthetic-testing medium such as the ASTM 'soil' can not mimic the effects of soil formation factors on soil properties. This could lead to overestimation or underestimation of the actual risk (Parmelee et al. 1997).

Future studies with our soil bioassay will focus on the measurement of metals within the soil solution rather than the amount spiked into the soil. In this manner, we hope to investigate the relationships between soil sorption and lethality of metals. To further validate our bioassay, we will also compare the toxic effects of different contaminants to *C. elegans* and other nematode species. Sub-lethal endpoints of toxicity are also being examined to provide a more sensitive indicator of soil toxicity.

Acknowledgments

We are grateful to the University of Georgia's Agricultural Experiment Station for financial support of this research. The nematode strain used in this work was provided by the *Caenorhabditis* Genetics Center, which is funded by the NIH National Center for Research Resources (NCRR).

References

Anderson, G. L., Boyd, W. A., and Williams, P. L., 2001, "Assessment of Sub-Lethal Endpoints for Toxicity Testing with the Nematode *Caenorhabditis elegans*," *Environmental Toxicology and Chemistry*, In press.

Blaxter, M., 1998, "*Caenorhabditis elegans* is a Nematode," *Science*, Vol. 282, pp. 2041-2046.

Boyd, W. A., Anderson, G. L., Dusenbery, D. B., and Williams, P. L., 2000, "Computer Tracking Method for Assessing Behavioral Changes in the Nematode *Caenorhabditis elegans*," *Environmental Toxicology and Risk Assessment: Recent Achievments in Environmental Fate and Transport: Ninth Volume, ASTM STP 1381*, F. T. Price, K. V. Brix, and N. K. Lane, Eds., American Society for Testing and Materials, West Conshohocken, PA, pp. 225-238.

Brenner, S., 1974, "The Genetics of *Caenorhabditis elegans*," *Genetics*, Vol. 77, pp. 71-94.

Caenorhabditis elegans Sequencing Consortium, 1998, "Genome Sequence of the Nematode *C. elegans*: A Platform for Investigating Biology," *Science*, Vol. 282, pp. 2012-2017.

Cressman, C. P. III and Williams, P. L., 1997, "Reference Toxicants for Toxicity Testing Using *Caenorhabditis elegans* in Aquatic Media," *Environmental Toxicology and Risk Assessment: Modeling and Risk Assessment (Sixth Volume), ASTM STP 1317*, F. James Dwyer, Thomas R. Doane, and Mark L. Hinman, Eds., American Society for Testing and Materials, West Conshohocken, PA, pp. 518-532.

Dhawan, R., Dusenbery, D. B., and Williams, P. L., 1999, "Comparison of Lethality, Reproduction, and Behavior as Toxicological Endpoints in the Nematode *Caenorhabditis elegans*," *Journal of Toxicology and Environmental Health*, Part A, Vol. 58, pp. 451-462.

Donkin, S. G., 1997, "Graphical Determination of Metal Bioavailability to Soil Invertebrates Utilizing the Langmuir Sorption Model," *Environmental Toxicology and Risk Assessment: Modeling and Risk Assessment (Sixth Volume), ASTM STP 1317*, F. James Dwyer, Thomas R. Doane, and Mark L. Hinman, Eds., American Society for Testing and Materials, West Conshohocken, PA, pp.28-43.

Donkin, S. G. and Dusenbery, D. B., 1993, "A Soil Toxicity Test Using the Nematode *Caenorhabditis elegans* and an Effective Method of Recovery," *Archives of Environmental Contamination and Toxicology*, Vol. 25, pp. 145-151.

Donkin, S. G. and Dusenbery, D. B., 1994, "Using The *Caenorhabditis elegans* Soil Toxicity Test to Identify Factors Affecting Toxicity of Four Metal Ions in Intact Soil," *Water, Air, and Soil Pollution*, Vol. 78, pp. 359-373.

Donkin, S. G., Eiteman, M. A., and Williams, P.L., 1995, "Toxicity of Glucosinolates and Their Enzymatic Decomposition Products to *Caenorhabditis elegans* ," *Journal of Nematology*, Vol. 27, No. 3, pp. 258-262.

Donkin, S. G. and Williams, P. L., 1995, "Influence of Developmental Stage, Salts, and Food Presence On Various End Points Using *Caenorhabditis elegans* for Aquatic Toxicity Testing," *Environmental Toxicology and Chemistry*, Vol. 14, No. 12, pp. 2139-2147.

Freeman, M. N., Marse, T. J., and Williams, P. L., 1998, "Establishment of Quality Assurance Procedures for Aquatic Toxicity Testing with the Nematode *Caenorhabditis elegans*," *Environmental Toxicology and Risk Assessment: Seventh Volume, ASTM STP 1333*, E. E. Little, A. J. DeLonay, and B. M. Greenberg, Eds., American Society for Testing and Materials, West Conshohocken, PA, pp. 45-59.

Freeman, M. N., Peredney, C. L., and Williams, P. L., 1999, "A Soil Bioassay Using the Nematode *Caenorhabditis elegans*," *Environmental Toxicology and Risk Assessment: Eighth Volume, ASTM STP 1364*, D. S. Henshel, M. C. Black, and M. C. Harrass, Eds., American Society for Testing and Materials, West Conshohocken, PA, pp. 305-318.

Kammenga, J. E., van Gestel, C. A. M., and Bakker, J., 1994, "Patterns of Sensitivity to Cadmium and Pentachlorophenol among Nematode Species from Different

Taxonomic and Ecological Groups," *Archives of Environmental Contamination and Toxicology*, Vol. 27, pp. 88-94.

Khanna, N., Cressman, C. P. III, Tatara, C. P., and Williams, P. L., 1997, "Tolerance of *Caenorhabditis elegans* to pH, Salinity and Hardness in Aquatic Media," *Archives of Environmental Contamination and Toxicology*, Vol. 32, pp. 110-114.

Lökke, H. and van Gestel, C. A. M., Eds., 1998, *Handbook of Soil Invertebrate Toxicity*, John Wiley & Sons, Ltd, New York, pp. 21-32.

Parmelee, R.W., Phillips, C.T., Checkai, R.T., and Bohlen, P.J., 1997, "Determining the Effects of Pollutants on Soil Faunal Communities and Trophic Structure Using a Refined Microcosm System," *Environmental Toxicology and Chemistry*, Vol. 16(6), pp. 1212-1217.

Peredney, C. L. and Williams, P. L., 2000, "Comparison of the Toxicological Effects of Nitrate versus Chloride Metallic Salts on *Caenorhabditis elegans* in Soil", *Environmental Toxicology and Risk Assessment: Recent Achievments in Environmental Fate and Transport: Ninth Volume, ASTM STP 1381*, F. T. Price, K. V. Brix, and N. K. Lane, Eds., American Society for Testing and Materials, West Conshohocken, PA, pp. 256-268.

SAS Institute Inc., 1989, *SAS/STAT® User's Guide, Version 6, Fourth Edition, Volume 2,* Cary, NC.

Sparks, D. L., 1995, *Environmental Soil Chemistry*, Academic Press, Inc., San Diego, CA, pp. 130-134.

Tatara, C. P., Newman, C. N., McCloskey, J. T., and Williams, P. L., 1997, "Predicting Relative Metal Toxicity with Ion Characteristics: *Caenorhabditis elegans* LC50," *Aquatic Toxicology*, Vol. 39, pp. 279-290.

Tatara, C. P., Newman, C. N., McCloskey J. T., and Williams, P. L., 1998, "Use of Ion Characteristics to Predict Relative Toxicity of Mono-, Di- and Trivalent Metal Ions: *Caenorhabditis elegans* LC50," *Aquatic Toxicology*, Vol. 42, pp.255-269.

West Inc. and Gully, D., 1994, *TOXSTAT® Documentation,* Western Ecosystems Technology, Inc., Cheyenne, WY.

Williams, P. L. and Dusenbery, D. B., 1988, "Using *Caenorhabditis elegans* to Predict Mammalian Acute Lethality to Metallic Salts," *Toxicology and Industrial Health*, Vol. 4, No. 4, pp. 469-478.

Williams, P. L. and Dusenbery, D. B., 1990, "Aquatic Toxicity Testing Using the Nematode *Caenorhabditis elegans*," *Environmental Toxicology and Chemistry*, Vol. 9, No. 4, pp. 1285-1290.

Wood, W.B., Ed., 1988, *The Nematode Caenorhabditis elegans*, Monograph 17, Cold Spring Harbor Laboratory, Plainview, NY.

Gladys L. Stephenson,[1] Juliska I. Princz,[2] Nicola Koper,[3] and Peter G. Miasek[4]

Terrestrial Toxicity Testing with Volatile Substances

Reference: Stephenson, G. L., Princz, J. I., Koper, N., and Miasek, P. G., "**Terrestrial Toxicity Testing with Volatile Substances,**" *Environmental Toxicology and Risk Assessment: Science, Policy, and Standardization – Implications for Environmental Decisions: Tenth Volume, ASTM STP 1403*, B. M. Greenberg, R. N. Hull, M. H. Roberts, Jr., and R. W. Gensemer, Eds., American Society for Testing and Materials, West Conshohocken, PA, 2001.

Abstract: The toxicity of volatile hydrocarbons to terrestrial organisms is currently being investigated. It was found that toxicity test methods required procedural modification during test soil preparation to minimize the loss of the test substance due to volatilization. A series of tests was initiated with an artificial and field-collected reference soil to investigate alternative test-soil, preparation, methodologies for evaluating motor gasoline (mogas) as it predominantly contains highly volatile low-end carbon components (≤C5-C13). The proposed approaches to minimize volatilization losses included the application of mogas at concentrations sufficiently high to accommodate the percentage lost during test soil preparation; the modification of test soil preparation methods; and the modification of the nature of test units. The analyses of benzene, toluene, ethylbenzene, xylene (BTEX) compounds, total purgeable hydrocarbons (TPuH), total extractable hydrocarbons (TEH), and total petroleum hydrocarbons (TPH) from soil samples quantified the losses of these mogas constituents at each stage of preparation. The constituents of the mogas were found to volatilize at different rates and the losses were to some extent, concentration dependent. Amending test soils at higher concentrations than required for an adverse effect compensated for the rate of the losses due to volatilization. Significant amounts of the mogas were lost regardless of the methods used to prepare the test soils. Alternative "closed" (minimized air exchange) test units were considered useful and acceptable, as they optimized exposure of the test organism to mogas and did not compromise their survival. The test methods developed to assess the toxicity of mogas in terrestrial organisms may be equally applicable to the toxicity testing of other highly volatile substances.

Keywords: motor gasoline, toxicity, volatilization, test methods, soil

---

[1] Ph. D. Candidate, Department of Environmental Biology, University of Guelph, Guelph, Ontario, Canada N1G 2W1.

[2] Toxicologist, ESG International Inc., 361 Southgate Dr., Guelph, Ontario, Canada, N1G 3M5.

[3] Ph.D, Candidate, Department of Renewable Resources, University of Alberta, Edmonton, Alberta, Canada T6G 2M7.

[4] Senior Environmental Advisor, Imperial Oil, 90 Wynford Dr., North York, Ontario, Canada, M3C 1K5.

Introduction

The Canada-wide standards (CWS) for petroleum hydrocarbons (PHC) are currently being developed pursuant to the 1998 Canada-wide Accord on Environmental Harmonization of the Canadian Council of Ministers of the Environment (CCME) and its Canada-wide Environmental Standards Sub-agreement. The goal for development of the Canada-wide standards for PHC is to provide a consistent approach to managing PHC-contaminated sites across the country and to protect human health and the environment by determining the acceptable risk associated with exposure to these substances in soils.

A number of research programs were initiated to provide supporting documentation in the form of toxicity data to aid in the CWS development process. The Petroleum Technology Alliance Canada (PTAC) and the Canadian Association of Petroleum Producers (CAPP) provided support for a multi-year, two-phase research program. Phase I aimed to develop a fraction-based approach to support ecologically-relevant, risk-based, soil quality criteria for the protection of environmental health. The test battery for Phase I of the PTAC project included both short-term and longer-term exposures to potentially lethal and sub-lethal concentrations, respectively, of Alberta Federated crude oil and its four fractions. Fraction 1 (F1) comprised petroleum hydrocarbons ranging from >C5 to nC10, Fraction 2 (F2) comprised >nC10 to nC16, Fraction 3 (F3) comprised >nC16 to nC34, and Fraction 4 (F4) comprised all hydrocarbons ≥C35. The aim of Phase II of the project was to examine the ecotoxicological properties and risks, if any, of weathered hydrocarbon residuals exceeding 1000 μg/g in agricultural soils.

A comparable two-phase research program, supported by the Canadian Petroleum Producers Institute (CPPI) and the Centre for Research in Earth and Space Technology (CRESTech), was initiated to assess the toxicity of additive-free motor gasoline (mogas) to terrestrial organisms. The composition of the mogas fell into the hydrocarbon range spanned by F1 and, in part, F2 of the crude oil. The mogas project was also divided into two phases. Phase I was designed to determine the toxicity of mogas to a terrestrial test-species battery which was comparable to that used in the PTAC project. Phase II was designed to examine the implications of sequestration on bioavailability and toxicity of mogas in soil to terrestrial organisms.

Phase I of the mogas project involved a series of preliminary toxicity tests with earthworms, plants, and springtails, and an artificial soil and a field-collected reference soil to investigate alternative test-soil preparation methodologies for evaluating the fate and effects of mogas as it predominantly contains highly volatile low-end carbon components. Since mogas losses can occur at different stages of test soil preparation, the initial nominal exposure concentration might differ from the actual (i.e., measured) concentrations of mogas to which the organisms are exposed. The proposed approaches to minimize the losses due to volatilization included the application of mogas at concentrations sufficiently high to accommodate the percentage lost during test soil preparation; the modification of the test soil preparation methods (amendment and mixing procedures); and the modification of the nature of the test units. The potential influence of test soil preparation methods on the results of the toxicity tests were also investigated.

There are two fundamental approaches used to prepare test soils for toxicity assessment. A batch of soil can be amended with a test substance at a relatively high concentration and subsequently proportionally diluting the soil with a clean control soil to produce a series of test soils (e.g., treatments) along a concentration gradient. Alternatively, each treatment (e.g., each exposure concentration) can be prepared independently by amending (e.g., spiking) individual batches of soil, that are sufficient in size to satisfy the test replicate requirement for that treatment, with the test substance. We compared the fate and behavior of mogas in the two types of soil using these two test-soil preparation approaches.

There are two ways to incorporate a test substance into a control soil or to mix the chemicallyspiked soils with the control soils. We compared the fate and effects of these two mixing procedures which included mechanically mixing the amended test soil with an electronic mixer and a stainless steel spoon for 3 to 5 minutes, or using a tumbling device whereby the test soils were placed into sealed glass containers and tumbled end-over-end for 24 h.

The third procedural modification included the use of "open" and "closed" test units. Traditionally, test units with terrestrial organisms allow the exchange of air. This air exchange was believed essential to the survival and well-being of the test organisms. However, the use of these "open" test units was thought to contribute to volatile losses of the hydrocarbons from soil. Therefore, the use of "closed" test units (i.e., those that did not permit air exchange) was compared with "open" test units. The results of these preliminary studies are presented with recommendations for testing with volatile substances.

The test methods and modifications briefly described herein are discussed in greater detail elsewhere (ESG International 2000). Additional toxicity data for a larger test battery and mogas in other types of soils are also available (ESG International 2000).

Materials and Methods

Production and Characterization of Mogas

The Environmental Technology Group (ETG) of the Imperial Oil (IOL) Research Department provided the additive-free, refinery blend of motor gasoline. Ten litres of mogas from each of five Ontario refineries were collected in May 1999 before the refineries had switched to a summer blend. All refinery samples were stored in a cold room (0-10°C) until preparation to limit the volatilization during handling. The 10-L samples were placed into a 100-L drum and agitated for five minutes to form a 50-L composite sample. The 50-L sample was then divided among fourteen, 4 L, aviation fuel containers, purged with nitrogen and returned to the cold room for storage. Subsamples were sent for compositional analyses to the IOL Research Analytical laboratory (Sarnia, Ontario, Canada) and the Philip Analytical Services Corp. (PASC) laboratory (Halifax, Nova Scotia, Canada). IOL characterized the mogas according to the Canadian General Standards Board procedure CAN/CGSB-3.0 No. 14.3-94 of the analytical protocol titled Standard Test Method for the Identification of Hydrocarbon Components in Automotive Gasoline Using Gas Chromatography. The PASC laboratory characterized the mogas using procedures recommended by the US TPH Criteria Working Group and the Atlantic Partners in RBCA Implementation (PIRI) titled Aliphatic and Aromatic Fractionation of

Petroleum Hydrocarbons. The mogas samples were analyzed in duplicate by each methodology to assess variability in the analytical procedures.

Test Soil Preparation

Control Soils – Two types of soil, an artificial and a field-collected reference soil, were used for the test method development and subsequent toxicity tests. The artificial soil (AS) was formulated in the laboratory as described by Stephenson et al. (1997).

The field-collected, reference soil (referred to as sandy loam reference or SLR) originated from an area that had been cultivated regularly for organic crop production but not subjected to pesticide application. The soil was classified as a fine sandy-loam in texture, and represented a "worse" case scenario with respect to mogas toxicity because it maximized bioavailability of the mogas to the organisms. It was collected in June 1999 from Beauchamp Farms (Eramosa, Wellington County, Ontario) and subsequently sieved (5-mm and 2-mm mesh), allotted to buckets, and placed in cold storage (4°C). The AS was comparable in texture, but had a higher organic matter content, and a greater percentage of clay resulting in a higher water holding capacity.

Amendment Procedures

A study was designed to compare the two fundamental approaches to test soil preparation described earlier (proportional dilution of a mogas-spiked soil with a clean control soil, and spiking individual treatments).

Proportional Dilution - A relatively large quantity of AS, sufficient to produce a series of test soils along a concentration gradient, was weighed into a stainless steel bowl. The batch of soil was then quantitatively amended, in increments, with sufficient mogas to achieve 100% saturation. Subsequent to each addition, the soil was mixed with a hand-held mechanical mixer in order to evenly incorporate the mogas into the soil. For each treatment, the mogas-amended soil was proportionally diluted (on a dry weight basis) with the clean control AS, and a pre-calculated amount of deionized water was added to achieve a moisture content of 35%. The contents were then mixed with the hand-held mechanical mixer and a stainless steel spoon for approximately three minutes, until homogeneity (i.e., uniform in texture and color) was achieved.

Spiking Individual Treatments - Each treatment (e.g., each concentration of the test substance in soil) was prepared independently by amending individual batches of AS, sufficient in size to satisfy the test replicate requirement for that treatment, with the mogas. Each batch of AS was prepared in a stainless steel bowl. Holes were "poked" into the soil with a gloved finger, and the pre-calculated amount of mogas was equally distributed (by volume) among these holes with the use of a pipette. The holes were then covered up with the surrounding soil to minimize volatilization. Deionized water was added in increments, and the contents of the bowl were then mixed for approximately three minutes with a hand-held mixer and a stainless steel spoon until the mixture was visibly homogenous.

Subsequent to test soil preparation, the toxicity of these test soils to earthworms (Eisenia fetida) was evaluated. Five clitellate E. fetida were placed into a 500-mL glass mason jar filled with 270 g wet weight (w.w.) of test soil. The test units were placed into cardboard boxes and ventilated in a fumehood at room temperature (19–25 °C) with a photoperiod of constant fluorescent illumination. Mortality was assessed on days 7 and 14 of the acute test, whereby the contents of each test unit were placed onto a tray, sorted with forceps, and the earthworms reported as either dead or alive. Mortality was determined as failure to respond (e.g., contract) upon gentle prodding with a glass rod. Dead worms were seldom observed due to the rapid rate of earthworm tissue decomposition. If repeated measurements were to be made, the contents on the tray were returned to the test unit and the earthworms placed onto the surface of the soil. Otherwise, the test soils were discarded. Sub-samples of the test soils were collected from both methods of test-soil preparation and analyzed for BTEX compounds, total purgeable hydrocarbons (TPuH, includes BTEX levels), total extractable hydrocarbons (TEH), and total petroleum hydrocarbons (TPH) by PASC (Burlington, Ontario, Canada). The soil sub-samples that were submitted consisted of the saturated batch of soil; test soils immediately after dilution, or spiking, and mixing; test soils immediately upon addition to the test units; and one sample from each of the control soils. The nominal exposure levels were equivalent to 0, 6.27, 12.53, 24.99, 51.79, 102.52, and 200.95 mg/g soil dry weight (d.w.). Sub-samples for chemical analyses were collected from treatments 6.27, 102.52, and 200.95 mg mogas/g soil d.w.

Mixing Methods

A study was designed to compare the effects of the two previously described mixing methods on the fate and effects of mogas in soil.

Mechanical Mixing – Individual quantities of AS, sufficient to satisfy the test replicate requirement for each treatment, were weighed into 1-L glass mason jars, and refrigerated for approximately 12 h at 6±3°C. Subsequently, each batch of soil, contained in the 1-L glass mason jar, was transferred to a stainless steel bowl and prepared by spiking individual treatments, and mixing 3 to 5 minutes with a hand-held mixer until homogeneity of soil texture and color was observed. The soils were then quantitatively distributed (by wet mass) among the test units within the appropriate treatment. Each treatment was prepared in order of increasing concentration. The prepared test units were refrigerated for an additional 24 h, and then acclimated to room temperature for approximately 3 hours before use in a seedling emergence toxicity test.

Tumbling – Individual quantities of AS, sufficient to satisfy the test replicate requirement for each treatment, were weighed into 1-L glass mason jars and refrigerated for approximately 12 h at 6±3°C. After the 12-h refrigeration period, the soil in each glass jar was quantitatively amended (by volume) with mogas and deionized water. The mogas and water were placed into holes in the soil that had been made with a glass stirring rod. The lids of the jars were then replaced, and the jars were transported to Canviro Analytical Laboratories (Kitchener-Waterloo, Ontario, Canada) where they were placed into a tumbling device, which tumbled the jars end-over-end at a rate of 10 rpm for 24 h. After the tumbling was complete, the contents of each jar (e.g., the treatment) were transferred into a sealed polyethylene zip-lock bag (Glad Zipper™) and 'hand-kneaded' until uniform in texture and color. Thereafter, 150 g w.w. of the test soil were added to each appropriate test unit, and the seeds planted.

The plant species used for these tests was *Zea mays* (corn) with nominal mogas exposure levels of 0, 1, 2, 3, 5, 6, 8, 12, 15, 25, 50, and 100 mg/g soil d.w. Five seeds were planted per test unit in a circular pattern with one seed planted in the middle to a depth that was twice that of the width of the seed; the planted seeds were then covered with the test soil. The test units were randomly placed into an environmental growth chamber with a photoperiod of 16 h light (24 ± 2°C): 8 h dark (16 ± 2°C). The light intensity was on average 400 μmoles/m^2/s. At the end of the 7-day test, the visible concentration-response of the plants was photographed before the test units were processed. Processing each test unit entailed separating the plants from the soil, spraying the roots with water to remove any adhering soil particles, measuring the shoot and root lengths, and determining the shoot and root wet masses. The shoots and roots were transferred to separate aluminium weigh-boats, which were then placed into a drying oven at 90°C for 48 h. Thereafter, the dry masses were determined. The treatments from which the sub-samples were collected for BTEX, TEH, TPuH, and TPH analyses for each of the procedures were 0, 1, 15, and 100 mg mogas/g soil d.w.

Test Unit Modification

Toxicity of mogas to plants (barley) and two species of soil invertebrates (earthworm and springtail) was evaluated in both open and closed test units.

Plants - Artificial test soils were prepared by spiking individual treatments with mechanical mixing. The "open" plant test units consisted of five *Hordeum vulgare* (barley) seeds planted into 70 g w.w. of soil in a glass petri dish (100 x 15 mm). The petri dish was then placed into an inverted 1-L polypropylene container (i.e. the petri dish was placed onto the plastic lid of the container). The containers were temporarily removed when the plants were watered. The "closed" test units consisted of covered glass petri dishes with the edges sealed with parafilm for the first 48 h. Thereafter, the parafilm and the glass petri dish lids were removed, and the test units were treated as "open" test units.

Throughout the duration of the tests, the integrity of the plastic 1-L containers was compromised at the higher concentrations; the plastic became warped and more malleable. Since the plastic containers were apparently permeable to and reactive with the volatile compounds, sealed 1-L glass parfait jars with hinged lids were investigated as alternative test units. Soil, 150 g w.w. for acute (short-term, 7-day) tests and 650 g w.w. for definitive (longer-term, 14- to 21-day) tests, was placed into the bottom of the jar, and the seeds planted within. The lids remained closed for the duration of the acute toxicity tests, and for the first 7 days of the definitive tests. These test units were subjected to the same test conditions as described earlier for corn.

Invertebrates - Toxicity tests with *Eisenia fetida* were performed in both the AS and SLR, and subjected to both "open" and "closed" conditions. The test units consisted of 270 g w.w. of soil placed into a 500-mL glass mason jar covered with aluminium foil fastened with a metal screw ring. The nominal exposure concentrations were 0, 0.5, 1, 2, 3, and 5 mg/g soil d.w. The "open" test units had four holes poked into the aluminium foil to allow for exchange of air; the "closed" test units had no holes.

Test soils were prepared on Day −1 by spiking individual treatments using mechanical mixing methodology, and quantitatively added to the appropriate test units. The test units were sealed tightly, to minimize volatilization, and acclimated to room temperature for an equilibration period of 24 h. On day 0, the earthworms were removed from the cultures, washed with de-ionized water to remove any adhering soil particles, and placed into a tray lined with paper towel. Five clitellate worms were added to each test unit, across treatment levels. The test units were subjected to the same test conditions, and adult survival was assessed on both Day 7 and 14, as previously described.

Test units for the springtail (*Onychiurus folsomi*) 7-day toxicity tests consisted of 30 g w.w. of soil placed into a 125-mL glass mason jar with the metal cap and screw-ring. The lids were screwed on tightly and "closed" for the duration of the acute toxicity tests. Test soils were prepared and equilibrated comparable to those of the earthworm toxicity tests. Ten adults were transferred from a single culture, using the moistened hairs of a finely bristled paintbrush, to each of the test units across treatments. Maturity was judged by the appearance of an enlarged, rounded abdomen, and a body length of 2 mm or more. The test units were subjected to the same test conditions as the earthworm toxicity tests. At the end of the 7-day test, the springtails were floated, due to their hydrophobic outer integument, with tap water, counted and removed with a finely bristled paintbrush. Adult mortality was assessed as total cessation of movement of any body part. Toxicity to springtails of mogas in both types of soil (AS and SLR) was assessed.

Loss of Mogas from Test Soils

Subsamples of test soils were collected from two of the toxicity tests to assess the extent of mogas degradation over a period of 14 days. One of the tests consisted of an acute screening test with corn where the test soils, made with AS, were prepared by spiking methodology and mechanically mixing or tumbling in closed containers. Independent replicate test units were established for chemical analyses and subjected to "closed" conditions. Subsamples of soil were collected from the test units of nominal treatments 1, 15, and 100 mg mogas/g AS d.w., on days 0, 3, and 7, and analyzed for BTEX, TEH, TPuH, and TPH levels.

The second test was an acute 7-day test with the springtail, *O. folsomi*, exposed to mogas-spiked AS and SLR soils in closed test units. Independent replicate test units were prepared for chemical analyses with an extra set of replicates for sampling on day 14. The nominal exposure concentrations were 0, 0.5, 1, 2, 3, 8, and 10 mg/g soil d.w. Soil subsamples were collected from time-independent replicates in treatments 0, 1, 3, and 8 mg mogas/g AS and SLR d.w., on days 0, 1, 3, 7, and 14, and analyzed for BTEX, TEH, TPuH and TPH levels.

Soil subsampling consisted of completely filling, to eliminate headspace, two 50-mL amber bottles; one was archived, and the other was used to determine the concentration of the petroleum hydrocarbons in the soil. The expected soil concentrations of the mogas constituents were calculated based on the percent composition of these constituents present in the mogas from compositional analyses. Expected soil concentrations were calculated using a percentage composition for benzene of 1.5%, toluene of 5.1%, ethylbenzene of 1.5%, o-xylene of 1.65%, m,p-xylene of 5.55%, TPuH of 81.3%, and TEH of 17.6%.

Statistical Analysis

The plant toxicity data were analyzed using nonlinear regression procedures (Stephenson et al. 2000) that had been re-parameterized to include ICp estimates and their associated 95% confidence limits. The residuals were examined to ensure all assumptions were met, including homogeneity of variance among treatments. If data showed heteroscedasticity among treatments, data were weighted with the inverse of the variance of each treatment (Myers 1986). Analysis of variance procedures and a one-tailed Dunnett's test (SPSS 1997) were applied to the emergence data. The results of the invertebrate toxicity tests were analyzed to determine the LC50 using the Probit, the Moving Average, and the Trimmed Spearman-Karber methods of linear regression analysis (Stephan 1989).

Results and Discussion

Production and Characterization of Mogas

The relative percent deviation (RPD) for the IOL duplicate samples was less than 2%, which indicates that the methodology was reliable and that there was little variation between the samples. The RPD for the PASC duplicate samples varied between 0 and 23%, which meets the industry standard for acceptability for analytical duplicates. Table 1 summarizes the results of the two analytical approaches. The analytical results for the individual BTEX compounds for the IOL methodology were 1.5, 5.1, 1.5, and 7.2 wt% (weight by percentage), respectively. For the PASC methodology, they were 1.5, 4.7, 1.5, and 7.1 wt%, respectively. The corresponding % RPDs were 1.1, 8.5, 1.8, and 2.6%, respectively.

The variability between the two methodologies was minimal for the aromatic components. With the exception of the >C10-12 aromatic hydrocarbons (RPD = 59%), the two methods produced comparable results. However, the results for the aliphatic hydrocarbons were more variable with RPDs ranging from 28% to 92% at concentrations >1wt%.

Table 1 - *Comparison of the analytical results (% by weight) for the two methods of PHC analyses showing the RPD (%) for each carbon range.*

	Aromatics			Aliphatics		
Carbon Range	PASC Method (Atlantic PIRI)	IOL Method (CGSB)	% RPD	PASC Method (Atlantic PIRI)	IOL Method (CGSB)	% RPD
<C5	NA	ND	ND	NA	14	ND
C5-C6	NA	ND	ND	NA	23	ND
>C6-C8	NA[1]	NA[1]	0	39	29	-36
>C8-C10	6.5[2]	7.2[2]	10	<5	4	-28
>C10-C12	2.9	7.1	59	2	1	-92
>C12-C16	1.0	1.1	9	<1	<1	-415
>C16-C21	0.1	ND	ND	<1	ND	ND
>C21-C32	ND	ND	ND	ND	ND	ND
Total	25[3]	31[3]	19	<47	70	>33

[1]Excludes benzene and toluene (Philip=1.5 + 4.7 = 6.2 wt%, IOL = 1.5 + 5.1 = 6.6 wt %).
[2]Excludes ethylbenzene and xylenes (Philip = 1.5 + 7.1 = 8.6 wt%, IOL = 1.5 + 7.2 = 8.7 wt%).
[3]Includes BTEX (Philip = 15 wt%, IOL = 15 wt%).
NA Not Analysed.
ND Not Detected.

The most significant difference between the two analytical approaches was that the Philip Atlantic PIRI procedure does not measure aliphatic hydrocarbons ≤C6. The IOL CGSB procedure showed that approximately 36% of the total aliphatics in the mogas were ≤C6. The IOL CGSB method also showed that over 64% of the mogas was comprised of ≤C10 aliphatic hydrocarbons and 21% was comprised of ≤C10 aromatic hydrocarbons for a total of 85% of the constituents in mogas in the carbon range of ≤C10. This compositional resolution indicates that the majority of the unweathered gasoline components are quantified in the volatile petroleum hydrocarbon methodology of PASC. In this procedure the concentration of the aromatic components are determined using an average response to a multi-component aromatic and aliphatic blend, while the concentration of the aliphatic components is determined by subtraction. The differences noted between the two methods were attributed primarily to this estimation of the concentration. Given the significant differences discussed above, it was recommended that the IOL CGSB methodology be used to determine the composition of the mogas since it covers the entire boiling range of the gasoline and is accredited by the Canadian Standards Board.

Amendment Procedures

The nominal and the measured exposure concentrations of the test soils prepared using both amendment procedures are presented in Table 2. Test soil preparation by the proportional dilution method reduced the amount of volatilization at higher concentrations; however, at the lowest concentration, the spiking methodology minimized this loss. Upon comparison, approximately 68 to 91% of the mogas was lost due to volatilization during test soil preparation, regardless of the amendment method used. The reduction of volatilization varied with the constituent and the concentration and, as there was no clear pattern to this variability, one test soil preparation method could not be recommended as being better than the other.

Table 2–*Nominal and measured initial exposure concentrations of mogas in test soils prepared by proportional dilution or spiking individual treatments at 0, 6.27, 102.52, and 200.95 mg/g soil d.w. in artificial soil.*

Dilution Equivalent (% contamination)	Nominal Concentration (mg/g soil d.w.)	Measured Concentration (mg/g soil d.w.)	Percent of Nominal (%)	Percent Lost (%)
Dilution Methodology				
0	0	0.00055		
3	6.27	0.55	8.77	91.23
50	102.52	32	31.21	68.79
100	200.95	51	25.38[1]	74.62
"Saturated"[1]	200.95	86	42.80[2]	57.20
Spiking Methodology				
0	0	0.0016		
3	6.27	0.88	14.03	85.96
50	102.52	27	26.34	73.66
100	200.95	36	17.91	82.09

[1]The difference between "saturated" and "100% dilution" was temporal (≈10 min) during which the "saturated" batch of soil with mogas remained in a covered container. The "saturated" subsample of soil was collected for analyses immediately after the mogas was added to the batch of control soil.

Mixing Methods

The exposure concentrations, nominal and measured, are presented in Table 3 for both types of the mixing methodologies. It was observed that the losses were greater, on average, for the BTEX compounds when using mechanical mixing procedures. However, the losses of TPuH and TEH at the lower concentrations were greater using the tumbling device. At higher concentrations, a reduction in the loss of volatiles was evident with the use of the tumbling device, when used in conjunction with the spiking methodology. However, the use of the tumbling device resulted in the build up of mogas vapors, and a film of gasoline was apparent on the outside of the jars spiked at the higher concentrations, indicative that some of the vapors had escaped during the tumbling. The loss could, perhaps, be further reduced by tumbling at a lower temperature (e.g., 4-10°C) rather than at room temperature, and enclosing the test soils in high-density polypropylene bags in the jars.

Plants - The IC50s and IC20s for each of the plant tests are presented in Table 4. In terms of toxicity, there were no apparent differences between the effects on plant growth using the two methods of mixing. The results indicate that much of the mogas was lost. regardless of the mixing methodology.

Table 3 - *Exposure concentrations of mogas in artificial soil at 1000, 15 000 and 100 000 mg/kg soil d.w. over the course of a 7-d acute toxicity test with Zea mays.*

Nominal Concentration (mg/kg soil d.w.)	Measured Parameter	Measured Concentration (mg/kg soil d.w.) Day 0	Day 3	Day 7
Mechanically mixed soils				
AS-1000	BTEX	12.2	5.8	<D.L.[1]
AS-15000		70.6	15.0	5.14
AS-100000		8420	5760	5950
AS-1000	TPuH	67	5.8	<D.L.
AS-15000		310	380	51
AS-100000		12000	14000	11000
AS-1000	TEH	110	35	<D.L.
AS-15000		1200	640	220
AS-100000		17000	14000	11000
AS-1000	TPH	177	40.8	<D.L.
AS-15000		1510	1020	271
AS-100000		29000	28000	22000
Tumbled soils				
AS-1000	BTEX	12.4	4.6	<D.L.
AS-15000		936	110.9	14.4
AS-100000		8630	11320	6410
AS-1000	TPuH	12	4.6	<D.L.
AS-15000		3800	520	80
AS-100000		16000	21000	9000
AS-1000	TEH	53	27	14
AS-15000		1300	890	430
AS-100000		14000	15000	12000
AS-1000	TPH	65	31.6	14
AS-15000		5100	1410	510
AS-100000		30000	36000	21000

[1]<D.L. less than the detection limit of the analytical method.

Use of Open Versus Closed Test Units

Plants – The IC50s for the different measurement endpoints for the barley in open and closed test units in AS are presented in Table 4. It was determined that the original polypropylene test containers were inappropriate for use with mogas in soil because the material was permeable to, and reactive with, the volatile constituents. The test units warped in the headspace region and not where the soil was in contact with the test unit. The alternative glass test units (parfait jars with lids) obviated this problem. The use of these glass test units during 7-day acute exposures was acceptable in that, when closed, they did not adversely affect seedling emergence or growth and the soils did not require the addition of water during the test period. It terms of toxicity, the corn was marginally less sensitive than barley, and the IC50s produced from the use of closed test units were marginally lower than those produced from the use of open test units. The toxicity of mogas to barley and corn was not affected by the test soil preparation methodologies.

Table 4-*Effects of mogas (mg/g soil d.w.) on short-term (7 days) growth of corn and barley in artificial soil.*[1]

Species	Variable	Model	IC50	LCL	UCL	IC20	LCL	UCL	W?
Barley (S, M, O)	Shoot Length	Gompertz	7.24	6.22	8.25	4.43	3.17	5.68	N
	Shoot Wet Mass	Gompertz	7.86	5.85	9.86	5.53	2.68	8.39	N
	Shoot Dry Mass	Gompertz	7.79	5.97	9.62	5.74	3.17	8.31	N
	Root Length	Gompertz	4.48	4.13	4.84	2.31	1.94	2.67	N
	Root Wet Mass	Gompertz	4.31	2.94	5.67	2.18	0.77	3.58	N
	Root Dry Mass	Gompertz	4.78	3.63	5.93	2.32	1.20	3.44	N
Barley (S, M, C)	Shoot Length	Logistic	5.00	4.33	5.66	2.85	2.18	3.52	N
	Shoot Wet Mass	Gompertz	5.50	4.72	6.27	4.39	3.47	5.31	N
	Shoot Dry Mass	Logistic	5.44	5.00	5.88	3.56	2.99	4.12	N
	Root Length	Logistic	2.76	2.46	3.05	1.59	1.26	1.93	N
	Root Wet Mass	Gompertz	3.66	2.74	4.58	1.93	0.84	3.01	N
	Root Dry Mass	Gompertz	3.59	2.78	4.40	1.62	0.76	2.48	N
Corn (S, M, C)	Shoot Length	Logistic	4.65	4.13	5.18	3.08	2.30	3.86	Y
	Shoot Wet Mass	Logistic	9.25	7.87	10.63	6.67	5.43	7.91	N
	Shoot Dry Mass	Gompertz	9.62	8.19	11.05	6.25	4.76	7.74	N
	Root Length	Exponential	2.70	2.42	2.99	1.00	0.77	1.23	Y
	Root Wet Mass	Logistic	8.93	7.36	10.49	6.75	5.34	8.16	N
	Root Dry Mass	Gompertz	8.44	6.44	10.45	5.47	3.32	7.61	N
Corn (S, T, C)	Shoot Length	Hormesis	4.88	4.49	5.27	3.23	2.80	3.66	N
	Shoot Wet Mass	Logistic	7.59	7.28	7.91	5.26	4.50	6.01	Y
	Shoot Dry Mass	Gompertz	7.71	6.58	8.83	4.23	3.00	5.46	N
	Root Length	Logistic	3.14	2.86	3.43	1.92	1.43	2.41	Y
	Root Wet Mass	Hormesis	9.09	7.13	11.06	6.83	5.64	8.02	N
	Root Dry Mass	Hormesis	9.61	6.81	12.40	6.73	4.95	8.50	N

[1]W? Indicates if data has been weighted; M Mechanical Mixing Methodology; T Tumbling Methodology
LCL Lower Confidence Limit; Y Yes; C Closed Test Units
UCL Upper Confidence Limit; N No
S Spiking Methodology; O Open Test Units

Earthworms – The 14-day Spearman-Karber LC50, with the lower and upper 95% confidence limits, for *E. fetida* exposed to mogas in AS in the "open" test units was 1.86 (1.56 – 2.21) mg/g AS d.w. and 1.15 (0.88 – 1.49) mg/g AS d.w. for "closed" test units. The 14-day Spearman-Karber LC50s in the SLR were 0.71 (95% confidence limits unavailable) and 0.40 (0.32 – 0.50) mg/g SLR d.w. for "open" and "closed" test units, respectively. The LC50s were slightly lower in the "closed" test units relative to the "open" test units. The use of "closed" test units for acute exposure durations reduced the volatilization of mogas constituents and, the lack of air exchange did not compromise the survival of the test organisms in the control treatments. Mogas was more toxic to the earthworms in the SLR than in the AS.

Springtails - The 7-day LC50, with the lower and upper 95% confidence limits, for *Onychiurus folsomi* exposed to mogas in AS was 5.96 (5.34-6.66) mg/g AS d.w. in closed test units. The 7-day LC50, with the lower and upper 95% confidence limits, for

Onychiurus folsomi exposed to mogas in SLR was 4.19 (3.68-4.77) mg/g SLR d.w. in closed test units. Sensitivity to mogas increased when the springtails were exposed to the contaminant in the sandy loam as compared to the artificial soil (Fig. 1).

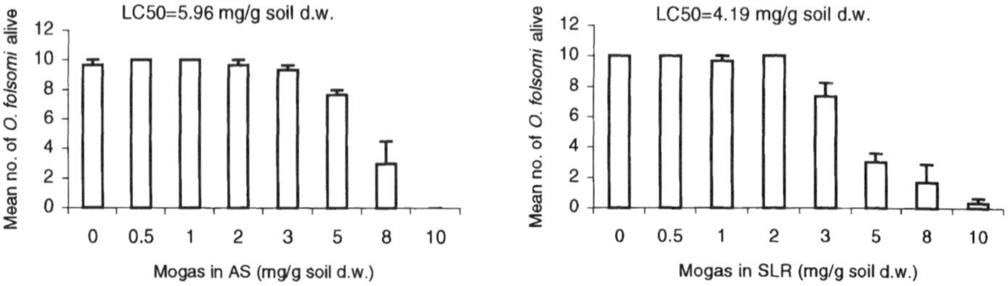

Figure 1 - *Survivorship of adult springtails (Onychiurus folsomi) following a 7 day exposure to mogas in artificial (AS) and sandy loam reference (SLR) soil. Bars indicate the standard error for survivorship in the treatment.*

Loss of Mogas from Test Soils

The results of the chemical analyses of the acute corn toxicity tests are presented in Table 3. The BTEX compounds dissipated rapidly from the soils at the lower concentrations (e.g., <15, 000 mg/kg soil d.w.), but were detectable at the higher concentrations (e.g., ≥15, 000 mg/kg soil d.w.). Similar results were observed in the acute toxicity tests with *O. folsomi* in both the AS and the SLR (Table 5), with most of the mogas constituents dissipating after 7 days to below detection limits on Day 14. The rate of dissipation appeared to be constituent and concentration dependent.

Soil properties such as texture, porosity, water content, and organic carbon content influence the rate of diffusion of volatiles through soil (Johnson and Perrott 1991). The AS was observed to retain a greater amount of the mogas at the lower concentrations (i.e., ≤3000) when compared to the SLR. This could have been due to a greater organic matter (present as peat) and silt content, which could increase the adsorption of the gasoline to the soil particles. In addition, the moisture content affects the available pore space, with increased saturation decreasing the amount of air-filled pores thus reducing volatilization (Sanders and Talimcioglu 1997). The moisture content of the SLR (18%) was increased to 60% of its full water-holding capacity to help reduce volatilization before the soil structure visibly degraded. The moisture content of the AS (35%) was between 70-80% of its water-holding capacity.

In general, the relationship between the expected initial nominal exposure concentrations, calculated as TPH based on the proportional representation, and the actual measured values, suggest that 66 – 93% of the mogas (as TPH) was lost during test soil preparation. These results emphasize the necessity of measuring the initial exposure concentrations at t=0 (i.e., those concentrations to which the organism are exposed) in order to quantify the volatility losses and differentiate between the actual and the nominal exposure concentrations. Toxicity estimates derived with nominal concentrations will be inaccurate.

The initial measured exposure concentrations, for all of the available chemistry data in all of the toxicity tests performed, were regressed, on logarithmic scales, against the nominal concentrations as TPH (Fig. 2). Despite the magnitude of the losses that occurred during test soil preparation, there was a strong ($r^2 = 0.98$) relationship between the nominal and measured concentrations, indicating high predictability of actual exposure concentrations from the equation of the line ($y = 1.232x - 1.762$; Fig. 2). Therefore, the equation of the line could be used to adjust the statistical endpoints (i.e., LC50s or ICps) to reflect more realistically the PHC levels. Comparable results were found with the independent regression, using the same technique, of the acute toxicity tests ($r^2 = 0.98$) and the definitive toxicity tests ($r^2 = 0.99$).

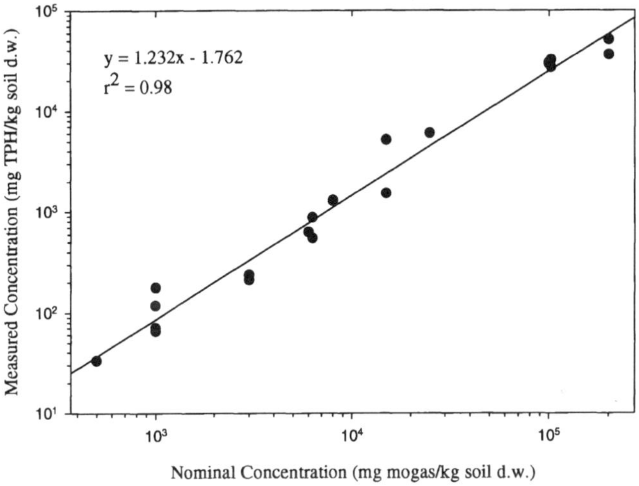

Figure 2–*Regression of the initial (t=0) nominal exposure concentrations of mogas in soil versus the actual measured concentrations of mogas as TPH in soil. The regression incorporated data from all of the tests performed (acute and definitive) in both the artificial and the sandy-loam reference soil*

Table 5-*Measured concentrations of mogas in soil (mg/kg soil d.w.) over the course of 14 days[1] in a 7-d toxicity test with O. folsomi exposed to mogas in artificial soil and the sandy loam reference soil. Test soils were prepared by spiking and mechanical mixing.*

Nominal Concentration (mg/kg d.w)	Calculated Nominal Concentration (mg/kg d.w.)	Measured Parameter	Measured Concentration (mg/kg d.w.)				
			Day 0	Day 1	Day 3	Day 7	Day 14
Artificial Soil							
AS-0	0	BTEX	<D.L.[2]	<D.L.	<D.L.	<D.L.	<D.L.
AS-1000	153		17.0	6.6	0.7	<D.L.	<D.L.
AS-3000	459		40.4	11.4	3.0	<D.L.	<D.L.
AS-8000	1224		34.5	88.1	36.6	1.5	<D.L.
AS-0	0	TPuH	<D.L.	<D.L.	<D.L.	<D.L.	<D.L.
AS-1000	813		58	11	<D.L.	<D.L.	<D.L.
AS-3000	2439		41	11	3.0	<D.L.	<D.L.
AS-8000	6504		690	140	100	1.5	<D.L.
AS-0	0	TEH	<D.L.	<D.L.	<D.L.	<D.L.	<D.L.
AS-1000	176		60	38	18	20	<D.L.
AS-3000	528		170	110	190	40	15
AS-8000	1408		590	350	250	120	59
AS-0	0	TPH	<D.L.	<D.L.	<D.L.	<D.L.	<D.L.
AS-1000	989		118	49	18	20	<D.L.
AS-3000	2967		211	121	193	40	15
AS-8000	7909		1280	490	350	121.5	59
Sandy-loam Reference							
SLR-0	0	BTEX	<D.L.	0.5	<D.L.	<D.L.	<D.L.
SLR-1000	153		15.5	1.0	<D.L.	<D.L.	<D.L.
SLR-3000	459		67.5	8.6	1.33	<D.L.	<D.L.
SLR-8000	1224		467.0	88	26.9	8.3	<D.L.
SLR-0	0	TPuH	<D.L.	0.5	<D.L.	<D.L.	<D.L.
SLR-1000	813		16	1.0	<D.L.	<D.L.	<D.L.
SLR-3000	2439		67	8.6	7.6	<D.L.	<D.L.
SLR-8000	6504		580	180	270	170	57
SLR-0	0	TEH	<D.L.	<D.L.	<D.L.	<D.L.	<D.L.
SLR-1000	176		55	30	17	14	<D.L.
SLR-3000	528		170	79	54	29	<D.L.
SLR-8000	1408		710	570	190	160	64
SLR-0	0	TPH	<D.L.	0.5	<D.L.	<D.L.	<D.L.
SLR-1000	989		71	31	17	14	<D.L.
SLR-3000	2967		237	87.6	61.6	29	<D.L.
SLR-8000	7909		1290	750	460	330	121

[1]Extra test units were prepared to include soil for analysis on day 14.
[2]<D.L. less than the detection limit of the analytical method.

Conclusions

Volatile substances present a unique problem during formulation of test soils because of the losses from volatilization. Amendment procedures can be modified to minimize this loss, however, the losses are only slightly reduced. Test soil preparation by proportional dilution reduced the amount of volatilization at higher concentrations when compared to spiking individual batches of soil for each treatment. However, at lower concentrations, the spiking procedure minimized this loss. The use of a tumbling device, instead of the traditional mechanical mixing to mix the test soils, also helped to reduce the loss of some of the volatiles when used in conjunction with the spiking methodology. However, as there was no clear pattern to the variability of volatilization, one test soil preparation method could not be recommended as being better than the other.

The "closed" test units were considered useful and acceptable because they did not compromise the test organisms in the control treatments, they optimized exposure of test organisms to mogas, and they obviated watering of plants. In order to minimize the loss of the volatile constituents in mogas from test soils during the test, it was recommended that "closed" test units be used for the 7-day acute tests and the first 5-7 days of the tests with longer durations.

The constituents of the mogas were found to volatilize at different rates and the loss was to some extent concentration dependent. Approximately 70-90% of the mogas was lost as a result of volatilization during test soil preparation, regardless of the methodology used. As a result, it is essential to measure the initial exposure concentrations in order to quantify the loss and to determine the actual concentration to which the organisms are exposed. Despite the magnitude of losses that occur, the relationship between the actual and nominal concentrations can be used to adjust the statistical effect values to reflect more realistically the PHC effect levels.

Acknowledgments

The authors would like to acknowledge Imperial Oil, the Canadian Petroleum Products Institute, the Centre for Research in Earth and Space Technology, the Canadian Network of Toxicology Centres, the University of Guelph, and ESG International Inc. for logistical and financial support. We thank J. McCann, N. Feisthauer, N. Mackintosh, J. Kirk, and J. Qui for their technical assistance. P. Walsh (IOL) is recognized for supplying the motor gasoline, characterization of the mogas, and for the technical advice on safe storage and handling of the material. We also recognize and thank Dr. L. Martel for his suggestion regarding the use of the parfait jars for plant testing. Dr. P. Miasek served as the technical advisor to this study and his thoroughness and continued support were greatly appreciated. We would also like to express our appreciation to the members of the CCME EcoTAG for their recommendations and technical comments.

References

ESG International, 2000, *Final Report on the Acute Screening and Definitive, Chronic Toxicity Tests with Motor Gasoline.* Prepared for the Canadian Petroleum Producers Association, Ottawa, Ontario, Canada, 33 pp.

Myers, R. H., 1986, *Classical and Modern Regression with Applications*, Prindle, Weber and Schmidt Publishers, Massachusetts, CN.

Johnson, R.L., and Perrott, M., 1991, "Gasoline Vapor Transport through a High-Water-Content Soil," *Journal of Contaminant Hydrology*, Vol. 8, pp. 317-334.

Sanders, P.F., and Talimcioglu, N.M., 1997, "Soil-to-Indoor Air Exposure Models for Volatile Organic Compounds: the Effect of Soil Moisture," *Environmental Toxicology and Chemistry*, Vol. 16, No. 12, pp. 2597-2604.

SPSS, 1997, "*SYSTAT 7.0.1*", Chicago, IL, USA.

Stephan, C. E., 1989, *Software to calculate LC50 values with confidence intervals using probit, moving averages, and Spearman-Karber procedures.* Modified by R. G. Clements and M. C. Harrass. United States Environmental Protection Agency, Duluth, MN.

Stephenson, G. L., Solomon, K. R., Hale, B., Greenberg, B. M., and Scroggins, R. P., 1997, "Development of Suitable Test Methods for Evaluating the Toxicity of Contaminated Soils to a Battery of Plant Species Relevant to Soil Environments in Canada," *Environmental Toxicology and Risk Assessment: Modeling and Risk Assessment (Sixth Volume), ASTM STP 1317*, F. J. Dwyer, T. R. Doane, and M. L. Hinman, Eds, American Society for Testing and Materials, West Conshohocken, PA, 1997, pp. 474-489.

Stephenson, G. L., Koper, N., Atkinson, G. F., Solomon, K. R., and Scroggins, R. P., 2000, "Use of Nonlinear Regression Techniques for Describing Concentration-Response Relationships for Plant Species Exposed to Contaminated Site Soil, " *Environmental Toxicology and Chemistry*, Vol. 19, No. 12, pp. 229-242.

Jason B. Wells[1] and Roman P. Lanno[2]

Passive Sampling Devices (PSDs) as Biological Surrogates for Estimating the Bioavailability of Organic Chemicals in Soil

---

Reference: Wells, J. B., and Lanno, R. P. "**Passive Sampling Devices (PSDs) as Biological Surrogates for Estimating the Bioavailability of Organic Chemicals in Soil,**" *Environmental Toxicology and Risk Assessment: Science, Policy, and Standardization - Implications for Environmental Decisions: Tenth Volume, ASTM STP 1403*, B. M. Greenberg, R. N. Hull, M. H. Roberts, Jr., and R. W. Gensemer, Eds., American Society for Testing and Materials, West Conshohocken, PA, 2001.

Abstract: Organic chemical exposure in soil toxicity tests and in ecological risk assessment of terrestrial systems is usually expressed as the total chemical measured. Possible alternatives to total chemical measures of organic chemical bioavailability and exposure include body residues in test organisms, soil extraction with selective solvents, and passive sampling devices (PSDs) as biological surrogates. Semipermeable membrane devices (SPMDs) offer potential as a biological surrogate in soil systems. Solid-phase microextraction (SPME) fibers are a rapid and sensitive means for detecting PAHs in soil and have the advantage of not requiring solvent extraction of soil. The objective of this study was to compare chemical uptake and residues in earthworms, SPMDs, and SPMEs exposed in artificial soil spiked with phenanthrene (PHE). Bioavailable PHE, as assessed by mortality and PHE body residues, varied dramatically with soil organic matter content. Both SPMEs and SPMDs could discriminate differences in PHE availability between treatments. However, PHE levels measured using SPMEs were more precise and allowed discrimination between toxic and non-toxic levels of PHE, while PHE levels in SPMDs were too variable for use as a predictive tool.

Keywords: bioavailability, phenanthrene, earthworms, passive sampling devices, semipermeable membrane devices, solid-phase microextraction

[1]Research assistant and [2]Associate professor, Department of Zoology, Oklahoma State University, 430 Life Sciences West, Stillwater, OK 74078.

Bioavailability is key to determining the toxicity of a chemical in the environment, yet it is a problematic parameter to measure. Bioavailability may be described as the interaction between a biological receptor and a chemical that has the capacity to interact with the receptor. Bioavailability of a contaminant is specific to the exposure matrix, duration of exposure, route of entry, and receptor (e.g., invertebrate, microbe). Figure 1 presents the concept of bioavailability in a schematic fashion (as modified from Landrum et al. 1994).

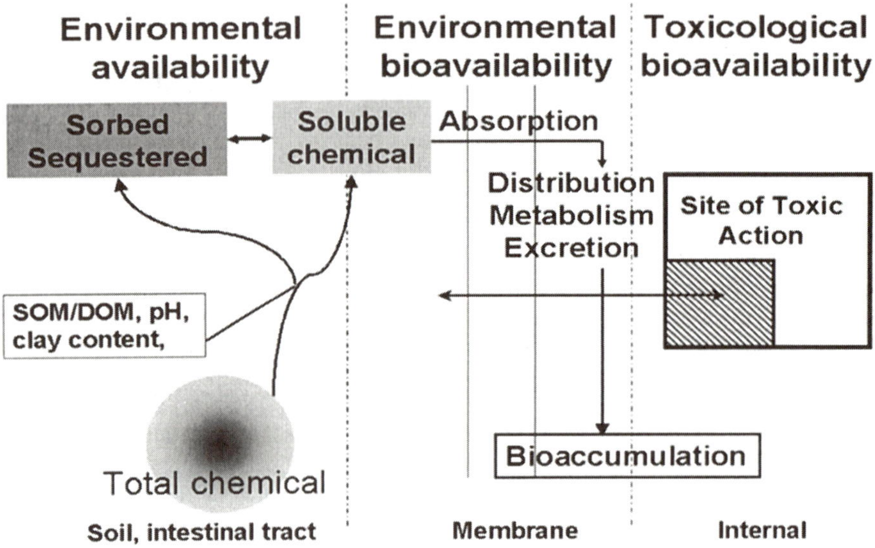

Figure 1 – *Schematic representation of bioavailability*

For example, as PAHs enter the terrestrial environment, immediately upon contact they interact with specific soil components (e.g., soil organic matter, SOM), with the nature of these interactions dependent upon the form of chemical introduced, the physical/chemical constitution of the soil, and the duration of interaction. Each interaction between a chemical and specific environmental phases is characterized by a different equilibration period. For example, the surficial adsorption of PAHs to SOM is relatively rapid (days) and results in the removal of some portion of PAHs from soil solution. However, intra-particle diffusion of PAH molecules, and possibly other processes such as entrapment in SOM or micropores, will continue over time (days to years), further reducing the environmentally available fraction of PAHs (Reid et al. 2000). PAHs remaining in the soil solution are available for interactions with other environmental components and the portion of this chemical fraction that interacts with organisms can be defined as environmentally bioavailable. Although microbes may be in contact with essentially all PAHs in soil solution, soil macroinvertebrates will only come in contact with a small portion of the environmentally available PAHs. Environmentally bioavailable chemicals may adsorb to membrane or cuticle surfaces and remain bound external to the organism. They may also be absorbed across membranes and transported via the vascular system to another site in the organism where interactions with biomolecules may occur. Metabolic processes may detoxify the chemical, or it may interact with an essential molecule associated with a site of toxic action. Interactions between absorbed chemicals and site(s) of toxic action can be referred to as toxicological bioavailability. Chemicals may also bioaccumulate, not resulting in any apparent toxicity.

Total chemical measures have little relevance to biological observations in soil and sediment systems (Landrum et al. 1994), and have even been described as inappropriate as measures of exposure in soil systems (Conder and Lanno 2000). Soil constituents (e.g., humic substances), coupled with soil pore-spaces of varying sizes and shapes, compete for binding of lipophilic contaminants (Carmichael et al. 1997, Burgos et al. 1999). Soil matrices can be highly variable in composition and heterogeneous in structure, and, unlike aquatic systems, soil heterogeneity may not be predicted or modeled effectively. This heterogeneous mixture of soil components coupled with environmental modifying factors such as temperature, moisture content, and organic matter content makes theoretical toxicity prediction very difficult for risk assessments in soil systems (Lanno and McCarty 1997; Sijm et al. 2000). Thus, total chemical concentrations are not appropriate estimates of exposure when accounting for the influence of so many modifying factors.

Any chemical measure in the exposure medium, including measurements using biomimetic samplers, is only a surrogate for toxicological bioavailability, or the dose at the site of toxic action inside the organism (McCarty et al. 1992). The expression of exposure in ecotoxicology, especially as a total chemical level, has led to a great deal of confusion in assessing the relative sensitivity of test species and the relative potency of different chemicals, especially in matrices as heterogeneous as soils. In contrast to measuring environmental levels of organic chemicals, critical body residues (CBRs), or body burdens explicitly consider bioavailability and provide a more precise estimate of the actual dose of chemical present at the site of toxic action (McCarty and Mackay 1993). This approach has been used successfully to examine the effects of modifying factors (e.g., soil type, temperature, test species) on the toxicity of some organic chemicals in soil systems (Fitzgerald et al. 1996, Belfroid et al. 1996, Lanno et al. 1998).

By definition, bioavailability can only determined by living organisms (Van Brummelen et al. 1998, Weston and Mayer 1998). Any chemical estimates of bioavailability must be correlated with biological measures of bioavailability or toxicological bioavailability. Weak solvent extractions have been used with limited success as surrogates for bioavailability of PAHs due to the analyte or medium-specificity of solvent extraction systems and poor correlation with biological responses or bioaccumulation (Kelsey et al. 1997, Tang and Alexander 1999). Passive sampling devices (PSDs) may mimic organisms (biomimetic) by providing a solid phase for chemical partitioning. PSDs are specific to classes of contaminants (e.g., non-polar organics) but not specific to individual contaminants within a class. If properly correlated with biological responses, chemical determination using PSDs may predict toxicity as a screening tool in the first tier of ecological risk assessment, providing an alternative for or replacing conventional chemical and biological methods. Two technologies being investigated for use as PSDs in soil are semipermeable membrane devices (SPMDs) and solid phase microextraction (SPME) fibers.

SPMDs are composed of lay-flat low-density polyethylene (LPDE) dialysis tubing filled with a known mass of triolein. The dialysis tubing has been shown to effectively mimic bipolar lipid membranes in the uptake of lipophilic environmental contaminants and the triolein represents storage lipid (Huckins et al. 1990). SPMDs have been used to detect and accumulate lipophilic contaminants from aquatic and atmospheric media, but application in soil systems is limited (Petty et al. 1993, Huckins et al. 1996). SPMDs have been applied in terrestrial systems to monitor compost fortified with various congeners of PCBs (Strandberg et al. 1997) and soil vapor for chlorohydrocarbons, where SPMDs were buried in contaminated lakeshore soil (Rantalainen et al. 1998). Neither of these studies related SPMD chemical levels to any biological responses.

Solid phase microextraction (SPME) fiber technology, a completely solventless extraction method (Zhang et al. 1994), may also be useful in estimating chemical bioavailability in soil. SPME devices are constructed of an optical fiber (1 cm in length) coated with a non-polar phase (7 μm thick), such as polydimethyl siloxane (PDMS). The fiber adsorbs analytes by diffusion from the substrate by exploiting the fugacity of the compounds of interest. This sampling technology has the benefit of no liquid chemical extractions or concentration procedures with the ability to derivatize samples as collected. Analysis entails insertion of the fiber into the heated injection port of a gas chromatograph (GC), followed by thermal desorption of analytes and separation by conventional thermal gradient programming followed by suitable detection methods. Desorption times vary from seconds to minutes depending on the fiber coating and analyte of interest. Direct contact measurements using SPME fibers have only been made for aquatic and atmospheric media. Soil and tissues have been sampled by headspace analysis only. The direct measurement of soil contaminants has been investigated with limited success (Parkerton and Stone 1998, Prosen 1998, Tugulea et al. 1998).

The experimental approach for this study was to conduct two experiments exposing earthworms and biomimetic PSDs (SPMDs and SPMEs) to phenanthrene (PHE)-spiked artificial soil. The objective of this study was to determine how modifications of soil organic matter content affects PHE bioavailability by earthworms and to compare uptake of PHE by SPMDs and SPME fibers. Relationships between PHE residues in PSDs and earthworms were examined to determine if PSDs could be used as surrogate measures to estimate bioavailability and predict toxicity of PHE in soil.

Methods and Materials

General Experimental Design

Treatments comprised two levels of soil organic matter (10% OM and 1% OM, as peat moss) and three nominal concentrations (0.31, 2.05, and 3.10 mmol/kg dry mass soil) of PHE with an acetone solvent control (in triplicate) for each soil type. The choice of using two levels of organic matter was to compare the ASTM Guide for Conducting Laboratory Soil Toxicity or Bioaccumulation Tests With Lumbricid Earthworm *Eisenia fetida* (E1676-97) protocol (10% OM) with more relevant field SOM levels (~1% OM).

Exposures included earthworms (*Eisenia fetida)*, semipermeable membrane devices (SPMDs), and soil-only which was used for physical/chemical analyses and solid-phase microextraction (SPME) fiber determinations. Independent replicates were prepared for each treatment-time combination, with earthworm and soil-only treatments sampled at 0, 2, 4, 8, and 16 d and SPMD treatments at 0, 4, 8, 16, and 32 d. Exposure durations for the control soil containers were 0 and 16 d. Earthworms were exposed independently and simultaneously to SPMDs and were not fed during the test. These tests followed ASTM Guide for Conducting Laboratory Soil Toxicity or Bioaccumulation Tests With Lumbricid Earthworm *Eisenia fetida* (E1676-97) with the following variations. The PHE concentrations and exposure durations were chosen based on two unpublished rangefinder mortality tests using *E. fetida* and a rangefinder uptake of PHE using the SPMDs in 3.10 mmol PHE/kg-10% OM artificial soil. Selection of earthworms for this assay was based on an initial minimum fresh mass of 250 mg without regard to sexual maturity. Earthworms were hand-sorted from a mass culture and placed on moistened filter paper to allow depuration of gut contents for 24 h at 24±1 °C. They were then randomly separated into groups of 12 worms per replicate test container, weighed, and placed in test containers after test soil moisture equilibration was complete (24 h). Earthworms determined to be dead (no response from stimulation with blunt probe) were removed from the containers and rinsed with reagent grade water (RGW, pH 7.0, Type I ASTM, resistivity 18MΩ), wrapped in *n*-hexane-rinsed aluminum foil, sealed in Ziplock® bags and frozen (-20 °C). Any earthworms remaining alive at end of the test were sacrificed and frozen as above.

Experimental Organisms

Earthworms (*E. fetida*) were obtained from Granny's Hillside Farms, Gore, OK, and cultured in antibiotic-free composted horse manure (24-27 °C) at Oklahoma State University-Ecotoxicology and Water Quality Research Laboratory (OSU-EWQRL). Bedding moisture was maintained by spraying weekly with reconstituted moderately hard water. Cocoons were separated from bedding material and hatched to provide synchronized earthworm cultures.

Artificial Soil Preparation

The standard (10% OM) artificial soil in this experiment was composed (% dry weight) of 69% silica sand (60 mesh, Blasting Specialties, Tulsa, OK), 20% pulverized EPK Kaolin clay (Tomorrow's Treasures, OKC, OK), 10% *Sphagnum* peat (passed through a 2-mm sieve, Wal-Mart, Stillwater, OK), and 1% calcium carbonate ($CaCO_3$, Fisher Scientific). Composition of the low (1% OM) artificial soil was 76.67 % silica sand, 22.23 % Kaolin clay, 1 % *Sphagnum* peat (2-mm sieved), and 0.1 % $CaCO_3$. Before the preparation of artificial soil, the water content of the sieved peat was determined and the amount of peat used to prepare the artificial soil was adjusted for moisture content. Each test container was prepared individually, yielding 258 experimental units. Sand was measured into test containers and spiked using a stock solution of PHE dissolved in acetone. The acetone was allowed to evaporate from the sand overnight in a darkened fume hood. Once acetone had evaporated, all artificial soil components (200 g, dry mass) were combined into test containers and mixed in a rotary mixer (25 rpm) for one hour.

Moisture content for both soil types was adjusted to 125% field moisture capacity by adding RGW and mixing until uniform in color and texture (with an acetone-rinsed stainless steel impeller, 5-cm dia., attached to ¾-hp drill press at 190 RPM). This was done to ensure that both soil types contained the same proportion of free soil water. Field capacity of both soil types was assessed following ASTM Method for Capillary-Moisture Relationships for Coarse- and Medium-Textured Soils by Porous-Plate Apparatus D2325-68 (1994). Artificial soil (saturated with RGW for 48 h) was placed into support rings on a primed ceramic pore plate within a pressure plate apparatus (Soil Moisture, Inc.). Pressure was applied (0.3 atm) and expelled water was collected for 36 h or when steady state was reached. The soil was removed and moisture content determined (percent difference by dry mass, Topp 1993). Temperature and moisture of the test containers was allowed to equilibrate for 24 h in a Percival Scientific environmental chamber (24±1 °C) in continuous light before the addition of earthworms or SPMDs. Following moisture equilibration and at the completion of the test, soil moisture (Topp 1993), and pH (10 g dry mass soil/20 mL 0.01M $CaCl_2$, Hendershot et al. 1993) were evaluated (Table 1).

Table 1 - *Soil moisture and pH of 1% OM and 10% OM test soils 125% field moisture capacity with respect to days after soil moisture equilibration.*[a]

	1% OM	10% OM
Percent Moisture		
Day 0	17.10 (1.03)	27.05 (1.22)
Day 16	18.77 (4.18)	26.94 (1.22)
pH		
Day 0	7.10 (0.03)	7.41 (0.02)
Day 16	6.92 (0.04)	7.45 (0.05)

[a] Values are means and standard deviations, n=3.

Semipermeable Membrane Device (SPMD) Deployment

SPMDs (2.54 cm x 5.08 cm, 0.0556 g triolein, Environmental Sampling Technologies (EST), St. Joseph, MO) were received from the manufacturer in hexane-rinsed, sealed tin cans. One SPMD was deployed per 200 g (dry soil) replicate. SPMDs were deployed in a static manner, independently and simultaneous to the earthworm test, and buried in the soil with no disturbances during the exposure period. SPMDs were removed from respective test containers after exposures of 4, 8, 16, and 32 d (n=3 at each exposure period). Acetone control SPMDs were removed after 16 d (n=3). After removal from the soil, each SPMD was rinsed with RGW to remove any soil, sealed in its original can, and frozen (-20 °C) until dialysis. Trip blank, manufacture blank, and spike-recovery SPMDs were used. Trip blanks were opened at various intervals during deployment. Manufacturer blanks were not opened until dialysis. Spike recovery was done by injecting 100 µL of PHE certified standard (Chem Service F81MS, 100 µg/mL) through the membrane and resealing the membrane. Spike recovery for PHE was 80% and PHE was not detected in blank SPMDs.

Chemical Analyses

SPMD Dialysis and Residue Analysis - Dialysis and gel permeation cleanup of SPMDs was conducted by EST using methods described elsewhere (Huckins et al. 1996). SPMD extracts were received from EST in 5-mL ampules and quantitatively transferred to 15-mL glass graduated conical-centrifuge tubes (Baxter, ± 0.05 mL) and adjusted to analytical volume. Dialysates were analyzed for PHE residues using high performance liquid chromatography (HPLC). A Supelcosil LC-PAH (Supelco), 5 cm x 4.6 mm ID x 3 µm reversed-phase analytical column was used at ambient temperature for PHE quantification. Acetonitrile (Optima grade, Fisher Scientific) and RGW were used as the mobile phase in a gradient mixture initially 60:40 acetonitrile:water, 0.3 min hold and then ramped to 100 % acetonitrile at 4.0 min accomplished with a Dionex GP-50 quaternary pump (Dionex Corp., Sunnyvale, CA) at a flow rate of 3.0 mL/min. Injections were 25 µL with a Dionex LC-10 autoinjectior from a Dionex AS-40 autosampler. PHE was detected using a Waters™ 484 deuterium arc lamp UV/VIS detector. Integrations were conducted at 254 nm with an optical bandwidth of 8 nm. Peaks from samples were identified by comparison of retention times with a certified reference standard (Chem Service, F81MS, 100 µg/mL). Concentrations were determined by peak area from standard curves. Calibration standards were checked using the certified reference standard. Results were expressed as mass PHE/SPMD surface area. All data collection and chromatogram analysis was done using Dionex Peaknet® software ver. 4.2 and 5.1 (Dionex 1995-1999).

Solid Phase Microextraction (SPME) Fiber Analyses – The goal of SPME analysis was to determine the potentially bioavailable fraction of PHE in the soil rather than total PHE. Solid phase microextraction fibers (SPME, 7µm polydimethyl siloxane (PDMS) with manual holders, Supelco, Bellefonte, PA) were used to assess uptake of PHE directly from the aqueous phase of soil at the earthworm toxicity test temperature (24 ±1 °C). Ten SPME fiber assemblies were used in this study. Each determination was made using 0.500 g freeze-dried artificial soil. Freeze-dried, spiked artificial soil (0.500 g, collected at 0 and 16 d post moisture equilibration from the soil only exposure regime), 15 mL RGW, and a Teflon®-coated magnetic stir bar (0.3 cm x 1.3 cm) were placed in screw-top amber SPME vials (15 mL headspace with Teflon septum, Supelco). A ten-place magnetic stirrer (1200 RPM, IKA) was used with ten sample vials and ten SPME fiber assemblies to obtain steady-state data for PHE concentrations in soil suspensions. A support stand was constructed to hold ten SPME manual holders simultaneously during exposure. The needle of the SPME apparatus was inserted through the Teflon septum of the sample vial when the fiber was deployed. Each vial was aligned on the magnetic stirrer for optimum stirring velocity (~1 000 rpm). Each SPME fiber was exposed (until steady state was achieved - 5 h). This was verified during method development by monitoring PHE uptake at 4, 8, 12, and 16 h. No differences were found between any of the exposure durations ($p \geq 0.05$, $\alpha = 0.05$, $n = 2$). Residue analysis was accomplished by gas chromatography (Tracor 565 GC-FID, megabore fused silica capillary column (DB-5, 30 m X 0.53 mm ID X 1.5 µm, J&W Scientific), 0.75-mm ID SPME-inlet liner (Supelco), JADE septum-less injector with SPME adapter (0.56 mm ID, Alltec)). Helium (High Purity, Sooner Airgas) was used as the carrier and makeup gas. The flow rate for the carrier gas was set to 35 cm/sec linear velocity and make-up flow rate was set to 45 mL/min. Hydrogen (fuel for FID, High Purity, Sooner Airgas) flow rate was 35 mL/min and breathing air (oxidant, Grade D, Sooner Airgas) flow rate was 350 mL/min. The temperature program for direct injection GC analysis was: injection port temp-290 °C, detector temp-300 °C, initial oven temp-160 °C (5 minute hold) with 35 °C/min ramp to 210 °C (7 minute hold).

Thermal desorption and conditioning of the SPME fiber was accomplished by exposing the fiber while inserted into the heated injection port (290 °C) of the GC for five minutes. This resulted in adequate desorption followed by blank analyses of each fiber to ensure no carryover problems existed. SPME fiber performance was determined before and after each soil determination by measuring a reference standard solution (1 mg PHE/L RGW). Integration of peaks was done by external calibration using injections from PHE standards with a certified PHE check standard (Chem Service, F81MS). Chromatogram data was collected and analyzed using PeakNet® chromatography software (Version 5.1, Dionex 1999).

Earthworm Body Burden Analysis – Baseline residue analysis was conducted using 12 unexposed earthworms from the OSU-EWQRL culture population. Exposed test earthworms were randomly selected for body burden analysis at each observation time from each exposure concentration. Earthworms were removed from storage (-20 °C), thawed to room temperature, placed into 20-mL glass vials, fresh mass recorded (± 0.00005 g, Mettler-Toledo Model AT261, Columbus, Ohio) and freeze-dried for 12 h (<100 μg Hg, Lyph-Lock 12, Labconco). Individual, freeze-dried earthworms were then transferred to 10-mLTeflon Oakridge centrifuge tubes with sealing cap assemblies (VWR Scientific) and 3 mL of RGW was added. Mechanical tissue homogenization of the whole earthworm was conducted for two minutes with a TH115 tissue homogenizer (OMNI International, Warrenton, VA). Three mL *n*-hexane (95%, Fisher Scientific) was added to the homogenate and ultrasonic extraction was done for two minutes at 40% duty cycle (Fisher M300). Following sonication, rotary extraction was conducted for one hour in total darkness (Rotamix, ATR Inc. Laurel, MD, 40 rpm). Extracts were then centrifuged to separate hexane from RGW (Sorvall RC2-B Superspeed, 5000 *g* for 5 min.). The hexane layer was removed using *n*-hexane-rinsed Pasteur pipettes, and concentrated to 2.0 mL using a gentle stream of N_2 for silica-gel cleanup. Solid phase extraction cartridges (SPE, 500 mg silica gel, 3-mL volume, BakerBond J.T.Baker, Phillipsburg, NJ) topped with a 1-cm layer of sodium sulfate (Na_2SO_4, Fisher Scientific) were used for cleanup of earthworm extracts. SPE columns were conditioned before use by rinsing with three column volumes of *n*-hexane. Following column conditioning, the sample was quantitatively transferred to the SPE column. Three column-volumes of *n*-hexane were used to elute the sample from the SPE cartridge. The eluate was collected in 40-mL glass graduated centrifuge tubes (± 0.05 mL, Kontes), solvent replaced to acetonitrile and subsequently concentrated to analytical volume using a gentle stream of N_2. One cartridge was used per sample. Earthworm whole body extracts were analyzed for PHE residues using HPLC as described above for SPMDs. Results were expressed as moles PHE/earthworm wet mass. Spike recovery was conducted by adding 100 μL PHE certified standard (Chem Service F81MS, 100 μg/mL) to reference worm homogenates and subjecting to treatment and chemical analysis as above. Blank analyses were conducted to correct for any impurities encountered. Earthworm body residues were not corrected for spike recovery of PHE (86.5%, 16.5, SD, n=8).

Total Chemical Analysis –Total PHE levels in soil (Table 2) were determined using accelerated solvent extraction (ASE by Dionex, 1:1 methylene chloride:acetone) followed by quantification by HPLC as above for SPMDs. Actual PHE levels were 42-67% of nominal and did not differ between day 0 and day 16. Recovery of a PHE spike added to the soil just prior to extraction was 103%. All values in the results and discussion are presented as nominal concentrations.

Table 2 – *Total PHE concentrations (mmol/kg; mean with SD in parentheses) measured in test soils by ASE (Accelerated Solvent Extraction) with $MeCl_2$:Acetone, 1:1.*[a]

	PHE	% of nominal
Controls (1%, 10%)	BDL[b]	-
10%-0.31 mmol/kg	0.21 (0.01)	66
10%-2.05 mmol/kg	1.3 (0.04)	63
10%-3.1 mmol/kg	2.1 (0.04)	67
1%-0.31 mmol/kg	0.13 (0.01)	42
1%-2.05 mmol/kg	0.93	45
1%-3.1 mmol/kg	1.7 (0.01)	56

[a] The reported values for ASE are the means of three soil replicates.
[b] BDL – below detection limit of 0.02 mmol/kg.

Statistical Analyses

Data interpretation was done using SAS® (Statistical Analysis System version 6.12, SAS Institute, Inc. 1989-1996), Origin® (Version 6.0, Microcal™1991-1999), and Excel 2000 (Version 9.0.2720, Microsoft® 1983-1999). Standard descriptive statistics, ANOVA, and linear and nonlinear regression techniques were used. Earthworm LD_{50} values were estimated by probit analysis (SAS PROC PROBIT). SPMD data was analyzed by two-way regression (SAS PROC REG) and three-way ANOVA (SAS PROC MIXED) to examine relationships of soil organic matter, soil PHE concentration, and duration of exposure. SPME fiber data was examined by three-way ANOVA (SAS PROC MIXED) to examine relationships of soil organic matter, soil PHE concentration, and duration of exposure of PHE residues between days zero and 16.

Results

Mortalities differed between soils with 10% OM and 1% OM at similar PHE concentrations (Figures 2 and 3). Mortality reached 100% in 96 h for worms exposed to 2.05 and 3.10 mmol PHE/kg, and 95% within 192 h in groups exposed to 0.31 mmol PHE/kg in soil containing 1% OM. Mortality in soils containing 10% OM was much reduced, with only 61% mortality in groups exposed to 3.10 mmol PHE/kg, 7% at 2.05 mmol/kg, and 0% at 0.31 mmol/kg. Probit analysis of PHE residues in live and dead earthworms yielded an LD_{50} of 0.114 (0.072-0.172, 95% fiducial limits) mmol PHE/kg, wet mass.

SPMDs accumulated PHE from all spiked soils (Figures 4 & 5). Over a 32-day period, PHE concentrations in the SPMDs appeared to reach a steady state, except for those exposed to 3.10 mmol PHE/kg-10% OM (Figure 5). PHE concentrations in these SPMDs appeared to reach a maximum level at 16 d and then decreased. All earthworm mortality occurred within the first eight days of exposure, during the linear phase of PHE uptake by the SPMDs (Figures 2-7). Uptake of PHE by SPMDs in both soil types containing 0.31 mmol PHE/kg were similar and not significantly different from zero (control). Due to the variability in PHE residues at this exposure concentration, it was not possible to discriminate between SPMD residues associated with lethal PHE exposure levels (1% OM) and non-lethal PHE exposure levels (10% OM) ($p>0.05$) (Figures 6 & 7). The uptake of PHE by all SPMDs exposed to the two higher concentrations of PHE was significantly different from zero (control) ($p<0.05$).

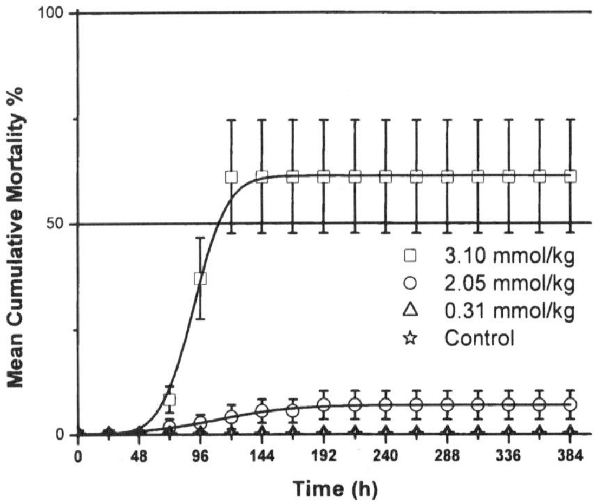

Figure 2 – *Percent cumulative mortality of E. fetida exposed to PHE during an acute toxicity test in artificial soil containing 10% OM. Values are mean ± SEM (n=3).*

In contrast, PHE measurements employing SPME fibers enabled discrimination between PHE levels of 0.31 mmol/kg in soils of differing organic matter content (Figure 8). Within each soil type, a clear increase in environmentally available PHE was observed as PHE concentrations increased, with lower levels of PHE measured by SPME in the soil containing 10% OM. Determination of PHE by SPME showed no significant differences in PHE concentrations between day zero and day sixteen ($p>0.05$, $n=2$), so data were pooled for further statistical analysis.

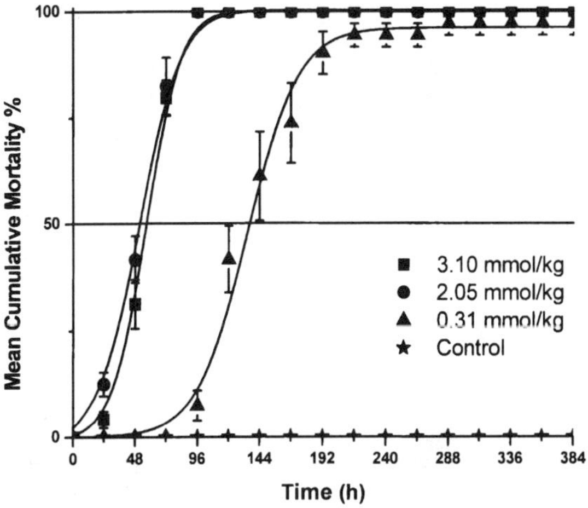

Figure 3 – *Percent cumulative mortality of E. fetida exposed PHE during an acute toxicity test in artificial soil containing 1% OM. Values are mean ± SEM (n=3).*

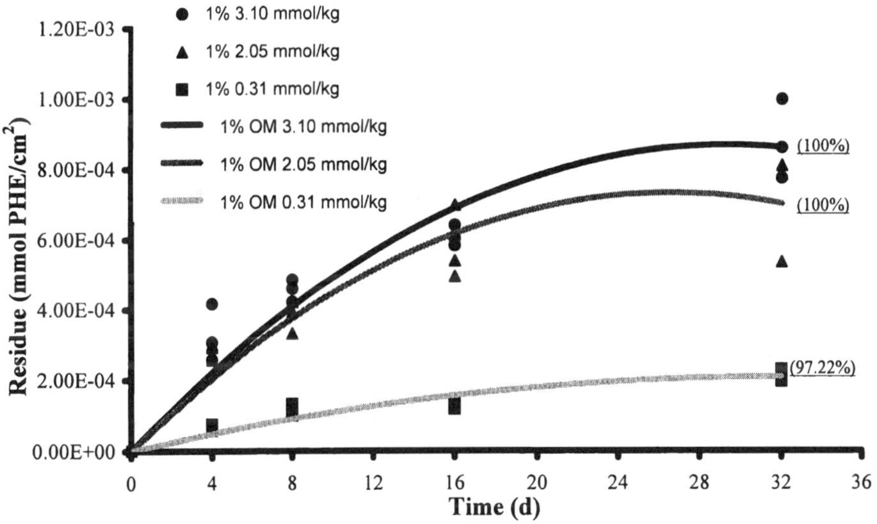

Figure 4– *Semipermeable membrane device uptake of PHE over 32 d in 1% OM artificial soil. Numbers in parentheses indicate the percentage of E. fetida mortality observed in the respective soil concentrations.*

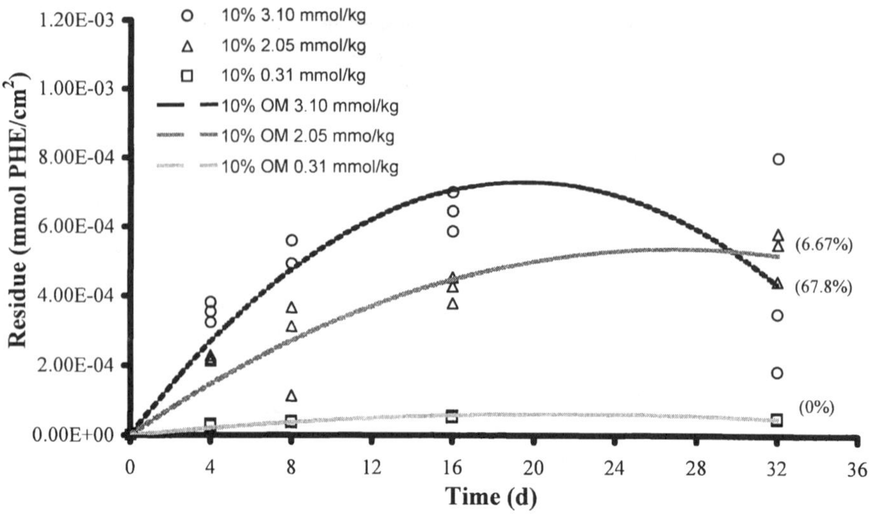

Figure 5 – *Semipermeable membrane device uptake of PHE over 32 d in 10% OM artificial soil. Numbers in parentheses indicate the percentage of E. fetida mortality observed in the respective soil concentrations.*

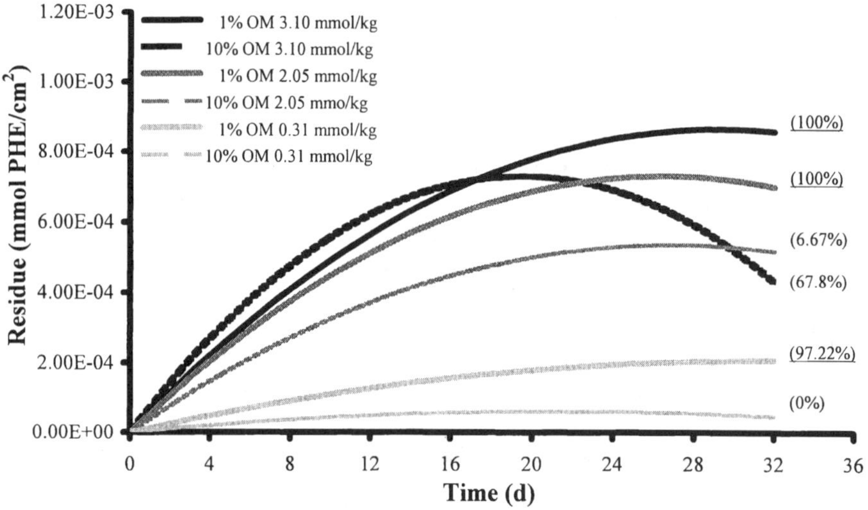

Figure 6 – *Semipermeable membrane device uptake of PHE over 32 d in both soil types. Numbers in parentheses indicate the percentage of E. fetida mortality observed in the respective soil concentrations.*

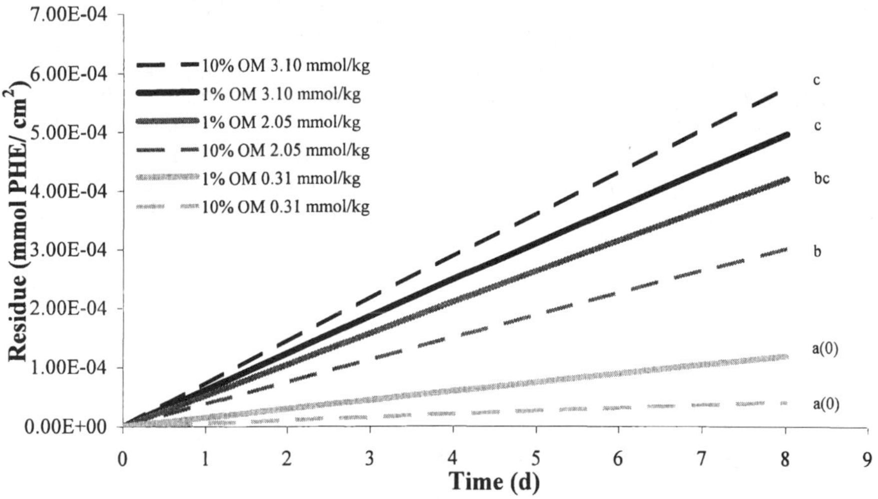

Figure 7 – *Linear phase uptake by SPMDs over 8d. Common letters indicate no significant differences ($p \geq 0.05$). PHE uptake by SPMDs exposed to 0.31 mmol PHE/kg in 1% OM or 10% OM was not significantly different from zero (control).*

Discussion

The bioavailability of PHE to earthworms was greatly reduced in artificial soil containing 10% OM compared to artificial soil containing 1% OM. This observation is supported by biological responses of the earthworms (lethality), by bioimimetic measurements of environmental availability, and by actual measures of bioavailability as PHE residues in earthworms. In soils containing 1% OM, mortality was high (95-100%) regardless of PHE concentration, suggesting that a sufficient amount of PHE was bioavailable to result in acute toxicity at all PHE levels. Test soils containing 1% OM appeared to have insufficient organic matter to bind PHE and reduce the bioavailable fraction below acutely toxic levels. In soils containing 10% OM, mortality of earthworms was reduced in a dose-dependent manner with only 61% mortality at the highest PHE level.

The observed trends in mortality were supported by PHE residues measured in whole earthworms. Regardless of whether earthworms were exposed to PHE in soil containing 1% or 10% OM, the PHE residues were within two standard deviations of the LD_{50} (0.114 mmol PHE/kg, wet weight). This residue represents a median lethal critical body residue (CBR_{50}), and most live earthworms from soil containing 10% OM had PHE residues that were below the lower fiducial limit of the CBR_{50}. The reduced accumulation of PHE by live worms suggests that PHE bioavailability was reduced by increasing the SOM. In contrast, PHE in the 1% OM soil was much more bioavailable, as reflected by bioaccumulation of PHE in earthworms to a lethal level.

Both biomimetic measures of bioavailability, SPMEs and SPMDs, were able to detect differences in the environmentally available fraction of PHE in soils. However, SPMDs only allowed statistical resolution between the highest and lowest PHE concentrations in soil (Figures 6 & 7). In contrast, PHE uptake by SPMEs was much less variable, resulting in significant differences in environmentally available PHE at many concentrations in soil, and specifically between PHE levels associated with earthworm mortality in the 0.31 mmol PHE/kg-1% OM treatment and the non-lethal 0.31 mmol PHE/kg-10% OM treatment (Figure 8). Due to increased variability, PHE uptake by SPMDs in the 0.31 mmol/kg treatments was not significantly different from controls, suggesting that SPMDs are not able to discriminate between lethal and non-lethal environmentally available PHE concentrations (Figures 6 & 7).

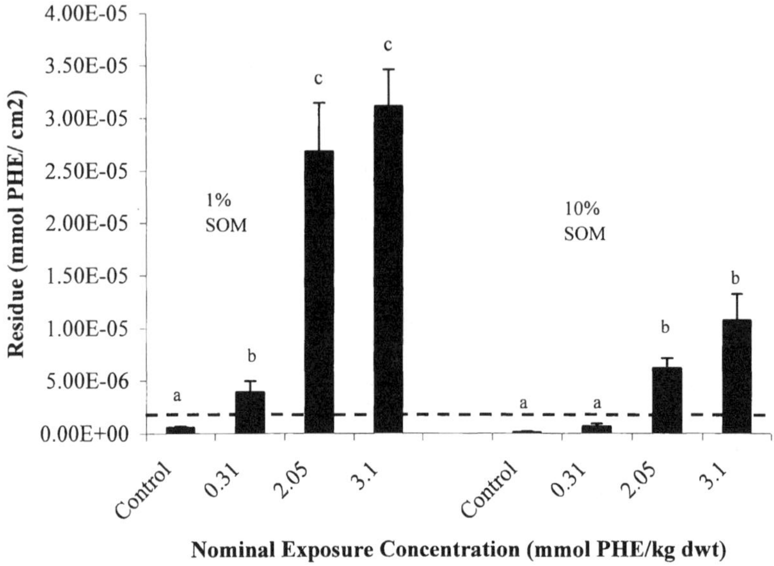

Figure 8 – *Solid phase microextraction (SPME) fiber analysis of 1% OM and 10% OM artificial soil (pooled from Day-0 [n=2] and Day-16 [n=2]) spiked with PHE at various concentrations. Residues above the dashed line indicate soil concentrations where mortality was observed for E. fetida. Values are means ± SEM (n=4). Common letters indicate no significant differences ($p \geq 0.05$, $\alpha = 0.05$).*

SPME fibers appear to be the more promising of the two PSD technologies examined during this study as a tool for the prediction of the environmental availability and toxicity of PHE in soil. SPME determinations of PHE are more precise than SPMD estimates and are able to resolve differences between low levels of PHE and discriminate between lethal and non-lethal levels of PHE. Although subject to greater variability, SPMDs may still have specific applications in assessing the environmental availability of lipophilic organic compounds in soil. SPME fibers represent point-in-time estimates of environmental availability, since determinations are made on a subsample of soil. However, SPMDs have been exposed in a soil for up to 32 days and provide a temporal integration of chemical accumulation, more closely representing the dermal uptake of hydrophobic contaminants by earthworms.

Both SPMEs and SPMDs have limitations as surrogates for the uptake of chemicals by organisms. These PSDs only measure the parent compound available for accumulation since chemical metabolism does not take place within the samplers. These devices are also fragile, and in field applicatons, susceptible to damage, theft, and vandalism.

More studies are needed to understand and optimize soil conditions that may affect chemical uptake by PSDs. Preliminary data (Wells and Lanno, unpublished) suggest that accurate comparisons of chemical accumulation kinetics between soil types using SPMDs may require that soil moisture content be standardized to some proportion of the field moisture capacity of the soils. Sufficient time (>16 d) is also required to accumulate quantifiable levels of chemicals, and in some cases, SPMD extracts may even need to be pooled to obtain detectable contaminant levels.

Many types of solid phases exist for SPME fibers and phases may be selected to best match the fugacity of the organic chemical of interest. Fibers incorporating a bonded phase are more durable for use in soil slurry applications requiring replacement less often.

In summary, both PSDs used in this study were able to detect differences in the environmentally available fraction of PHE in soils differing in organic matter content. However, measurements made with SPMEs were much more precise, allowing discrimination between lethal and non-lethal PHE concentrations. SPME fibers appear to be a promising screening tool that may be used to predict potential toxicity associated with the environmentally available fraction of organic chemicals in soil.

Acknowledgements

The authors wish to thank the Gas Technology Institute (formerly Gas Research Institute) for financial assistance; Dave Nakles, ThermoRetec Inc., for administrative support; Sherry LeBlanc, Matthew TenEyck, Sarah Coughlin, Karen Bradham, Jason Conder, Brad Knight, and Elaine Stebler for their support and technical assistance on this project; and James Huckins, USGS-CERC Columbia, MO, for his supportive discussions on the intricacies of SPMDs.

References

Belfroid, A. C., Sijm, D. T. H. M., and Van Gestel, C. A. M., 1996, "Bioavailability and Toxicokinetics of Hydrophobic Aromatic Compounds in Benthic and Terrestrial Invertebrates," *Environmental Reviews*, Vol. 4, pp. 276-299.

Burgos, W. D., Munson, C. M., and Duffy, C. J., 1999, "Phenanthrene Adsorption-Desorption Hysteresis in Soil Described Using Discrete-Interval Equilibrium Models," *Water Resources Research*, Vol. 35, pp. 2043-2051.

Carmichael, L. M., Christman, R. F., and Pfander, F. K., 1997, "Desorption and Mineralization Kinetics of Phenanthrene and Chrysene in Contaminated Soils," *Environmental Science and Technology*, Vol. 31, pp. 126-132.

Conder, J. M., and Lanno, R. P., 2000, "Evaluation of Surrogate Measures of Cadmium, Lead, and Zinc Bioavailability to *Eisenia fetida*," *Chemosphere*, Vol. 41, pp. 1659-1668.

Fitzgerald, D., Warner, K. A., Lanno, R. P., and Dixon, D. G., 1996, "Assessing the Effects of Modifying Factors on Pentachlorophenol Toxicity to Earthworms: Applications of Body Residues," *Environmental Toxicology and Chemistry*, Vol. 15, pp. 2299-2304.

Hendershot, W. H., Lalande, H., and Duquette, M., 1993, "Soil Reaction and Exchangeable Acidity," *Soil Sampling and Methods of Analysis*, M. R. Carter, Ed. Lewis Publishers, Boca Raton, FL, USA, pp. 141-145.

Huckins, J. N., Tubergen, M. W., and Manuweera, G. K., 1990, "Semipermeable Membrane Devices Containing Model Lipid: A New Approach to Monitoring the Bioavailability of Lipophilic Contaminants and Estimating their Bioconcentration Potential," *Chemosphere*, Vol. 20, pp. 533-552.

Huckins, J. N., Petty, J. D., Lebo, J. A., Orazio, C.E., Prest, H. F., Tillitt, D. E., Ellis, G. S., Johnson, T. B., and Manuweera, G. K., 1996, "Semipermeable Membrane Devices (SPMDs) for the Concentration and Assessment of Bioavailable Organic Contaminants in Aquatic Environments," *Techniques in Aquatic Toxicology,* G. K. Ostrander, Ed., CRC Press, Boca Raton, FL, pp. 625-656.

Kelsey, J. W., Kottler, B. D., and Alexander, M., 1997, "Selective Chemical Extractants to Predict Bioavailability of Soil-Aged Organic Chemicals," *Environmental Science and Technology*, Vol. 31, pp. 214-217.

Landrum, P. F., Hayton, W. L., Lee, H., McCarty, L. S., Mackay, D., and McKim, J. M., 1994, "Synopsis of Discussion Session on the Kinetics Behind Environmental Bioavailability," *Bioavailability*, J. L. Hamelink, P. F. Landrum, H. F. Bergman, and W. H. Benson, Eds., CRC Press, Boca Raton, FL, pp. 203-219.

Lanno, R. P., and McCarty, L. S., 1997, "Earthworm Bioassays: Adopting Techniques from Aquatic Toxicity Testing," *Soil Biology and Biochemistry,* Vol. 29, pp. 693-697.

Lanno, R. P., LeBlanc, S. C., Knight, B. L., Tymowski, R., and Fitzgerald, D. G., 1998, "Application of Body Residues as a Tool in the Assessment of Soil Toxicity," *Advances in Earthworm Ecotoxicology*, S. Sheppard, J. Bembridge, M. Holmstrup, and L. Posthuma, Eds., SETAC Press, Pensacola, FL, pp. 41-53.

McCarty, L. S., Mackay, D., Smith, A. D., Ozburn, G. W., and Dixon, D. G., 1992, "Residue-Based Interpretation of Toxicity and Bioconcentration QSARs from Aquatic Bioassays: Neutral Narcotic Organics," *Environmental Toxicology and Chemistry*, Vol. 11, pp. 917-930.

McCarty, L. S., and Mackay, D., 1993, "Enhancing Ecotoxicological Modeling and Assessment: Body Residues and Modes of Toxic Action," *Environmental Science and Technology*, Vol. 27, pp.1719-1728.

Parkerton, T. F., and Stone, M. A., 1998, "Ecotoxicity on a Stick: A Novel New Analytical Method for Assessing the Toxicity of Hydrocarbon-Contaminated Samples," Bioavailability Workshop Proceedings, Pinawa, Manitoba. (In press).

Petty, J. D., Huckins, J. N., and Zajicek, J. L., 1993, "Application of Semipermeable Membrane Devices (SPMDs) as Passive Air Samplers," *Chemosphere*, Vol. 27, pp.1609-1624.

Prozen, H., and Zupanecic-Kralj, L., 1998, "Use of Solid-Phase Microextraction in Analysis of Pesticides in Soil," *ACTA Chimica Slovania*, Vol. 45, pp. 1-18.

Rantalainen, A., Paasivirta, J., and Herve, S., 1998, "Uptake of Chlorohydrocarbons From Soil by Lipid-Containing Semipermeable Membrane Devices (SPMDs)," *Chemosphere*, Vol. 36 pp. 1415-1427.

Reid, B.J., Jones, K.C., and Semple, K.T., 2000, "Bioavailability of Persistent Organic Pollutants in Soils and Sediments-a Perspective on Mechanisms, Consequences, and Assessment," *Environmental Pollution*, Vol. 108, pp. 103-112.

Sijm, D., Kraaij, R., and Belfroid, A., 2000, "Bioavailability in Soil or Sediment: Exposure of Different Organisms and Approaches to Study it," *Environmental Pollution*, Vol. 108, pp. 113-119.

Strandberg, B., Wagman, N., Bergqvist, P. A., Haglund, P., and Rappe, C., 1997, "Semipermeable Membrane Devices as Passive Samplers to Determine Organochlorine Pollutants in Compost," *Environmental Science and Technology*, Vol. 31, pp. 2960-2965.

Tang, J., and Alexander, M., 1999, "Mild Extractability and Bioavailability of Polycyclic Aromatic Hydrocarbons in Soil," *Environmental Toxicology and Chemistry*, Vol. 18, pp. 2711-2714.

Topp, G. C., 1993, "Soil Water Content," *Soil Sampling and Methods of Analysis*. M. R. Carter, Ed., Lewis Publishers, Boca Raton, FL, USA, pp. 541-557.

Tugulea, A., Sarna, L. P., and Webster, G. R., 1998, "Solid Phase Microextraction (SPME) of the Herbicide Atrazine in Aqueous Soil Suspensions" *International Journal of Analytical Chemistry*, Vol. 68, pp. 137-153.

Van Brummelen, T. C., Van Hattum, B., Crommentuijn, T., and Kalf, D. F., 1998, "Bioavailability and Ecotoxicity of PAHs," *The Handbook of Environmental Chemistry*, Vol. 3 part J. A. H. Neilson, Ed. Springer-Verlag, New York, NY, USA, pp. 205-245.

Weston, D. P., and Mayer, L. M., 1998, "In Vitro Digestive Fluid Extraction as a Measure of the Bioavailability of Sediment-Associated Polycyclic Aromatic Hydrocarbons: Sources of Variation and Implications for Partitioning Models," *Environmental Toxicology and Chemistry*, Vol. 17, pp. 820-829.

Zhang, Z., and Pawliszyn, J. 1994, "Solid-phase microextraction," *Analytical Chemistry*, Vol. 66, pp. 844A-853A.

Xiao-Dong Huang,[1] Bernard R. Glick,[2] and Bruce M. Greenberg[2]

Combining Remediation Techniques Increases Kinetics for Removal of Persistent Organic Contaminants from Soil

Reference: Huang, X.-D., Glick, B. R., and Greenberg, B. M., "**Combining Remediation Techniques Increases Kinetics for Removal of Persistent Organic Contaminants from Soil,**" *Environmental Toxicology and Risk Assessment: Science, Policy, and Standardization - Implications for Environmental Decisions: Tenth Volume, ASTM STP 1403*, B. M. Greenberg, R. N. Hull, M. H. Roberts, Jr., and R. W. Gensemer, Eds., American Society for Testing and Materials, West Conshohocken, PA, 2001.

Abstract: A number of techniques, both mechanical and biological, have been investigated for the remediation of persistent organic contaminants from soils. However, most of these techniques have been applied independently. As a consequence of using only one process, remediation usually is slow for persistent organic contaminants. To improve remediation, multiple techniques that complement different aspects of contaminant removal have been applied to soils in combination. This resulted in an enhanced multi-process phytoremediation system that improved and accelerated the overall remediation resulting in removal of 95% of total PAHs. The remediation system includes physical (volatilization), photochemical (photooxidation), microbial degradation and plant growth (phytoremediation) processes. The techniques applied to realize these processes are land farming (aeration and light exposure), microbial remediation (introduction of contaminant degrading bacteria) and phytoremediation (plant growth with plant growth promoting rhizobacteria). This system was very effective at removal of persistent, strongly bound contaminants from soil. It appears that the combination of these components may be a viable solution for remediating persistent organic contaminants from soils.

Keywords: phytoremediation, photooxidation, rhizobacteria, PAHs, persistent organic contaminants

Large amounts of hazardous waste have been released into aquatic and terrestrial environments due to industrial activities and energy consumption (Neff 1979; Cooke and Dennis 1983; Safe 1984). Many organic contaminants are toxic, mutagenic and carcinogenic. They are persistent in the environment posing a significant hazard to ecosystems and human health (Neff 1979; Safe 1984). Because of their hazardous nature and persistence in the environment, it is expensive to remediate contaminated tracts of land for new usage. In many cases, it could take decades to clean up these sites. Therefore, research and development of remediation technologies for these types of contamination are needed.

[1]Research Associate and [2]Professor respectively, Department of Biology, University of Waterloo, Waterloo, On N2L 3G1 Canada.

Many techniques have been advanced to remediate persistent organic contaminants from soil (Cookson 1995; Mcnicoll and Baweja 1995; Alexander 1999). However, many are costly and/or inefficient. Physical removal and washing of contaminated soil with solvents is expensive and has met with mixed results. Land farming has been used for *in situ* remediation. However, the practice is primarily effective for removal of small, volatile chemicals. To improve the effectiveness of land farming, nutrient supplements, such as nitrogen and phosphorus, have been applied to enhance natural microbial degradation of contaminants (Amada et al. 1993). However, this is generally still limited to relatively small chemicals. Microbial bioremediation with organisms that are capable of degrading contaminants has been investigated extensively. For instance, "bioreactors" have been attempted, but the contaminated soils must be brought to the reactor for cleanup. This is expensive and can damage the soil. Alternatively, *in situ* bioremediation, usually inoculation of contaminant degrading microorganisms at contaminated sites, has been attempted. However, it is difficult to generate sufficient biomass in natural soils to allow an acceptable rate of sequestration and degradation of hydrophobic molecules (Alexander 1999). A further problem is that few microorganisms can use high molecular weight contaminants as a sole carbon source. Therefore, a readily degradable organic carbon source often must be supplied for co-metabolism of high molecular weight compounds (Cookson 1995; Alexander 1999).

For bioremediation to be effective, the throughput must be very high. A route for achieving this is by increasing biomass. For this reason, phytoremediation has recently received considerable attention (McCutcheon 1996; Rock 1996; McIntire and Lewis 1997; Raskin 1997). Plants have extensive root systems that explore a large volume of soil and assimilate contaminants over a wide area. As well, roots can enhance microbial activity by supplying substrates and nutrients. Phytoremediation has been successfully used to remediate a variety of contaminants in soil and groundwater. For instance, *Brassica* plants have been used effectively to take up heavy metals such as cadmium, zinc, copper, and nickel (Raskin 1997; Burd et al. 2000). Hybrid poplar trees have been used for removal of herbicides, such as atrazine (Burken and Schnoor 1997). Many other plants have been used to take up and/or degrade various organic contaminants in soils (Shann and Boyle 1994; Cunningham et al. 1996; Siciliano and Germida 1997; McIntire and Lewis 1997). The advantages of phytoremediation are: 1) it preserves the natural structure and texture of soil; 2) it is driven by solar energy and is suitable to most regions and climates; 3) it is low in cost and technically feasible; 4) it has the potential to be rapid by providing large amounts of biomass.

Although using plants for remediation of persistent organic contaminants holds advantages over other methods, many limitations exist for current application on a large scale (McCutcheon 1996; Drake 1997; Rock 1997). For instance, when contaminant concentrations in the soil are high, many plants will not grow enough to provide sufficient biomass for successful remediation. In many cases, contaminated soils are poor in nutrients, which will limit plant growth, slowing the remediation process. Further, microbial populations in contaminated soils are often depressed both in diversity and abundance (Baldwin 1922) and contaminated soils do not contain the appropriate microorganisms for the efficient degradation of the contaminants. This further limits the effectiveness of remediation. Therefore, phytoremediation processes are, in general, slow and the time scale for complete remediation is often unacceptably long (McCutcheon 1996; Drake 1997; Rock 1997). To address this problem, we have developed a multi-component phytoremediation system for the removal of recalcitrant organic contaminants from soil. This paper presents a theory of using kinetics of multiple processes for remediation of PAH compounds.

Multi-Process Strategy for Remediation

Three common types of kinetics may be used to describe remediation processes. They are zero order, first order and second order kinetics (Fig. 1). In zero order kinetics,

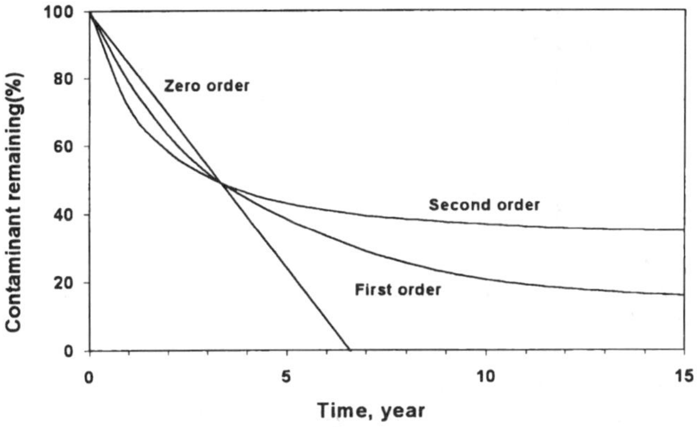

Figure 1 *Three common types of kinetics observed for contaminant remediation. Zero order: -dC/dt/=k; first order: -dC/dt=kC; second order: -dC/dt=kC²*.

contaminant concentration decreases by linear relation with time. That is, the rate of contaminant removal is concentration independent (i.e., -dC/dt=k). In first order kinetics, an exponential decay of contaminant concentration is observed as a function of time (i.e., -dC/dt=kC). In this case, the rate of contaminant uptake is proportional to contaminant concentration. In second order kinetics, a higher order exponential decay is observed. This means the rate of contaminant removal is proportional to the square of contaminant concentration or on the product of two contaminant concentrations (i.e., $-dC/dt=kC^2$ or $-dC/dt=kC_1C_2$).

Remediation rates for *in situ* bioremediation of persistent organic contaminants usually follow first or second order kinetics (Alexander 1999). Because of the exponential relationship between time and contaminant concentration in soil, it takes a long time for a single remediation process to completely remove persistent organic contaminants. However, the initial remediation rates are nearly linear (zero order) for all three types of kinetics. Although remediation rates can be accelerated by optimizing environmental factors for a single process, it is very difficult, if not impossible, to change the overall kinetics of degradation. However, if the initial remediation rates are combined in a multi-process system, the remediation kinetics can remain approximately linear (i.e., pseudo zero order), and faster for a greater fraction of the degradation process (Fig. 2).

Therefore, the time required for complete remediation can be shortened by several folds. Furthermore, it might even become possible for rapid and complete removal of the

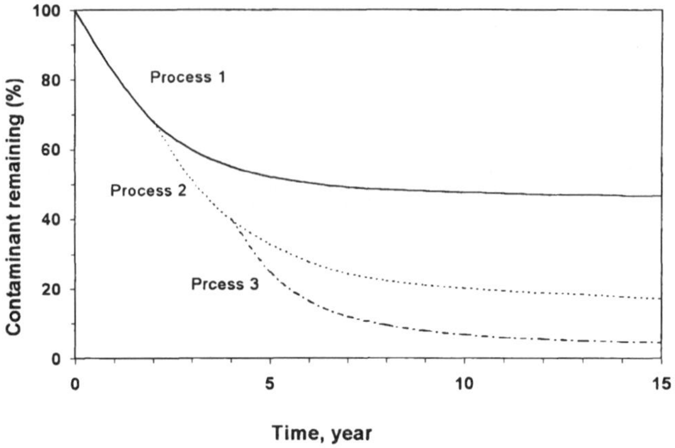

persistent organic contaminants from soils.

Figure 2 *Kinetics of multi-process for contaminant remediation. Successive application of three processes can allow for pseudo-zero order kinetics.*

To complicate matters, contaminated sites usually contain complex mixtures of contaminant chemicals. For example, PCBs are composed of 209 congeners and most PCBs contaminated sites contain more than 50 congeners. Petroleum hydrocarbon contaminants are also a large group of chemicals containing hundreds of different compounds. For instance, creosote, as a common source of polycyclic aromatic hydrocarbon (PAHs) contamination, contains more than 100 chemicals, most of which are aromatics. It is very difficult, if not impossible, to use a single technique to remove rapidly and completely all the components of such complex mixtures. Therefore, by knowing the contaminating components, and understanding their properties, and treating them strategically with selected multiple remediation processes, it may become feasible to remove them rapidly and completely. By combining multiple techniques, and optimizing each remediation process, the overall remediation process can be improved greatly and the time required for removal of persistent organic contaminants from soils can be shortened significantly.

A Case Study of Creosote (PAHs) Contaminants

Polycyclic aromatic hydrocarbons (PAHs) are a particularly recalcitrant group of contaminants (Neff 1979; Cooke and Dennis 1983). There are many sources for soil contamination by PAHs including creosote, fossil fuels and steel production (Neff 1979; Cooke and Dennis 1983). Not surprisingly PAHs are one of the most prevalent soil contaminants worldwide. At the present time, the techniques used to remediate PAH contaminated soils are inefficient and costly (McNicoll and Baweja 1995; Rock 1997). PAHs are composed of hundreds of compounds. For instance, the regulated priority list of

PAH compounds in the environment contains 16 compounds. They are different in size (2 to 6 benzene rings), shape, structure, and properties. Small compounds, such as naphthalene, acenaphthene, and acenaphthylene, are volatile or semi-volatile. Many are subject to photooxidation. Many of the smaller and less hydrophobic PAHs are subject to microbial degradation. Others (i.e., benzo(a)pyrene, dibenzo(a,h)pyrene, benzo(g,h,i)perylene, and indo(1,2,3-c,d)pyrene) are highly hydrophobic and binding strongly to organic matter in soils. This later group is particularly recalcitrant to

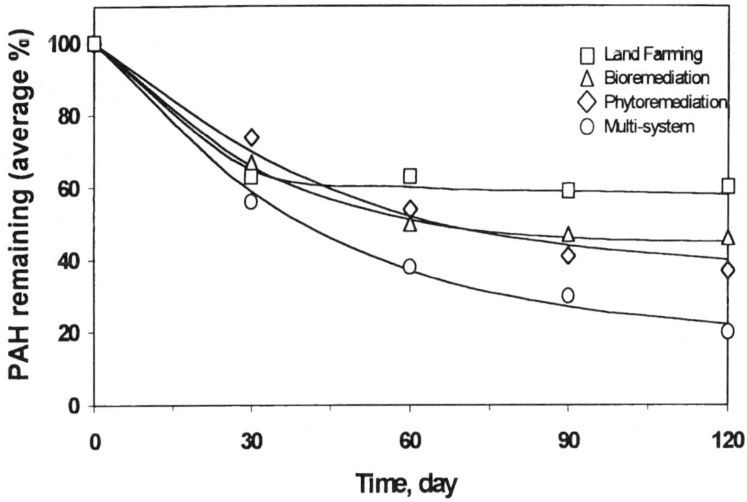

remediation.

Figure 3 *Comparison of PAH removal rates of single method with multi- component system.*

To make remediation effective and efficient for PAHs, different techniques are required for removal of different classes of these compounds. Based on properties of these mixtures, a multiple technique remediation system was developed that involved land farming, light exposure, microbial inoculation and plant growth with plant growth promoting rhizobacteria (PGPR). These four remediation processes resulted in volatilization, photochemical oxidation, microbial degradation and phytoremediation. They provide four complementary kinetic processes that we hoped to remove completely all classes of PAHs from soil. This multiple technique system was tested in the laboratory to assess its efficiency.

Land farming was chosen because it is a fast and effective method for removal of volatile chemicals such as naphthalene, acenaphthene, and acenaphthylene. It also aerates the soil, resulting in an increase in the potential for redox reactions in the soil. Further, it exposes buried chemicals to sunlight for photooxidation. One problem with degrading intact PAHs is that the first oxidation step is difficult for most biological organisms. This is because the π-orbital structures of intact PAHs provide great thermodynamic stability.

However, PAHs are readily photooxidized by sunlight to quinones and hydroxyl quinones (McConkey et al. 1997). Therefore, the soil was tilled before bioremediation treatment so a new layer of soil was exposed to light. Land farming was performed by turning the soil twice per week. When this was done, approximately 40% of the PAHs were lost from the soil due to volatilization and photooxidation to new products (Fig. 3).

Microbial remediation with bacteria might be more efficient if some of the PAHs have first been photooxidized making them more amendable to metabolism. The bacterial species that were used to inoculate soil were selected from an old creosote contaminated site and acclimated with PAHs in the laboratory for 10 weeks. This bacterial mixture contains strains of *Pseudomonas putida, Flavobacterium sp., Pseudomonas aeruginosa* and an unknown strain. The soil was inoculated with these bacteria following the land farming treatment. Inoculation with PAH degrading bacteria enhanced removal of PAHs from soil [Fig. 3]. In particular, fluoranthene, pyrene and benzo(a)anthracene, which can be used as a reduced carbon source for these bacteria (Trzesicka-Mlynarz 1993), were readily remediated (data not shown).

Growth of plants in soil without land farming or degradative bacteria resulted in removal of PAHs on par with bacteria (Fig. 3). However, removal of a larger fraction of the higher molecular weight PAHs was observed (data not shown). It was observed that plant growth was poor on the contaminated soil, which impaired remediation (see below). However, when a multi-component system was used, the plants grew much better (see below) and PAH removal was greatly improved (Fig. 3). This system included land farming and light exposures, followed by inoculation of the soil with the PAH degrading bacteria, followed by stimulation of plant growth with plant growth promoting rhizobacteria. In this case, plant growth was vigorous (see below) and efficient remediation was achieved (Fig. 3).

To summarize, a comparison of remediation rates of the multi-component phytoremediation system with the individual methods is shown in Figure 3. Land farming is the least effective technique used in these experiments, and the overall remediation efficiency for 16 PAHs was only 35%. The compounds removed by land farming were limited to the small PAH compounds such as naphthalene, acenaphthene, acenathylene, fluorene, phenanthrene, anthracene and benzo(a)anthracene. They are either volatile or subject to photooxidation. Land farming combined with bioremediation by inoculation with PAH degrading bacteria is more effective than land farming alone. Here, the total removal rate of PAHs was about 50%. This is comparable with phytoremediation following land farming treatment (55%) (Fig. 3). The advantage of phytoremediation over bacterial treatment was that it was more effective at removing the larger, more tightly soil bound PAHs (Huang et al in preparation). The multi-component remediation system had the greatest level for removal of PAH contaminants from soil, with an average removal for 16 PAHs at 80% and the total material removed at 95%. The greatest improvement was for the strongly soil bound PAHs. In the multi-component system, where the kinetics overall are first order, the pseudo-linear range is much longer than with any single method. Thus, one can estimate that if it takes 15 to 20 years to remediate a highly contaminated soil site by bioremediation or phytoremediation alone, it will only take the multi-component system three to six years to achieve the equivalent level of remediation.

One important reason for inoculation of plants with plant growth promoting bacteria is that growth of plants in contaminated soil is much improved with inoculation of PGPR. This allows more rapid and greater accumulation of biomass, particularly for roots in the soil (Tables 1 and 2). These bacteria are known to increase plant growth, reduce

Table 1 *Alfalfa germination efficiency grown on creosote contaminated soil.*

Creosote, g/kg	Untreated soil[1]	Landfarmed soil[2]	Lanfarmed soil with PGPR[3]
0	100.0	100.0	100.0
0.5	2.0	93.4	100.0
1.0	0	75.3	86.0
2.0	0	17.9	72.0
3.0	0	3.9	12.0

[1]Untreated soil, plant growth in contaminated soil without landfarming and PGPR.
[2]Landfarmed soil, plant growth in the contaminated soil that was landfarmed twice a week for a month prior to sewing seeds.
[3]Landfarmed soil with PGPR, plant growth with PGPR in the soil that was land farmed for a month prior to sewing seeds.

stress (Siciliano and Germida 1997; Shann et al. 1999, Burd et al 2000), including chemical toxicity. This allows vigorous plant growth, particularly in roots in the presence of chemical stressors (Siciliano and Germida 1997; Shah et al. 1999; Burd et al. 2000). Precisely how plant growth promoting bacteria alleviate stress is unclear. However, some of these bacteria contain the enzyme 1-aminocyclopropane-1-carboxylic acid deaminase that can lower the levels of stress ethylene in plants (Shah et al. 1999). It has previously

Table 2 *Germination efficiency of plant species grown on creosote contaminated soil.*

Creosote	Wild rye		Kentucky blue grass		Tall fescue	
g/kg	without	with PGPR	without	with PGPR	without	with PGPR
0	100.0	100	100.0	100.0	100	100.0
0.5	39.5	102.3	104.6	99.2	101.6	98.8
1.0	7.6	35.0	99.2	107.7	102.1	103.7
2.0	9.1	24.6	30.5	61.2	39.4	86.9
3.0	2.1	1.5	15.5	39.2	17.0	67.4

[1]Plants with or without inoculation of PGPR were grown on creosote contaminated soil.

been reported that plant growth promoting bacteria by lowering plant ethylene levels can reduce nickel toxicity to plants and can decrease the damage to plants from flooding and decrease the deleterious effects of certain pathogens (Glick 1995).

Plant growth promoting bacteria have an important role to play in bioremediation. Plants are effective at removing large amounts of persistent organic contaminants if they can accumulate large amounts of root biomass. Plants are then able to generate a large amount of root biomass in soil thereby facilitating the bacterial growth and allowing for enhanced microbial degradation of contaminants. Plant roots are also capable of acting as a sink for contaminants from soil. Also, plant roots can release enzymes into the soil that can degrade contaminants. Moreover, plant roots are capable of taking large amounts of water from soil and this water movement in soil will bring contaminants in contact with roots and bacteria surrounding the roots. Therefore, phytoremediation can be effective at removing large amounts of contaminants from soil, as long as good conditions for plant growth are maintained. This combined strategy of using plants, bacteria, and land farming shows a great potential to remediate large amounts of persistent organic contaminants from soil.

References:

Alexander, M., 1999, *Biodegradation and Bioremediation.* Academic Press, Inc. San Diego, USA. pp.71-98, pp.254-269.

Amada, A., Dickson, A.A. and Maate G.O., 1993, Remediation of Oil-polluted Soils: Effects of Organic and Inorganic Nutrient Supplements on the Performance of Maize. *Water Air Soil Pollut.* 66: 59-77.

Baldwin, I.L., 1922, Modification of Soil Flora Induced by Application of Crude Petroleum. *Soil Sci.* 14: 465-477

Burd G.I., Dixon, D.G. and Glick, B.G., 2000, Plant Growth Promoting Bacteria That Decease Heavy Metal Toxicity in Plants. *Can J. Microbiol.* 46:237-245.

Burken, J.G. and Schnoor, J.L., 1997, Uptake and Metabolism of Atrazine by Poplar Trees. *Environ. Sci. Technol.* 31:1399-1406.

Cooke, M. and Dennis, A.J., 1983, *Polycyclic Aromatic Hydrocarbons: Formation, Metabolism and Measurement* Battelle Press Inc.

Cookson, J.T., 1995, *Bioremediation Engineering: Design and Application.* McGraw-Hill, Inc. New York, USA. pp.51-92, 311-319.

Cunningham, S.D., Anderson, T.A., Schwab, A.P. and Hsu, F.C., 1996, *Advance in Agronomy.* 56: 55.

Drake, E., 1997. Phytoremediation of Soil: Current Prospects and Limitations for Industrial Application. *IBC Phytoremediation Conference.* Seattle, Washington. June 18.

Glick, B.R. The Enhancement of Plant Growth by Free Living Bacteria. *Can. J. of Microbiol.* **1995**, 41, 109.

Huang, X.-D., El-Alawi, Y.S., Glick, B., and Greenberg, B., 2000. Multi-component Phytoremediation System to Remove Polycyclic Aromatic Hydrocarbons from Contaminated Soil. In preparation.

McConkey, B., Duxbury, C., Dixon, D.G. and Greenberg, B.M., 1997. Toxicity of a PAH Photooxidation Product to the Bacteria *Photobacterium Phosphoreum* and the Duckweed *Lemna gibba*: Effects of Phenanthrene and its Primary Product, Phenanthrenequinone. *Environ. Toxico. Chem.* 16: 892.

McCutcheon, S., 1996. Workshop on Phytoremediation of Organic Contaminants. Fort Worth, Texas.

McIntire, T. and Lewis, G.M., 1997. The Advancement of Phytoremediation as Innovative Environmental Technology for Stabilization, Remediation and Restoration of Contaminated Sites *J. Soil Contam.* 6: 227.

McNicoll, D.M and Baweja, A.S., 1995 *Bioremediation of Petroleum-Contaminated Soils: an Innovative, Environmental Friendly Technology*, Environment Canada.

Neff, J.M., 1979. *Polycyclic Aromatic Hydrocarbons in the Aquatic Environments*. Appl. Sci. Pub. London.

Raskin, I., Smith, R.D. and Salt, D.E., 1997. Phytoremediation of Metals: Using Plants to Remove Pollutants from the Environment. *Curr. Opin. Biotechnol.* 8: 221-226.

Rock, S., 1996. Workshop on Phytoremediation of Organic Contaminants. Fort Worth, Texas. website: www.ibcusa.com/conf/phyto/

Rock, S., 1997. Phytoremediation of Petroleum in Soil and Groundwater. In *12th Annual Conference on Contaminated Soils - Analysis, Site Assessment, Fate, Environmental and Human Risk Assessment, Remediation and Regulation*, P T. Kostecki and E.J. Calabrese Eds.

Safe, S., 1984. Polychlorinated Biphenyls and Polubrominated Biphenyls: Biochemistry, Toxicology and Mechanisms of Action. *CRC Crit. Rev. Toxicol.* 13:319.

Shah, S., Li, J., Moffatt, B. A. and Glick, B.R., 1999. Isolation and Characterization of ACC Deaminase Genes from Two Different Plant Growth Promoting Rhizobacteria. *Can. J. of Microbiol.* In press.

Shann, J.R. and Boyle, J.J., 1994. Influence of Plant Species on In Situ Rhizosphere Degradation In *Biorem. through rihzospere Technol.* Anderson & Coats Eds, ACS Series 563. Washington DC. 71-81.

Siciliano, S.D. and Germida, J.J., 1997. Bacteria Inoculates of Forage Grasses Enhance Degradation of 2-Chlorobenzoiz acid in Soil. *Environ. Toxico. Chem.* 16:1098-1104.

Trzesicka-Mlynarz, D., 1993. *Biodegradation PAHs by A Mixed Culture of Bacteria Isolated from Contaminated Soil.* Thesis of University of Waterloo, Waterloo, ON Canada.

NEW DIRECTIONS IN ENVIRONMENTAL ASSESSMENT AND RECOVERY

Wayne G. Landis[1] and John F. McLaughlin[1]

If Not Recovery, Then What?

Reference: Landis, W. G. and McLaughlin, J. F., **"If Not Recovery, Then What?,"** *Environmental Toxicology and Risk Assessment: Science, Policy, and Standardization - Implications for Environmental Decisions: Tenth Volume, ASTM STP 1403*, B. M. Greenberg, R. N. Hull, M. H. Roberts, Jr., and R. W. Gensemer, Eds., American Society for Testing and Materials, West Conshohocken, PA, 2001.

Abstract: Recovery of ecological systems is an often-stated goal of activities associated with Superfund sites, toxic spills, and the restoration of habitats such as the Florida Everglades. Often recovery is associated with constructs related to ecosystem health, integrity, or sustainability. Return to an original state has been demonstrated empirically not to be an option. Integrity and sustainability are not defined in a quantitative fashion amenable to prediction. We present two alternative quantitative descriptions of the goals of restoration activities. The first uses surveys of supposedly unimpacted sites to define a multivariate description of the expected community given the specifications of the abiotic factors. The second uses stakeholder-desired characteristics of an ecological system to define the desired ranges for various ecosystem functions and/or structural characteristics and to form an assessment space. With these approaches, a risk assessment can determine the stressors causing the displacement of the system and management options to return to the assessment space. Management goals and actions can be directed at those variables and monitoring programs can be established to measure progress. Assessments about system status relate directly to the properties of concern and the management goals. The methodology does permit the reconstruction of important resources and other valued components of ecological systems.

Keywords: recovery, sustainability, restoration, multiple stressors

---

[1]Director, Institute of Environmental Toxicology and Chemistry, and professor, respectively, Huxley College, Western Washington University, Bellingham, WA 98225-9180, USA.

Introduction

In the preparation of a standard, we need to have a discussion or dialog concerning the goals of the engineering or management process that will use that methodology. There has been an increasing interest in the performance of ecological risk assessments and restoration of damaged sites as evidenced by recent American Society for Testing and Materials, United States Environmental Protection Agency, and Society for Environmental Toxicology and Chemistry symposia and workshops. Departing from the classical methods oriented paper, this short article examines the goal of risk assessment and restoration activities in light of current developments in ecology and environmental toxicology. We offer specific solutions and relate these methods to improvement in restoration efficiency and monitoring efficacy.

If Not Recovery....

Preventing degradation or restoring ecological integrity, health, and the balance of nature are often stated as risk assessment or restoration goals. In many cases a reference site is used as a comparison to the site under study. In this section we examine the reality of these goals in light of empirical observations and current ecological thought.

Ecological integrity and health are ambiguous terms that prevent a quantitative delineation of restoration goals. Often the definitions use the metaphor of an organism in attempting the definition. A typical definition is proposed by Haskell (1992):

> "An ecological system is healthy and free from "distress syndrome" if it is stable and sustainable -- that is, if it is active and maintains its organization and autonomy over time and is resilient to stress."

Karr (1992) has provided a definition even more tied to the organismal metaphor:

> "A biological system, whether individual or ecological, can be considered healthy when its inherent potential is realized, its condition is stable, its capacity for self-repair when perturbed is preserved, and minimal external support for management is needed."

Inherent potential is not defined. Self-repair is an organismal property generally comprised of the immune response and directed cell growth. Comparable processes are not known in ecological systems. Ideas of integrity and health are derived from a balance of nature model of community structure and response to disturbance.

The balance of nature is also a commonly used goal that is based on a Clementian ideal of ecological succession and community structure. The difficulties with this model have been extensively described (Kapustka and Landis 1998). The Clementian model assumes an optimal and stable community structure for each environment and that successional processes attempt to reach this optimal condition. Perturbations from the optimal community structure are counteracted by mechanisms following a prescribed sequence of taxa to restore the original condition.

The balance of nature and other model structures relying upon an intrinsic balance have been refuted experimentally and by field observation. Connell and Sousa (1983) found stability in populations to be a rare event. In a series of microcosm experiments Drake (1991) demonstrated the importance of assembly order in determining the response of ecological systems to disturbance. Constructed landscapes (Drake et al. 1996) also demonstrated patchiness determined by stochastic processes. The persistence of impacts following a chemical perturbation also has been demonstrated experimentally.

Blanck and colleagues (Blanck et al. 1988; Molander and Blanck 1992) demonstrated that algal communities develop via natural selection upon the populations' resistance to chemical stress. This adaptive response, pollution-induced community tolerance (PICT) is proposed as a common property of ecological systems. Kersting and Van Wijngaarden (1999) confirmed this pattern in a complex stream microcosm experiment with a herbicide stress on a macrophyte community. Upon the second exposure to afalon the community showed a reduced response compared to the initial stressor event.

Community conditioning is a broader ranging hypothesis to PICT. Community conditioning (Matthews et al. 1996, Landis et al. 1996) states that ecological systems preserve information about prior events, including impacts due to chemical stressors. Community conditioning does not suggest that an increase in tolerance is a necessary response to the stressor, but is perhaps one of many alterations to the dynamics and composition of ecological systems. A series of long-term microcosm experiments (Landis et al. 2000) have demonstrated the persistence of the effects first seen in shorter-term experiments (Landis et al. 1993a, 1993b).

PICT and community conditioning recognize the importance of history not predestination on the composition of ecological systems. The importance of history and dynamics has also been demonstrated for landscapes. Wu and Loucks (1995) have demonstrated that ecological systems are not stable at the local level, but instead that patchiness is important for persistence at a landscape level. Stochastic and deterministic processes are co-occurring, producing the spatial and temporal mosaic of ecological systems (Wu and Loucks 1995, Wu 1999). Patch dynamics and distribution, rather than a balance of nature approach, provide much more quantitative understanding of the distribution of species along a landscape.

Ecological Reality–Not the Balance of Nature

Research of last ten years has demonstrated that the current status of ecological systems is determined by the history of the site in combination with patterns within the landscape. Also important are the dynamics of the systems and how these are affected by a variety of constraints. The balance of nature does not exist as an intrinsic property of ecological systems. The question of what state should be the goal of restoration activities can not fall back upon the balance of nature as an effective model.

Then What?

Our goal is not to eliminate restoration as a management goal but to define what recovery means in a risk assessment or restoration context. There are at least two ways of defining a restoration or recovery goal that are not dependent upon the failed paradigms of the past. Each method requires a value-based determination of design criteria for the ecological system undergoing restoration.

Field-Derived Reference Space–It is possible to define the recovery goals based on a reference space-derived from sampling so-called unimpacted sites. Rosenberg et al. (1997) reviews a number of studies that use this approach and describes possible application to sediment toxicity evaluations and risk assessment. Essentially, hundreds of samples are taken from a variety of sites within a region that allegedly have little or no human (modern culture) influence. Samples from a site would describe the spatial and temporal variability of the site both biologically and with regard to the abiotic factors. Multivariate regression can provide equations that show a particular community composition should exist for a specified set of abiotic features. Confidence bounds can then be derived, describing a reference space for a particular abiotic setting. It may be that for certain combinations of abiotic factors that few examples exist, expanding the uncertainty of that specific prediction. In other parts of the reference space there may be numerous data points, narrowing the uncertainty. Comparing the reference space to the impacted site can then be done, requiring an appropriate sampling of the impacted site to appropriately judge sample error, spatial and temporal variability and other uncertainties (See Figure 1).

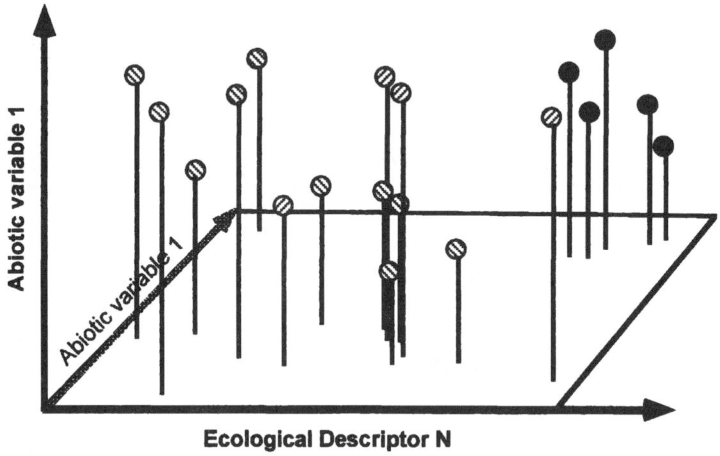

Figure 1–Mapping the relationship between an ecological descriptor and the abiotic variables. The black points are for the site of interest. The hatched points are for sites that exhibit ecological conditions are deemed desirable.

An approach such as that presented by Kersting (1988) would be a means of quantifying the differences between the impacted site and the sample-derived design space. The field research would describe a normal operating space (NOS) that represents the desired status of the ecological system and the expected or allowed range of variability (Figure 2). A distance is measured from the center of this space to the point under consideration for restoration (A). This distance is divided by the distance from the center of the NOS to its border (B) provides a measure denoted as ecosystem strain. If the ecosystem strain is ≤1, the site is within the desired NOS and restoration has been accomplished.

The societal value intrinsic to such an approach is the desire to have the impacted site resemble other sites that have had minimal impact due to human influences with the same abiotic factors. This is a value decision stating that the system described by the multivariate regression best fits the needs of the stakeholders. In many cases the restoration effort would require not only the cleanup of the contamination, but also the restoration of habitat and isolation of the area from future human influences.

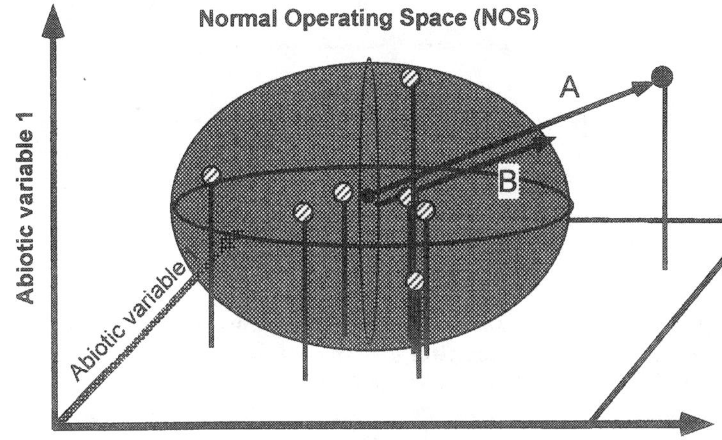

Figure 2–Normal operating space as a restoration goal. The hatched points decribe the position of biological communities with abiotic values similar to the contaminated site. The solid point represents the site under consideration for restoration.

Stakeholder-defined assessment volume. A different approach is to *a priori* describe an assessment space based upon the values of the stakeholders for the contaminated site (Figure 3). This approach has been described by Landis et al. (1994) and expanded on by Landis and McLaughlin (2000). Briefly, the stakeholders are polled to construct a list of specifications for a particular site. Landis, Luxon, and Bodensteiner (2000) constructed such a list of specifications for parts of the McKenzie and Willamette Rivers in western Oregon. In this instance the social values were derived from the Willamette Valley Livability Forum (WVLF). This forum, established by the Governor of Oregon, met to decide the environmental goals to be achieved by 2050. Environmental goals, such as maintaining sport salmonid fisheries and other recreational uses, are then tied to the quantitative values used by wildlife and resource management agencies as targets. The numerical values derived from the resource management agencies or interest groups provide the values for the box.

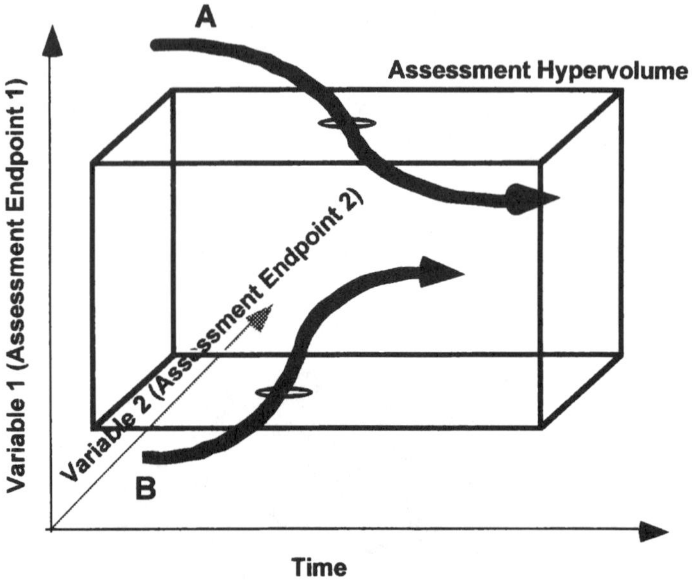

Figure 3–"The box." The axes are determined by quantitative descriptions of stakeholder values and the time axis is used to delineate rates of restoration or the persistence of the ecological system afterwards. The goal of the restoration effort is to move the ecological system from outside to inside the box regardless of its initial point (Lines A and B).

Typically, there are conflicting specifications, such as the use of water for irrigation and the preservation of sport salmonid habitat. Consultation among the stakeholders and the risk assessors or restoration team can help to resolve such issues, or different parts of the restored system set aside to meet each need. In regional level assessments these goals should be delineated within the area of concern.

Next, the time frame for return to the desired state and the persistence of the system within the box are specified. A rapid return to the assessment volume may require a massive engineering or cleanup effort compared to a more subtle restoration strategy. Once the system has moved to within the assessment box persistence needs to be delineated. In the case of the WVLF a 50-year time frame was specified. In other situations much shorter-term goals may be established. The critical aspect is that the specifications for a dynamic system have been completed when time is included.

A difficult issue will be in making predictions about time to recovery and the persistence of the system within the assessment hypervolume. Modeling can be a useful tool in this endeavor. Population models can be useful for projecting long-term trends. Spatial aspects of the distribution of the affected populations can be addressed and the dynamics calculated (McLaughlin and Landis 2000). One of the results of the patch dynamic modeling efforts is that contaminants and other stressors can affect populations occupying patches that are not contaminated.

Models are, at best, only simulations with associated uncertainties. An analysis of the uncertainties and a projection of accuracy of the forecast at specified time intervals should accompany a model prediction. Field data should be used to test the accuracy of the predictions and the accompanying assumptions. This incorporation of predictions about spatial and temporal dynamics is a critical aspect of defining recovery or restoration.

Discussion

Recovery as return to original state is not an option. However, this is not a loss as far as restoration activities are concerned. In fact, there are specific advantages.

1. Time is not wasted scouting for a prototypical reference site, identical to the contaminated site in all (or most aspects) except the chemical. In the reference space approach a general survey of the region is required, but such surveys are being attempted in many states. The goals established by the formation of the reference space will also help to ensure that data relevant to the construction of such a multidimensional space will be collected.
2. It is critical to not eliminate information by the use of indices such as the IBI to measure recovery. Such measures loose information because of the collapse of a variety of axes into a single number, with no measure of variability or uncertainty. Many different ecological states can provide the same numerical index value, and our objective is to as accurately as possible the status of the system of interest.
3. The goals of the restoration activity are very explicit and transparent when the approaches in this paper are used. The data used in the reference space approach, or the stakeholder decisions used in the box can be clearly documented and then presented to the decision makers.
4. Since the goals of restoration process can be so clearly described, monitoring programs to establish progress and to test hypotheses can be planned to provide the relevant information.
5. Both methods of establishing restoration goals can also be used to place bounds on acceptable uncertainty in both the measurement of current status and in predictive models.

Regardless of the method used, environmental scientists have important roles to play in the establishment and implementation of recovery goals. Obtaining and representing stakeholder values as assessment endpoints is critical to both approaches and social and biophysical scientists with the appropriate training should be employed.

Communication about the reality of restoration and recovery efforts is critical so that unattainable goals will not be perpetuated. Unattainable goals will lead to a perception of the failure of the restoration effort. Clearly defining the goals as outlined in both methods can aid in both the communication and expectation factors.

References

Blanck, H., Wangberg, S. A., and Molander, S., 1988. Pollution-Induced Community Tolerance: A New Ecotoxicological Tool. In J. Cairns, Jr. and J. R. Pratt, eds.

Functional Testing of Aquatic Biota for Estimating Hazards of Chemicals. STP 988. American Society for Testing and Materials. Philadelphia. PA. USA, pp. 219-230.

Connell, J. H., and Sousa, W. P., 1983, "On the Evidence Needed To Judge Ecological Stability or Persistence," *American Naturalist*, Vol. 121, No. 6, pp. 789-824.

Drake, J. A., 1991, "Community-Assembly Mechanics and the Structure of an Experimental Species Ensemble." *American Naturalist*, Vol. 137, pp. 1-26.

Drake, J. A., Flum, T. E., Witteman, G. J., Voskuil, T., Hoylman, A. M., Creson, C., Kenny, D. A., Huxel, G. R., Larue, C. S., and Duncan, J. R., 1993, "The Construction and Assembly of an Ecological Landscape," *Journal of Animal Ecology,* Vol. 62, pp.117-130.

Drake, J. A., Huxel, G. R., and Hewitt, C. L, 1996, "Microcosms as Models for Generating and Testing Community Theory," *Ecology,* Vol. 77, pp. 670-677.

Haskell, B. D., Norton, B. G., and Costanza, R, 1992, "Introduction: What Is Ecosystem Health and Why Should We Worry about It?" *Ecosystem Health: New Goals for Environmental Management,* Island Press, Washington, DC, pp. 3-20

Kapustka, L. A. and Landis, W. G, 1998, "Ecology: the Science Versus the Myth," *Human and Ecological Risk Assessment,* Vol. 4, pp. 829-838.

Karr, J. R., 1992, "Ecological integrity: Protecting Earth's Life Support Systems." *Ecosystem Health: New Goals for Environmental Management,* Island Press, Washington, DC, pp. 223-238.

Kersting, K., and Van Wijngaarden, P. A., 1999, "Effects of a Pulsed Treatment with the Herbicide Afalon (Active Ingredient Linuron) on Macrophyte-Dominated Mesocosms. I. Responses of Ecosystem Metabolism, " *Environmental Toxicology and Chemistry,* Vol. 18, pp. 2859-2865.

Kersting, K., 1988, "Normalized Ecosystem Strain in Micro-Ecosystems Using Different Sets of State Variables," *Verh. International. Verein. Limnology*, Vol. 23, pp. 1641-1646.

Landis, W. G., Luxon, M., and Bodensteiner, L.R., 2000. Design of a Relative Rank Method Regional-Scale Risk Assessment with Confirmational Sampling for the Willamette and McKenzie Rivers, Oregon. *Ninth Symposium on Environmental Toxicology and Risk Assessment: Recent Achievements in Environmental Fate and Transport, ASTM STP1381* F. T. Price, K. V. Brix and N. K. Lane, Eds., American Society for Testing and Materials, West Conshohocken, PA, pp 67-88.

Landis, W. G., Matthews, R. A., Markiewicz, A. J., Shough, N. A., and Matthews, G. B., 1993a, "Multivariate Analyses of the Impacts of the Turbine Fuel Jet-A Using a

Microcosm Toxicity Test," *Journal of Environmental Science*, Vol. 2, pp. 113-130.

Landis, W. G., Matthews, R. A., Markiewicz, A. J., and Matthews, G. B., 1993b, "Multivariate Analysis of the Impacts of the Turbine Fuel JP-4 in a Microcosm Toxicity Test with Implications for the Evaluation of Ecosystem Dynamics and Risk Assessment," *Ecotoxicology,* Vol. 2, pp. 271-300.

Landis, W. G., Matthews, G. B., Matthews, R. A., and Sergeant, A., 1994, "Application of Multivariate Techniques to Endpoint Determination, Selection and Evaluation in Ecological Risk Assessment." *Environmental Toxicology and Chemistry,* Vol. 12, pp. 1917-1927

Landis, W. G., Matthews, R. A., and Matthews, G. B., 1996, "The Layered and Historical Nature of Ecological Systems and the Risk Assessment of Pesticides," *Environmental Toxicology and Chemistry*, Vol.15, pp. 432-440.

Landis, W. G., Markiewicz, A. J., Matthews, R. A., and Matthews, G. B., 2000, "Confirmation of the Community Conditioning Hypothesis: Persistence of Effects in Model Ecological Structures Dosed with the Jet Fuel JP-8," *Environmental Toxicology and Chemistry,* Vol. 19, pp. 327-336.

Landis, W. G., and McLaughlin, J. F., in press 2000, "Establishing Specifications of Ecological Indicators for the Prediction of Sustainability," *Proceedings for Int. Congress on Ecosystem Health,* Univ. of California Davis.

Matthews, R.A., Landis, W. G., and Matthews, G. B., 1996, "Community Conditioning: An Ecological Approach to Environmental Toxicology, " *Environmental Toxicology and Chemistry,* Vol. 15, pp. 597-603.

McLaughlin, J. F. and Landis, W. G., 2000. Effects of Environmental Contaminants in Spatially Structured Environments. *Environmental Contaminants in Terrestrial Vertebrates: Effects on Populations. Communities, and Ecosystems.* Albers. P. H., et al., Eds., Society of Environmental Toxicology and Chemistry, Pensacola, FL.

Molander, S., and Blanck, H., 1992, "Detection of Pollution-Induced Community Tolerance (PICT) in Marine Periphyton Communities Established under Diuron Exposure," *Aquatic Toxicology,* Vol. 22, pp. 129-144.

Rosenberg, D. M., Reynoldson, T. B., Day, K. E., Resh, V. H., 1997, "Role of Abiotic Factors in Structuring Benthic Invertebrate Communities in Freshwater Systems," *Ecological Risk Assessment of Contaminated Sediments,* SETAC Press, Pensacola, FL.

Wu, J., 1999, "Hierarchy and Scaling: Extrapolating Information along a Scaling Ladder," *Canadian Journal of Remote Sensing,* Vol. 25, pp. 367-380.

Wu, J., and Loucks, O. L., 1995, "From Balance-of-Nature to Hierarchical Patch Dynamics: A Paradigm Shift in Ecology," *Quarterly Review of Biology*, Vol. 70, pp. 439-466.

Wu, J., and Levin, S. A., 1994, "A Spatial Patch Dynamic Modeling Approach to Pattern and Process in an Annual Grassland," *Ecological Monographs*, Vol. 64, pp. 447-464.

Geoffrey I. Sunahara,[1] Pierre Yves Robidoux,[2] Ping Gong,[3] Bernard Lachance,[2] Sylvie Rocheleau,[4] Sabine G. Dodard,[4] Manon Sarrazin,[4] Jalal Hawari,[5] Sonia Thiboutot,[6] Guy Ampleman,[7] and Agnès Y. Renoux[2]

Laboratory and Field Approaches to Characterize the Soil Ecotoxicology of Polynitro Explosives

---

Reference: Sunahara, G. I., Robidoux, P. Y., Gong, P., Lachance, B., Rocheleau, S., Dodard, S. G., Sarrazin, M., Hawari, J., Thiboutot, S., Ampleman, G., and Renoux, A. Y., **"Laboratory and Field Approaches to Characterize the Soil Ecotoxicology of Polynitro Explosives,"** *Environmental Toxicology and Risk Assessment: Science, Policy and Standardization – Implications for Environmental Decisions: Tenth Volume, ASTM STP 1403*, B. M. Greenberg, R. N. Hull, M. H. Roberts, Jr., and R. W. Gensemer, Eds., American Society for Testing and Materials, West Conshohocken, PA, 2001.

Abstract: Nitro-aromatic and heterocyclic compounds such as 2,4,6-trinitrotoluene (TNT), 1,3,5-trinitro-1,3,5-triazacyclohexane (RDX), 1,3,5,7-tetranitro-1,3,5,7-tetrazacyclooctane (HMX), have been identified worldwide in soil and groundwater, at sites related to military activities. Among these chemicals, the toxicology of TNT is better known; however, gaps of knowledge still exist. We characterized the soil ecotoxicology of these energetic polynitro substances and their degradation products. The toxicities of these chemicals on microbial, plants, and invertebrate (oligochaete) species, and to cultured mammalian cell systems were examined using spiked and field soil samples. A sensitivity distribution ranking the responses of species was assembled for establishing soil benchmarks for explosives such as TNT. Preliminary field studies were also carried out using earthworm mesocosms. These approaches will increase the toxicological understanding of energetic compounds and our ability to detect exposure/toxicities of these substances in the field, and aid in establishing environmentally acceptable criteria, which are of great interest to land managers.

Keywords: toxicity, TNT, RDX, HMX, explosives, ecotoxicity, cytotoxicity, soil, *Vibrio fischeri*, *Eisenia andrei*, V79 cells, field mesocosms

---

[1]Group Leader, Applied Ecotoxicology Group, [2]Research Officer, [3]Visiting Fellow, [4]Technical Officer, and [5]Group Leader, Analytical Chemistry Group, Biotechnology Research Institute, National Research Council of Canada, 6100 Royalmount Avenue, Montréal, Québec, Canada, H4P 2R2.

[6]Group Leader, Chemistry and Environment, and [7]Research Chemist, Defense Research Establishment Valcartier, Department of National Defense, 2459 Pie IX Boulevard, Val Bélair, Québec, Canada, G3J 1X5.

Introduction

2,4,6-Trinitrotoluene (TNT, CAS 118-96-7), 1,3,5-trinitro-1,3,5-triazacyclohexane (RDX, CAS 121-82-4), 1,3,5,7-tetranitro-1,3,5,7-tetrazacyclooctane (HMX, CAS 2691-41-0) and some of their degradation products are environmental contaminants identified in soil and groundwater at sites related to military and demolition activities. These sites are associated with the manufacturing, handling, testing and disposal of these substances. The chemical structures of these polynitro- substances are shown in Figure 1.

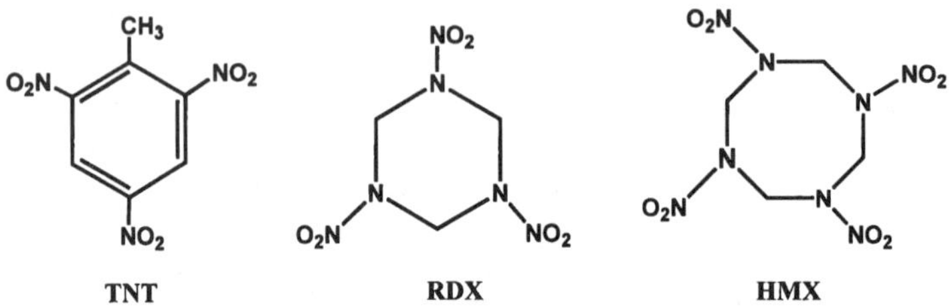

Figure 1 – *Chemical structures for 2,4,6-trinitrotoluene (TNT), 1,3,5-trinitro-1,3,5-triazacyclohexane (RDX), and 1,3,5,7-tetranitro-1,3,5,7-tetrazacyclooctane (HMX).*

Figure 2 shows the aerobic and anaerobic biotransformation products of TNT. The end product, TAT is only found under strictly anaerobic conditions, and is bound to the soil organic phase which limits its further degradation (Hawari et al. 1998).

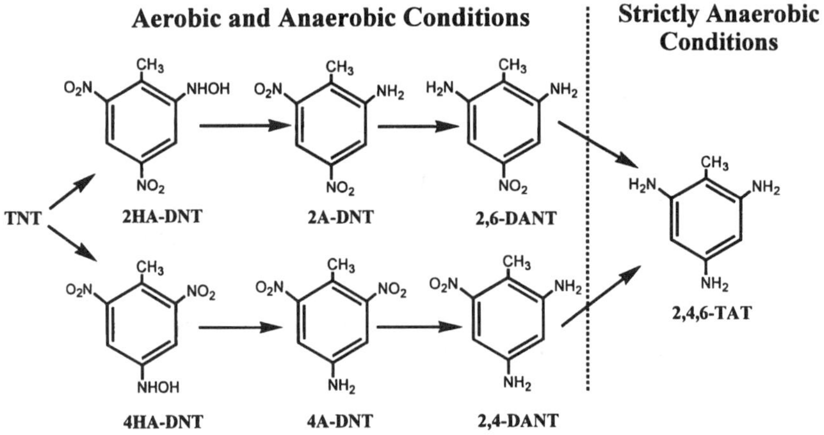

Figure 2 – *Chemical structures of TNT and some of its reduced biotransformation products. Abbreviations: TNT (2,4,6-trinitrotoluene), 2HA-DNT (2-hydroxyamino-dinitrotoluene), 2A-DNT (2-amino-DNT), 2,6-DANT (2,6-diaminonitrotoluene), 4HA-DNT (4-hydroxyamino-DNT), 4A-DNT (4-amino-DNT), 2,4-DANT (2,4-diamino-DNT), 2,4,6-TAT (2,4,6-triaminotoluene). Redrawn from Hawari et al. (1998).*

Concentrations of these explosives in soil may vary according to the type of the facility. For example, high concentrations (1 – 87 g/kg soil) may be found at production and handling sites (Simini et al. 1995) where effects include loss of vegetation and general degeneration of soil health. On the other hand, lower levels (< 10 mg/kg soil) may be found at unexploded ordnance (UXO) contaminated ranges at military training areas (Hawari 2000) and the ecological effects are often less obvious depending on the explosive.

In Canada, the Department of National Defense (DND) has about 100 training sites, most of which are contaminated by energetic materials but at relatively low concentrations (mainly below 10 mg/kg soil of TNT, RDX and HMX). Some of these sites will be decommissioned and alternative landuse will be considered by DND land managers. To achieve this, managers must consider the cost and time needed for decontamination, the quality and reusability of the site (alternative landuse), and the key overall question, "how clean is clean?" The (eco)toxicologist can assist the manager by providing information that could be used to decide if the soil on the contaminated site is acceptable for a specific use, or requires further rehabilitation. Toxicity tests can be used to : (1) provide toxicological data for ecological risk assessments (ERAs) of contaminated sites, and (2) generate soil quality criteria for explosives in soil, and (3) monitor the performance of environmental bioprocesses used for remediating explosives-contaminated soil.

The toxicological effects of these energetic compounds have been recently reviewed by Talmage et al. (1999). Although relatively well-characterized in mammalian and aquatic systems, scant toxicological data is available for terrestrial organisms. This information would be valuable for ecological risk assessments (ERAs) and for the development of terrestrial benchmarks (soil quality criteria) for sites contaminated with explosives. This chapter article describes an approach towards establishing ecotoxicologically based soil quality criteria for explosives and their degradation products. Although TNT is used as a model toxicant for soils at contaminated sites, it often occurs in soils at varying concentrations along with other explosives, RDX and HMX, as well as heavy metals. Data from single species toxicity tests with plants, earthworms, and microbes exposed to these energetic substances were examined and compared with the data from field studies. Ultimately, the data were used in a species-sensitivity rank order analysis to establish soil benchmarks for explosives. We have also conducted biochemical studies in parallel to the toxicity tests, to increase our understanding of the mechanisms underlying the toxicities of explosives.

Toxicity of Explosives to Microorganisms

In the 1940s, workers reported that TNT wastes reduced biochemical oxygen demand in sewage (Schott et al. 1943, Ruchhoft et al. 1945), implying that TNT might be toxic to microorganisms. Microbial toxicity of explosives and their related compounds was first evaluated in laboratory studies using pure compounds and pure-cultured microorganisms. Klausmeier et al. (1973) demonstrated that TNT (220 μM or greater) severely inhibited the growth of fungi, yeasts, actinomyces and gram-positive bacteria isolated from soil. Recently, Fuller and Manning (1997) further observed that the growth and TNT transformation capacity of gram-positive bacteria both exhibited 50% reduction at TNT levels as low as 44 μM. In contrast, many gram-negative bacteria grew well and degraded a substantial percentage of TNT in growth media with initial TNT up to 290 μM (Klausmeier et al. 1973, Fuller and Manning 1997). These findings consequently led to a conclusion that aerobic gram-positive bacteria are more sensitive to TNT than gram-negative bacteria. However, some exceptions do exist with regard to the general sensitivity of gram-positive bacteria to TNT. For example, some *Streptomyces* strains could grow at 330 or 440 μM TNT (Pasti-Grigsby et al. 1996), Vorbeck et al. (1994) observed transformation of 500 μM of TNT by *Mycobacterium* sp., and Vanderberg et al. (1995) reported growth of *Mycobacterium vaccae* in the presence of 200 μM of TNT.

Several laboratories have tested the toxicity of TNT, RDX, HMX and TNT degradation products, to a sensitive luminescent bacterium *Vibrio fischeri,* in order to examine the potential toxicity of explosives in soil leachates. Based on these type of studies (Table 1), TNT was the most toxic among these compounds (Drzyzga et al. 1995, Sunahara et al. 1998, Dodard et al. 1999). At their water solubility limits, RDX (181 μM) only caused about 20% inhibition of bioluminescence, whereas HMX (22 μM) was not toxic (Sunahara et al. 1998).

Table 1 - *Relative Microtox toxicity of pure explosives and related compounds.*

Compound	**Abbreviation**	**Relative toxicity [1] IC_{20}-15 min (μM)**
2,4,6-Trinitrotoluene	TNT	0.5
2-Amino-4,6-dinitrotoluene	2A-DNT	96
4-Amino-2,6-dinitrotoluene	4A-DNT	46
2,4-Diamino-6-nitrotoluene	2,4-DANT	119
2,6-Diamino-4-nitrotoluene	2,6-DANT	138
2,6-Dinitrotoluene	2,6-DNT	4.2
2,4-Dinitrotoluene	2,4-DNT	44
2,4,6-Triaminotoluene	TAT	172
1,3,5-Trinitro-1,3,5-triazacyclohexane	RDX	105
1,3,5,7-Tetranitro-1,3,5,7-tetraazacyclooctane	HMX	> 22

[1] Data taken from Sunahara et al. (1998) and Dodard et al. (1999).

Sunahara et al. (1998, 1999) used the U.S. EPA Method 8330 SW 846 acetonitrile-sonication extraction method, coupled with aquatic based Microtox tests (Microbics 1992) to assess the toxicity of TNT-spiked soils. Using a toxicity identification evaluation (TIE) approach, the toxicity of acetonitrile extracts of soil was compared with that of aqueous leachates of spiked- and field-contaminated soils, as well as pure TNT dissolved in water. A TNT-dependent inhibition of bioluminescence was observed with soil extracts, leachates and pure compound (Sunahara et al. 1999). Simini et al. (1995) also tested the toxicity of aqueous leachates of soils sampled from explosives-contaminated sites and found a significant correlation between TNT concentrations in soil and Microtox toxicity in leachates.

Studying microbial toxicity using indigenous microorganisms rather than a single marine bacterium is more relevant and the laboratory toxicity results can be extrapolated to impacts likely to occur in the field (Chapman 1995). Gong et al. (1999a) measured soil microbial activities such as potential nitrification activity (PNA), dehydrogenase activity (DHA) and heterotrophic nitrogen fixation activity (NFA). A TNT-dependent inhibitory response of soil microbial activities was established with IC_{50} values ranging from 39 to 533 mg TNT /kg soil, depending on indicators and soil types (Gong et al. 1999a). Winkel and Wilke (1997) also measured the effects of TNT on PNA and substrate-induced respiration (SIR) and found that addition of 50 mg TNT /kg soil (PNA) or 100 mg TNT/kg (SIR) could induce significant inhibition 1 to 22 d after spiking. In addition, our recent work indicated that RDX and HMX are much less toxic than TNT with no derivable IC_{50} values. RDX or HMX only reduced 10-15% of microbial activities (e.g. PNA as shown in Figure 3) at the highest exposure concentrations in soil (10,000 mg/kg soil).

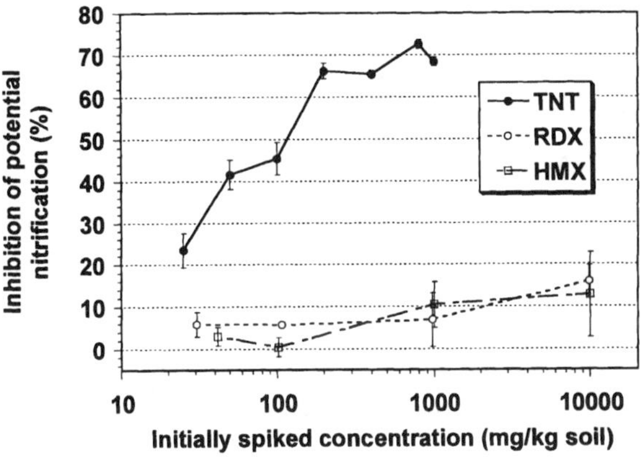

Figure 3 - *Effects of TNT, RDX and HMX on potential nitrification activity (PNA) in an uncontaminated garden soil. PNA was measured one week after explosives being spiked to the soil. Data are expressed as mean (point) ± standard deviation (error bar), n=4.*

Field studies can provide direct evidence for the *in situ* toxicity as site-specific conditions may modify the behavior of toxicants and thus alter their bioavailability. Gong et al. (1999a) assessed the response of indigenous microorganisms to TNT-contaminated field soil samples. Microbial toxicity as reflected by the inhibition of microbial activities (PNA, NFA and DHA) significantly correlated with TNT levels in soil. Although the estimated IC_{50}, LOEC and NOEC values are site- and indicator-specific, the lowest values were 51, 1, and 0.4 mg/kg, respectively, which is consistent and comparable with the results from laboratory spiking experiments (Gong et al. 1999a).

In another field study, Fuller and Manning (1998) investigated the effects of mixtures of TNT and other munitions on indigenous microbial communities in soils.

They measured specific sub-populations of soil microbial communities. TNT caused a shift from a gram-positive-dominated to a gram-negative-dominated community, which confirmed the results from early studies of Klausmeier et al. (1973). An important finding from this study was that chronic exposure to TNT dramatically altered soil microbial communities, with a greater number of TNT resistant bacteria isolated from highly contaminated soils (Fuller and Manning 1998).

Our recent work also confirmed this observation (Gong et al. 2000, Siciliano et al. 2000). Using a newly developed *in situ* respirometric technique (Witter et al. 2000), Gong et al. (2000) demonstrated that the glucose-utilizing microbial consortium in four field soils with long-term TNT-exposure history was more tolerant to TNT than that in two uncontaminated soils (Figure 4). By examining the utilization rate of thirty-one Biolog ECO substrates, Siciliano et al. (2000) observed that artificially added TNT in Biolog wells caused the greatest inhibition in the substrate utilization rate of microbial communities extracted from site soils with the lowest level of *in situ* exposure to TNT.

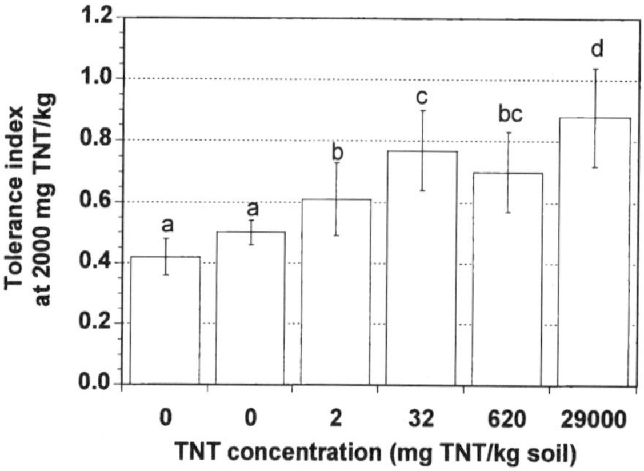

Figure 4 - *Tolerance of glucose-utilizing microbial consortium to the challenge of artificially added 2000 mg TNT /kg soil in six soils. Redrawn using data from Gong et al. (2000). The tolerance index for each soil was calculated as the ratio of the specific growth rate in TNT-added sub-sample to that in the non-TNT-spiked control sub-sample. Data are expressed as the mean (column) ± standard deviation (error bar) with n=12-16. Different letters above the bars indicate a significant difference at* $p \leq 0.05$.

Tolerance to TNT increased with the elevation of *in situ* TNT concentrations in soil (Gong et al. 2000, Siciliano et al. 2000). Together, these results indicate that pollution-induced microbial community tolerance is a sensitive indicator for soil contamination and can be used as a means of identifying those compounds that have exerted selective pressure on the community (Posthuma 1997, Gong et al. 2000, Witter et al. 2000).

At both the single species level (e.g. Microtox) and the community level, TNT is more toxic to microorganisms than RDX or HMX. TNT is often the predominant toxicant found in TNT-contaminated sites. In field sites where mixtures of TNT, RDX, HMX,

TNB and TNT degradation products exist, good correlations are often established between TNT levels and soil toxicity (Simini et al. 1995, Fuller and Manning 1998, Sunahara et al. 1999, Gong et al. 1999a, Siciliano et al. 2000).

It should be noted that microorganisms are able to transform TNT into less toxic intermediate degradation products such as the diamino-nitrotoluenes (Figures 2 and 3; Table 1). Even in pure cultures, the amended TNT can be rapidly transformed. Precautions should be taken with regard to the actual concentrations to which microorganisms are exposed. In the field, both toxicants and microorganisms are subjected to the influence of many biotic and abiotic factors (Domsch et al. 1983). Thus, for assessing the *in situ* toxicity it is advantageous to use ecotoxicological tools that are not influenced by confounding environmental factors. So far, pollution-induced community tolerance (PICT), a measurement independent of site-specific conditions and seasonal fluctuations, seems to be a potential tool that meets such requirements (Blanck et al. 1988, Posthuma 1997, Siciliano and Roy 1999, Gong et al. 2000, Siciliano et al. 2000).

Toxicity of TNT and RDX to Plants

Plants are an essential part of aquatic and terrestrial ecosystems. In recent years, phytotoxicity tests have been incorporated into ecological risk assessment for contaminated sites (Gong et al. 1999b). Several standardized tests such as the 96-h algae growth inhibition, seed germination, root elongation, and early seedling growth tests have been used for assessing the phytotoxicity of explosive compounds and explosives-contaminated environmental samples.

Studies on hydroponic or soil based phytotoxicity of explosives to higher plants are limited. At sublethal concentrations, TNT can induce morphologically abnormal development of roots. Gong et al. (1999b) and Peterson et al. (1996) observed sparse, short and abnormal root hairs of plants grown in TNT-amended soil or hydroponic solution. Compared to germination, seedling (shoot or root) growth is more sensitive, probably because seeds use the energy reserves in cotyledons for germination. TNT caused chlorosis in an aquatic plant, Eurasian Watermilfoil (*Myriophyllum spicatum*), at initial concentrations between 5.9 and 23 μM (Pavlostathis et al. 1998). It also inhibited root growth of a terrestrial plant, yellow nutsedge (*Cyperus esculentus* L.), at 22 μM and higher (Palazzo and Leggett 1986). TNT was also toxic to an aquatic plant duckweed (*Lemna minor*) at concentrations higher than 4.4 μM (Schott and Worthley 1974, Cataldo et al. 1989). Transpiration and biomass of hybrid poplar (*Populus* sp. *deltoides* × *nigra*, DN34) cuttings decreased when exposed to 22 μM of TNT (Thompson et al. 1998). Toussaint et al. (1995) derived an EC_{50} of 10 μM for the effect of TNT on root elongation of lettuce (*Lactuca sativa*). According to Peterson et al. (1996), germination and, root and shoot growth (length per day) of tall fescue (*Festuca arundinacea* Schreb.) decreased linearly with increasing TNT concentrations.

Gong et al. (1999b) investigated the effects of 25 to 1600 mg TNT /kg soil on four higher plant species. Among the four species tested, two dicotyledonous species, cress (*Lepidium sativum* L.) and turnip (*Brassica rapa* Metzg.), exhibited higher sensitivity to

TNT than did two monocotyledonous species, oat (*Acena sativa* L.) and wheat (*Triticum aestivum* L.). The derived lowest observable adverse effect concentration (LOAEC) was 50 mg TNT /kg soil with lower levels of TNT (5 to 50 mg/kg) stimulating seedling growth (Gong et al. 1999b). In a field study, Simini et al. (1995) evaluated the toxicity of soils contaminated with TNT, TNB, RDX, HMX and heavy metals to cucumber (*Cucumis sativus*) and radish (*Raphamus sativus*). TNT and TNB were found to account for most of the soil toxicity, and the LOEC of TNT was 7 to 19 mg/kg soil. Alfalfa (*Medicago sativa)* was not able to grow in soil contaminated with 100 mg TNT /kg whereas wheat and bush bean (*Phaseolus vulgaris*) could develop at 500 mg TNT /kg soil (Scheidemann et al. 1998). Oat can tolerate up to 1600 mg TNT/kg soil (Gong et al. 1999b). As for RDX, Simini et al. (1992) reported that concentrations ≥ 100 mg/kg soil significantly reduced the biomass of cucumber seedlings. Winfield et al. (1999) studied the toxicity of RDX (up to 4000 mg/kg soil) to 10 terrestrial plants, and found that exposure during early life stage elicited adverse responses in sensitive species with sunflower and sanfroin (dicots) being the most sensitive ones. Bean, wheat, and blando brome plants were grown in soil amended with 10 mg RDX /kg (Cataldo et al. 1989), and bush bean was also exposed to 10 mg/L RDX for 1 or 7 d (Harvey et al. 1991), but effects on growth were not reported.

Results from Gong et al. (1999b) and Winfield et al. (1999) suggest that dicots might be more sensitive to TNT and RDX than monocots. However, some other workers have found no indication of general difference in TNT sensitivity (Tucker et al. 1989) or TNT uptake and transformation (Scheidemann et al. 1998) between dicots and monocots. Görge et al. (1994) even reported that the dicot alfalfa grown in hydroponic solution containing TNT showed a higher tolerance to TNT than did the monocot chives (*Allium schoenoprasum*). Therefore, it is premature to generalize any principal difference in the sensitivity between dicots and monocots despite the existence of species-dependent tolerance to TNT and RDX (Görge et al. 1994, Scheidemann et al. 1998).

Chronic Toxicity of Explosives to Earthworms

Earthworm survival and reproduction tests are commonly used in terrestrial ecotoxicology to assess the toxicity of compounds in soil. We used these assays to examine the toxicity of explosives to soil invertebrates, specifically the composting earthworm *Eisenia andrei*. We chose this species as the laboratory test invertebrate species because of its very large toxicological literature database (particularly with respect to TNT) and its ease to culture and maintain under laboratory conditions. Furthermore, the size of these animals offered adequate quantities of tissue to allow quantification of TNT and its degradation products.

TNT is lethal to *Eisenia andrei* at concentrations ≥ 1.5 $\mu g/cm^2$ following 3 d on filter paper, and at concentrations ≥ 260 mg/kg after 7- and 14 d direct exposures in spiked soil (Phillips et al. 1993, Robidoux et al. 1999). The chronic and sublethal effects of explosives to *Eisenia andrei* were also demonstrated (Robidoux et al. 2000, 2001). Adult earthworms were exposed to TNT, RDX, or HMX in spiked artificial soils for 28 days after which time adults were removed and weighed. At the end of the test (56 d), the reproductive effects of these explosives were determined. The endpoints measured were the number of hatched and unhatched cocoons, and the number and biomass of juveniles.

TNT adversely affected reproduction in *E. andrei* (Figure 5). The number of cocoons produced and the number of hatched cocoons as well as the production of juveniles were significantly reduced at concentrations ≥ 220 mg TNT/kg soil d.w. The LOEC and NOEC for reproduction of earthworms (total juvenile biomass reduced) exposed to TNT were 110 mg/kg and 55 mg/kg dry soil, respectively (Figure 5). The reproductive toxicity of RDX- and HMX- spiked soil samples were also examined. In one study, the LOEC for reproduction of earthworms exposed to RDX was 95 mg/kg dry soil

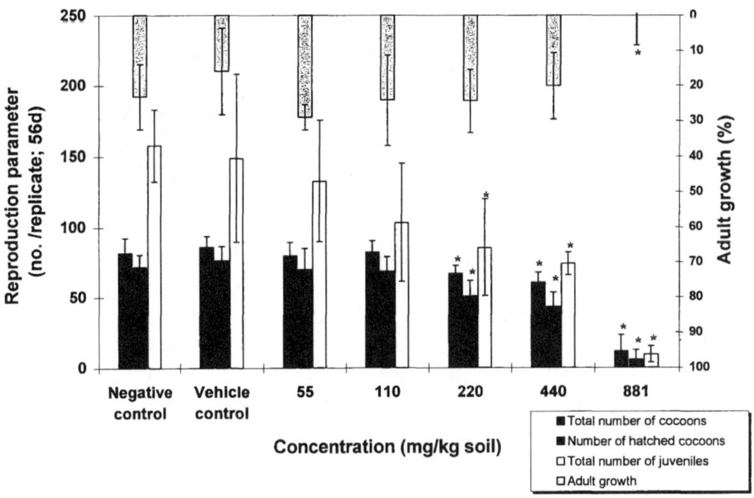

Figure 5 - *Effects of TNT in artificial soil on reproduction of E. andrei exposed during a 56-d earthworm toxicity test. Redrawn using data taken from Robidoux et al. (2000).*

(total number of juveniles, biomass, number of juveniles per hatched cocoon) and the NOEC was < 95 mg/kg (Robidoux et al. 2000). In another study (Robidoux et al. 2001), based on various reproduction parameters (total and hatched number of cocoons, number of juveniles and their biomass), the fecundity of earthworms was reduced at the different concentrations of HMX tested (from 280.0 ± 12.3 to 2502.9 ± 230.0 mg/kg dry soil) in spiked artificial soil (LOEC = 280.0 ± 12.3 mg/kg dry soil).

The growth (reflected by an increase of wet weight) of adult earthworms was also reduced when exposed to TNT-spiked soil at the highest tested concentration (881 mg/kg dry soil). RDX did not decrease earthworm growth, whereas HMX-spiked soil decreased the growth of animals at the different concentrations in soil mentioned above (Robidoux et al. 2001) and no effect on mortality was observed even at the highest concentration tested. Although differences in chemical structures and physico-chemical characteristics exist between TNT, RDX and HMX, we have noted that all of these compounds share a common property, i.e., reproductive toxicity at similar concentration ranges in soil. Further work is needed to understand the physiological and biochemical mechanisms underlying this phenomenon. Despite the lack of this information, the chronic toxicity of explosives to earthworms could be used to establish soil quality criteria and benchmarks for TNT.

Understanding the Mechanisms of Toxicity of Explosives

We are far from fully understanding the toxicological mechanisms underlying the hazardous effects of an environmental toxicant such as TNT. Fortunately, this chemical has a relatively strong toxicological base (including acute, sub-lethal, chronic and carcinogenicity, as well as cultured cell-based studies; Gordon and Hartley 1992, Lachance et al. 1999). In contrast, the mechanisms of toxicity on ecological targets are not well described. It is possible that certain toxicological mechanisms found in mammals may also be present in organisms inhabiting the soil. Our laboratory has recently addressed the question of the toxicokinetic mechanisms behind the bioavailability of TNT in the earthworm (Renoux et al. 2000). The following will briefly describe those studies and their implications.

Earlier results of the earthworm studies suggested that TNT, RDX and HMX are reproductive toxicants (Robidoux et al. 2000, 2001). Investigative studies were then conducted to advance our understanding of the mechanisms underlying these effects. As a first approach, the bioavailability and metabolism of these toxicants were studied using the earthworm and TNT as model organisms and toxicants, respectively. For this, TNT and its degradation products were measured in samples of TNT-spiked soils, as well as solvent extracts of earthworms previously exposed to TNT -spiked soil (Renoux et al. 2000). Analysis was carried out using U.S. EPA Method 8330 SW 846 for soil samples. Analyte concentrations were determined in a 14-day study carried out in the presence and absence of earthworms.

Concentrations of TNT in soil after 14-d exposure were compared to the initial soil TNT concentrations. Data indicates that TNT concentrations in spiked soil (having no earthworms added) are lower after 14 days compared to the start of the experiment, which decreased further if earthworms were added to the soil. In fact, the concentrations of TNT degradation products (2A-DNT and 4A-DNT) were greatly increased in soil samples supplemented with earthworms (Renoux et al. 2000).

Studies were then carried out to test whether the earthworm (*Eisenia andrei*) was capable of transforming TNT *in vivo*. Renoux et al. (2000) demonstrated the formation of 2A-DNT, 4A-DNT, 2,4-DANT as well as traces of 2,6-DANT in tissue homogenates of earthworms previously exposed to TNT on filter paper and in spiked soil. Similar findings have been reported by Johnson et al. (1999) who examined the body burdens of TNT in amphibians fed earthworms raised on TNT-contaminated soil. In addition, our laboratory showed that homogenates from non-exposed animals also exhibited TNT transformation potential *in vitro*. Taken together, these data suggest that earthworms may have enzymes (such as the nitroreductases) capable of partially metabolizing TNT to the monoamino- and diamino- degradation products (Figure 2). It is not known, however, whether the toxic action of TNT (upon a yet to be defined locus) is due to the parent compound and that formation of these degradation products represent detoxification products.

Alternatively, one can not rule out the possibility that the TNT degradation products detected in TNT-exposed earthworms may be equally or perhaps more toxic than the parent compound TNT (i.e., metabolic activation). Although confirmation is required using pure compounds, this possibility is doubtful based on the microbial toxicity data described above (Table 1). It is also not known if the transformation of TNT in earthworms is occurring intracellularly (i.e., within the earthworm cell) or is being carried out extracellularly by microbes associated within the lumen of the gut or the dermal surface of the earthworm. A metabolic role for these microbes would be consistent with the known microbial reductive metabolic pathways of TNT (Rieger and Knackmuss 1995, Sunahara et al. 1999).

Few studies are available to explain how TNT and its degradation products exert their toxic action on an organism (such as the earthworm). At the cellular level, TNT may be cytotoxic (lethal to earthworm cells) or perhaps genotoxic and lead to disturbances at levels regulating gene expression. Using mammalian cells, cytotoxicity ranking of selected explosive-related chemicals was carried out by Wellington and Mitchell (1991). These assays were carried out without external metabolic activation (S9 rodent liver homogenate), and generally showed that the primary TNT degradation products were less toxic than TNT. Honeycutt et al. (1996) assayed various TNT degradation products, and noted that the activities of these substances appeared within the same order of magnitude as that of TNT. These workers concluded that TNT toxicity is not mediated via metabolic activation. However, when expressed on a molar basis ("μM" instead of "ppm"), their data shows that the azoxy-degradation products are up to 14-times as toxic as TNT if tested using CHO cells.

Recently, Lachance et al. (1999) showed that following metabolic activation by a S9 fraction of rat liver homogenate, 2,4-DANT and 2,6-DANT were transformed into highly toxic species, whereas the toxicity of TNT itself was not changed. The significance of this finding for interpretation of TNT toxicity is still unclear, but suggests that metabolic activation (perhaps to hydroxylamine conjugate or amine oxide) by microsomal enzymes could be a necessary step of its toxicity. The same approach might be carried out for invertebrate cells, and could be followed by *in vivo* toxicity evaluation of the most important degradation products of TNT. In mammalian systems, mechanisms related to cytotoxicity and genotoxicity have been associated with abnormal tissue and organ development, e.g., chemically-induced carcinogenesis and reproductive diseases. Although the mechanisms of these effects may not have obvious implications in ecotoxicology, their role at the cellular and biochemical levels in wildlife and lower order species such as the microbes, plants and invertebrates can not be presently ruled out.

Field Approach: Mesocosm Experiments

Field studies are extremely useful for the validation of results derived from the laboratory. Mesocosm type experiments (described earlier by Svendsen and Weeks, 1997) were used to conduct a biological survey on invertebrates at an abandoned TNT factory. Blocks of soil were collected with a stainless steel tool (30 cm x 30 cm x 15 cm). Each block of soil was transferred into a separate nylon bag (9.4 L, 100-mesh) that was then returned to the location from which it was removed. Ten laboratory earthworms (*E. andrei*) and ten indigenous earthworms (single species obtained from soil near the study site and pre-acclimated for 24 h in OECD artificial soil) were placed inside the nylon bag containing the block of soil. The mesocosms were then closed and left in place for ten days; afterwhich, the surviving earthworms were counted. TNT and its degradation products were also estimated in the surviving animals, using the U.S. EPA Method 8330 SW 846.

Results of these preliminary mesocosm experiments indicated a TNT concentration-lethality response relationship similar to that obtained earlier in laboratory studies using *Eisenia andrei* (Robidoux et al. 1999). The survival of earthworms (*E. andrei* and indigenous species) decreased as the concentration of TNT (and the total nitroaromatic compounds) increased in the soil. Data indicated that earthworms (*E. andrei* and indigenous species) did not survive at concentration > 9000 mg TNT /kg soil. Most survivors were found at < 1200 mg TNT /kg soil. It was interesting to note that *E. andrei* tended to tolerate TNT concentrations as high as 4050 mg/ kg, but indigenous earthworms did not. The latter were only found at levels below 1150 mg TNT /kg soil. TNT seemed to be the primary toxicant, since mortality was not significantly correlated with the concentrations of other nitroaromatic compounds present in the soil. A parallel relationship between concentrations of 2,4-DNT (used in the synthesis of TNT) and TNT was noted. As the concentrations of 2,4-DNT concentrations in soil increased, so did those of TNT in the same soil sample. In addition, the concentrations of TNT and its degradation products in dried earthworms increased as concentrations of TNT (< 1200 mg/kg soil), 2-ADNT (< 150 mg /kg soil) and 4-ADNT (< 220 mg /kg soil), increased.

Establishing Ecotoxicological Screening Benchmarks for TNT

Ecotoxicologically based soil quality criteria for toxicants are sometimes called soil quality thresholds, generic environmentally acceptable criteria, or simply benchmarks (according to the application). In the absence of site-specific information, existing generic criteria are often used. A benchmark (expressed as a concentration of contaminant in the soil) is usually derived using published toxicity values that might include a number of different toxicological responses (increased lethality, decreased growth and/or fecundity, etc.) for a limited number of species. These criteria could then be used to evaluate the potential hazardous effects of a bioavailable contaminant (chemical stressor) on soil-borne organisms (receptors) present at the contaminated site.

The following describes one approach to estimating a soil benchmark for explosives (using TNT as a model toxicant). This benchmark can be used as a preliminary screening index for soil contaminated with TNT. Talmage et al. (1999) used a similar method that considered the lowest LOEC for plants, soil invertebrates, and soil heterotrophic processes. Soil microbial processes, including nitrification, nitrogen fixation and dehydrogenase activities, may be affected at 1 mg TNT/kg of soil (Gong et al. 1999a). Recent studies with earthworms (Robidoux et al. 1999, 2000) showed a LOEC of 110 mg/kg soil for TNT. If these data are taken with other results (LOECs reported in the literature), one can develop a sensitivity distribution of the sublethal effects of TNT on soil organisms. Compared to others, this method allows one to know the type and the relative proportion of organisms that may be affected by the contaminant.

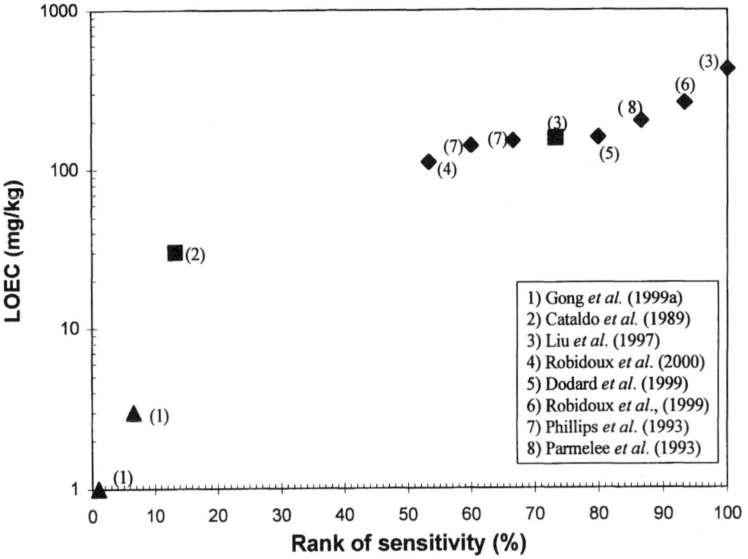

Figure 6 – *Terrestrial species sensitivity distribution to TNT. Symbols used: (▲) microorganisms, (■) plants and (◆) invertebrates. Numbers in brackets correspond to studies indicated in the inset and found in the references section.*

The LOECs generated from the chronic toxicity tests described earlier for plants, earthworms, and microbes, as well as, those from other sources, are listed in order of decreasing toxicity (*i.e.*, low to high values). The LOECs were then assigned ranks and the distribution of rank species sensitivity determined by dividing each rank value by the total number of available LOEC values and multiplying by 100. The percentage rank sensitivity was then plotted against log concentration (Figure 6). The benchmark is the concentration corresponding to the 10th percentile (Efroymson et al. 1997a, 1997b). Therefore, for TNT, the concentration corresponding to the 10th percentile is 2 mg/kg soil d.w. (Figure 6). This value is more than 10-times lower than those estimated by Talmage et al. (1999) who reported LOECs (mg/kg) of 30, 200 and > 20 for plants, soil invertebrates and soil microbes, respectively. Using sublethal endpoints (LOEC) described in this article, concentrations less than 2 mg/kg would protect more than 90% (an arbitrary level agreed upon *a priori*) of the soil organisms considered in this analysis.

These data also indicate that microorganisms were affected from 1 to 75 mg TNT/kg soil, whereas plants were sensitive to concentrations from 30 to 500 mg/kg, and invertebrates from 110 and 880 mg/kg. As described earlier in this article, studies using plants suggest that TNT has a LOEC of 30 mg/kg (Cataldo et al. 1989), but the general lack of phytotoxicity data weakens our confidence in this LOEC value and further work in this area is needed. Additional studies are required to determine the reference values of TNT specifically and explosives in general. No suitable studies were found for representative avian species. The benchmark approach may also be applied to other explosives such as RDX and HMX. However, more data is needed in order to compile a database sufficiently robust to estimate their ecologically based benchmark values.

Conclusions

Soil ecotoxicity test data generated from laboratory studies were used to derive a preliminary TNT benchmark at 2 mg TNT /kg soil. This benchmark was established to protect 90% of terrestrial species. Confidence in this value will depend on a number of factors including the quality of the ecotoxicity data (repeatability, reproducibility, and inter-laboratory validation), the technical conduct of the study, and the number of ecologically relevant species considered. A thorough understanding of the mechanisms underlying the ecotoxicological effects of TNT would also support our confidence in this benchmark value. To achieve this, one should identify the toxicant (TNT or its degradation products) in the target organism, the processes governing the bioavailability of the toxicant in soil and in the ecological receptors, as well as the physiological and biochemical mechanisms (toxicological loci) responsible for the toxic effect (acute and chronic responses). More work is needed to explain these effects at the cellular (cytotoxicity) and perhaps at the nuclear level (genotoxicity). A greater understanding of species-species associations such as microbes-earthworms may help to explain the fate of a toxicant (such as TNT) in the host organism and provide the necessary tools to predict possible detrimental ecological consequences of toxicant exposure in the field, such as the deterioration of the reproductive health of an earthworm population at a contaminated site. Evidence is provided to suggest that soil-earthworm interactions may also exist that would ultimately lead to changes in the concentrations of bioavailable TNT, and TNT degradation products in the soil matrix.

In view of the extent of sites contaminated with explosives worldwide, and their possible impact on surrounding ecosystems, there is a clear need for more work to achieve the above goals. TNT is only one example of an industrial and persistent environmental organic pollutant. Approaches such as those described in this article may also be used to improve our understanding (and prediction) of the ecotoxicology of other soil contaminants. The literature covering the soil ecotoxicology of RDX and HMX is scant and we are now pursuing our efforts in this area.

References

Blanck, H., Wängberg, S.-Å., and Molander, S., 1988, "Pollution-Induced Community Tolerance - A New Ecotoxicological Tool," *Functional Testing of Aquatic Biota for Estimating Hazards of Chemicals*, J. Cairns Jr. and J. R. Pratt, Eds., ASTM STP 988, American Society for Testing and Materials, Philadelphia, PA, pp. 219-230.

Cataldo, D. A., Harveys, S., Fellows, R. J., Bean, R. M., and McVeety, B. D., 1989, "An Evaluation of the Environmental Fate and Behavior of Munitions Material (TNT, RDX) in Soil and Plant Systems," *Report No. AD-A223 546*. Pacific Northwest Laboratories, Richland, OR.

Chapman, P. M., 1995, "Extrapolating Laboratory Toxicity Results to the Field," *Environmental Toxicology and Chemistry,* Vol. 14, pp. 927-930.

Dodard, S. G., Paquet, L., Robidoux, P. Y., Powlowski, J., Hawari, J., and Sunahara, G. I., 1998, "Ecotoxicological Effects of Recalcitrant Environmental Pollutants on Two Species of Soil Invertebrates (*Enchytraeus albidus* and *Eisenia andrei*)," *Proceedings of the 25th Annual Aquatic Workshop: October 18-21, 1998, Quebec City, Quebec*, R. van Coillie, P. Chassé, L. Hare, C. Julien, L. Martel, C. Thellen, and A. J. Nimi, Eds., Canadian Technical Report of Fisheries and Aquatic Sciences, No. 2260, p. 89.

Dodard, S. G., Renoux, A. Y., Hawari, J., Ampleman, G., Thiboutot, S., and Sunahara, G. I., 1999, "Ecotoxicity Characterization of Dinitrotoluenes and Some of Their Reduced Metabolites," *Chemosphere*, Vol. 38, pp. 2071-2079.

Domsch, K. H., Jagnow, G., and Anderson, T. H., 1983, "An Ecological Concept for Assessment of Side-Effects of Agrochemicals on Soil Microorganisms," *Residue Reviews*, Vol. 86, pp. 65-105.

Drzyzga, O., Gorontzy, T., Schmidt, A., and Blotevogel, K.-H., 1995, "Toxicity of Explosives and Related Compounds to the Luminescent Bacterium *Vibrio fischeri* NRRL-B-11177," *Archives of Environmental Contamination Toxicology,* Vol. 28, pp. 229-235.

Efroymson, R. A., Will, M. E., and Suter II, G. W., 1997a, "Toxicological Benchmarks for Contaminants of Potential Concern for Effects on Soil and Litter Invertebrates Heterotrophic Process," 1997 revision, ES/ER/TM-126/R2, Prepared for the U.S. Department of Energy, Oak Ridge National Laboratory, TN.

Efroymson, R. A., Will, M. E., Suter II, G. W., and Wooten, A. C., 1997b, "Toxicological Benchmarks for Screening Contaminants of Potential Concern for Effects on Terrestrial Plants," 1997 revision, ES/ER/TM-85/R3, Prepared for the U.S. Department of Energy, Oak Ridge National Laboratory, TN.

Fritsche, W., Scheibner, K., Herre, A., and Hofrichter, M., 2000, "Fungal Degradation of Explosives," *Biodegradation of Nitroaromatic Compounds and Explosives*, J. C. Spain, J. B. Hughes, and H.-J. Knackmuss, Eds., CRC Press, New York, NY, pp. 213-237.

Fuller, M. and Manning Jr., J. F., 1997, "Aerobic Gram-Positive and Gram-Negative Bacteria Exhibit Differential Sensitivity to and Transformation of 2,4,6-Trinitrotoluene (TNT)," *Current Microbiology,* Vol. 35, pp. 77-83.

Fuller, M. and Manning Jr., J. F., 1998, "Evidence for Differential Effects of 2,4,6-Trinitrotoluene and Other Munitions Compounds on Specific Subpopulations of Soil Microbial Communities," *Environmental Toxicology and Chemistry,* Vol. 17, pp. 2185-2195.

Gong, P., Gasparrini, P., Rho, D., Hawari, J., Thiboutot, S., Ampleman, G., and Sunahara, G. I., 2000, "An In-Situ Respirometric Technique to Measure Pollution-Induced Microbial Community Tolerance in Soils Contaminated with 2,4,6-Trinitrotoluene," *Ecotoxicology and Environmental Safety*, Vol. 47, pp. 96-103.

Gong, P., Siciliano, S. D., Greer, C. W., Paquet, L., Hawari, J., and Sunahara, G. I., 1999a, "Effects and Bioavailability of 2,4,6-Trinitrotoluene in Spiked and Field Contaminated Soils to Indigenous Microorganisms," *Environmental Toxicology and Chemistry,* Vol. 18, pp. 2681-2688.

Gong, P., Wilke, B.-M., and Fleischmann, S., 1999b, "Soil-Based Phytotoxicity of 2,4,6-Trinitrotoluene (TNT) to Terrestrial Higher Plants," *Archives of Environmental Contamination and Toxicology,* Vol. 36, pp. 152-157.

Gordon, L. and Hartley, W. R., 1992, "2,4,6-Trinitrotoluene," *Drinking Water Health Advisory: Munitions.* W. C. Roberts and W. R. Hartley, Eds, Lewis Publishers, Boca Raton, FL, pp. 327-398.

Görge, E., Brandt, S., and Werner, D., 1994, "Uptake and Metabolism of 2,4,6-Trinitrotoluene in Higher Plants," *Environmental Science and Pollution Research,* Vol. 1, pp. 229-233.

Harvey, S. D., Fellows, R. J., Cataldo, D. A., and Bean, R. M., 1991, "Fate of the Explosive Hexahydro-1,3,5-Trinitro-1,3,5-Triazine (RDX) in Soil and Bioaccumulation in Bush Bean Hydroponic Plants," *Environmental Toxicology and Chemistry,* Vol. 10, pp. 845-855.

Hawari, J., 2000, "Biodegradation of RDX and HMX: From Basic Research to Field Application," *Biodegradation of Nitroaromatic Compounds and Explosives,* J. C. Spain, J. B. Hughes, and H.-J. Knackmuss, Eds., CRC Press, New York, NY, pp. 277-310.

Hawari, J., Halasz, A., Paquet, L., Zhou, E., Spencer, B., Ampleman, G., and Thiboutot, S., 1998, "Characterization of Metabolites in the Biotransformation of 2,4,6-Trinitrotoluene with Anaerobic Sludge: Role of Triaminotoluene," *Applied and Environmental Microbiology*, Vol. 62, pp. 2200-2206.

Honeycutt, M. E., Jarvis, A. S. and McFarland, V. A., 1996, "Cytotoxicity and Mutagenicity of 2,4,6-Trinitrotoluene and its Metabolites," *Ecotoxicology and Environmental Safety*, Vol. 35, pp. 282-287.

Johnson, M. S., Franke, L. S., Lee, R. B., and Holladay, S. D., 1999, "Bioaccumulation of 2,4,6-Trinitrotoluene and Polychlorinated Biphenyls Through Two Routes of Exposure in a Terrestrial Amphibian: Is the Dermal Route Significant?" *Environmental Toxicology and Chemistry*, Vol. 18, pp. 873-878.

Klausmeier, R. E., Osmon, J. L., and Walls, D. R., 1973, "The Effect of Trinitrotoluene on Microorganisms," *Developments in Industrial Microbiology,* Vol. 15, pp. 309-317.

Lachance, B., Robidoux, P. Y., Hawari, J., Ampleman, G., Thiboutot, S. and Sunahara, G. I., 1999, "Cytotoxic and Genotoxic Effects of Energetic Compounds on Bacterial and Mammalian Cells *In Vitro*," *Mutation Research*, Vol. 444, pp. 25-39.

Liu, D., Spanggord, R., Bailey, H. C., Javizt, H., and Jones, D., 1983, *Acute Toxicity of LAP Wastewater and 2,4,6-Trinitrotoluene.* Vol. I, SRI International, Menlo Park, CA.

Microbics Corporation, 1992, *Microtox Manual: Microtox Basic Test Procedures*, Carlsbad, CA.

Palazzo, A. J. and Leggett, D. C., 1986, "Effect and Disposition of TNT in a Terrestrial Plant," *Journal of Environmental Quality,* Vol. 15, pp. 49-52.

Parmelee, R. W., Wentsel, R. S., and Phillips, C. T., 1993, "Soil Microcosm for Testing the Effects of Chemical Pollutants on Soil Fauna Communities and Trophic Structure," *Environmental Toxicology and Chemistry*, Vol. 12, pp. 1477-1486.

Pasti-Grigsby, M. B., Lewis, T. A., Crawford, D. L., and Crawford, R. L., 1996, "Transformation of 2,4,6-Trinitrotoluene (TNT) by Actinomycetes Isolated from TNT-Contaminated and Uncontaminated Environments," *Applied and Environmental Microbiology*, Vol. 62, pp. 1120-1123.

Pavlostathis, S. P., Comstock, K. K., Jacobson, M. E., and Saunders, F. M., 1998, "Transformation of 2,4,6-Trinitrotoluene by the Aquatic Plant *Myriophyllum spicatum*," *Environmental Toxicology and Chemistry,* Vol. 17, pp. 2266-2273.

Peterson, M. M., Horst, G. L., Shea, P. J., Comfort, S. D., and Peterson, R. K. D., 1996, "TNT and 4-Amino-2,6-Dinitrotoluene Influence on Germination and Early Seedling Development of Tall Fescue," *Environmental Pollution,* Vol. 93, pp. 57-62.

Phillips, C. T., Checkai, R. T., and Wentsel, R. S., 1993, "Toxicity of Selected Munitions and Munition-Contaminated Soil on the Earthworm (*Eisenia foetida*)," U. S. Army Chemical and Biological Defense Agency, Edgewood Research, Development and Engineering Center, Research and Technology Directorate, Aberdeen Proving Ground, MD.

Posthuma, L., 1997, "Effects of Toxicants on Population and Community Parameters in Field Conditions, and Their Potential Use in the Validation of Risk Assessment Methods," *Ecological Risk Assessment of Contaminants in Soil,* N. M. van Straalen and H. Løkke, Eds., Chapman & Hall, London, UK, pp. 85-117.

Renoux, A. Y., Sarrazin, M., Hawari, J., and Sunahara, G. I., 2000, "Transformation of 2,4,6-Trinitrotoluene in Soil in the Presence of the Earthworm *Eisenia andrei*," *Environmental Toxicology and Chemistry*, Vol. 19, pp. 1473-1480.

Rieger, P.-G., and Knackmuss, H.-J., 1995, "Basic Knowledge and Perspectives on Biodegradation of 2,4,6-Trinitrotoluene and Related Nitroaromatic Compounds in Contaminated Soil," *Biodegradation of Nitroaromatic Compounds*, J. C. Spain, Ed., Plenum, NY, pp. 1-18.

Robidoux, P. Y., Hawari, J., Thiboutot, S., Ampleman, G., and Sunahara, G. I., 1999, "Acute Toxicity of 2,4,6-Trinitrotoluene in Earthworm (*Eisenia andrei*)," *Ecotoxicology and Environmental Safety*, Vol. 44, pp. 311-321.

Robidoux, P. Y., Hawari, J., Thiboutot, S., Ampleman, G., and Sunahara, G. I., 2001, "Chronic Toxicity of Octahydro-1,3,5,7-Tetranitro-1,3,5,7-Tetraazocine (HMX) in Soil Determined using the Earthworm (*Eisenia andrei*) Reproduction Test," *Environmental Pollution*, Vol. 111, pp. 283-292.

Robidoux, P. Y., Svendsen, C., Caumartin, J., Hawari, J., Ampleman, G., Thiboutot, S., Weeks, J. M., and Sunahara, G. I., 2000, "Chronic Toxicity of Energetic Compounds in Soil Determined using the Earthworm (*Eisenia andrei*) Reproduction Test," *Environmental Toxicology and Chemistry*, Vol. 19, pp. 1764-1773.

Ruchhoft, C. C., LeBosquet, Jr., M., and Meckler, W. G., 1945, "TNT Wastes from Shell-Loading Plants," *Industrial and Engineering Chemistry,* Vol. 37, pp. 937-943.

Scheidemann, P., Klunk, A., Sens, C., and Werner, D., 1998, "Species Dependent Uptake and Tolerance of Nitroaromatic Compounds by Higher Plants," *Journal of Plant Physiology,* Vol. 152, pp. 242-247.

Schott, C. D., and Worthley, E. G., 1974, "The Toxicity of TNT and Related Wastes to an Aquatic Flowering Plant, *Lemma perpusilla*," *Technical Report 74016 AD-778158,* Edgewood Arsenal, Aberdeen Proving Ground, MD.

Schott, S., Ruchhoft, C. C., and Migregian, S., 1943, "TNT Wastes," *Industrial and Engineering Chemistry,* Vol. 35, pp. 1122-1127.

Siciliano, S. D., Gong, P., Sunahara, G. I., and Greer, C. W., 2000, "Assessment of 2,4,6-Trinitrotoluene Toxicity in Field Soils by Pollution Induced Community Tolerance (PICT), Denaturing Gradient Gel Electrophoresis (DGGE) and Seed Germination Assay," *Environmental Toxicology and Chemistry,* Vol. 19, pp. 2154-2160.

Siciliano, S. D. and Roy, R., 1999, "The Role of Soil Microbial Tests in Ecological Risk Assessment: Differentiating Between Exposure and Effects," *Human and Ecological Risk Assessment,* Vol. 5, pp. 671-682.

Simini, M., Rowland, R., Lee, E. H., and Wentsel, R. W., 1992, "Detection of Stress in *Cucumis sativus* Exposed to RDX using Chlorophyll Fluorescence," *SETAC 13th Annual Meeting Abstract Book,* 8-12 November 1992, Cincinnati, OH, p. 48.

Simini, M., Wentsel, R. S , Checkai, R. T., Phillips, C. T , Chester, N. A, Major, M. A., and Amos, J. C., 1995, "Evaluation of Soil Toxicity at Joliet Army Ammunition Plant," *Environmental Toxicology and Chemistry,* Vol. 14, pp. 623-630.

Sunahara, G. I., Dodard, S., Sarrazin, M., Paquet, L., Ampleman, G., Thiboutot, S., Hawari, J., and Renoux, A. Y., 1998, "Development of a Soil Extraction Procedure for Ecotoxicity Characterization of Energetic Compounds," *Ecotoxicology and Environmental Safety,* Vol. 39, pp. 185-194.

Sunahara, G. I., Dodard, S., Sarrazin, M., Paquet, L., Hawari, J., Greer, C. W., Ampleman, G., Thiboutot, S., and Renoux, A. Y., 1999, "Ecotoxicological Characterization of Energetic Substances using a Soil Extraction Procedure," *Ecotoxicology and Environmental Safety,* Vol. 43, pp. 138-148.

Svendsen, C. and Weeks, J. M., 1997, "Relevance and Applicability of a Simple Earthworm Biomarker of Copper Exposure: II. Validation and Applicability Under Field Conditions in a Mesocosm Experiment with Lumbricus rubellus," *Ecotoxicology and Environmental Safety,* Vol. 36, pp. 80-88.

Talmage, S. S., Opresko, D. M., Maxwell, C. J., Welsh, C. J. E., Crettella, F. M., and Reno, P. H., 1999, "Nitroaromatic Munition Compounds: Environmental Effects and Screening Values," *Reviews of Environmental Contamination and Toxicology,* Vol. 161, pp.1-156.

Thompson, P. L., Ramer, L. A., Guffey, A. P., and Schnoor, J. L., 1998, "Decreased Transpiration in Poplar Trees Exposed to 2,4,6-Trinitrotoluene," *Environmental Toxicology and Chemistry,* Vol. 17, pp. 902-906.

Toussaint, M. W., Shedd, T. R., van der Schalie, W. H., and Leather, G. R., 1995, "A Comparison of Standard Acute Toxicity Tests with Rapid-Screening Toxicity Tests," *Environmental Toxicology and Chemistry,* Vol. 14, pp. 907-915.

Tucker, W. L., Banwart, W. L., Branato, T. C., and Hassett, J. J., 1989, "Screening for Plant Tolerance to TNT," *Report for USATHAMA,* by CERL and the University of Illinois.

Vanderberg, L., Perry, J., and Unkefer, P., 1995, "Catabolism of 2,4,6-Trinitrotoluene by *Mycobacterium vaccae*," *Applied Microbiology and Biotechnology,* Vol. 43, pp. 937-945.

Vorbeck, C., Lenke, H., Fischer, P., and Knackmuss, H., 1994, "Identification of a Hydride-Meisenheimer Complex as a Metabolite of 2,4,6-Trinitrotoluene by a *Mycobacterium* strain," *Journal of Bacteriology,* Vol. 176, pp. 932-934.

Wellington, D. R. and Mitchell, W. R., 1991, "*In vitro* Cytotoxicity of Certain Munition Nitroaromatic Compounds," *Chemosphere*, Vol. 23, pp. 363-373.

Winfield, L. E., Rodgers Jr., J. H., D'Surney, S. J., and Lee, C. R., 1999, "Phytotoxicity of RDX Exposure (<12 days) to Selected Terrestrial Plants," *SETAC 20th Annual Meeting Abstract Book: Sustaining Global Environmental Integrity*, Philadelphia, PA, p. 158.

Winkel, B. and Wilke, B.-M., 1997, "Wirkung von TNT (2,4,6-Trinitrotoluol) auf Bodenatmung und Nitrifikation," *Mitteilungen der Deutschen Bodenkundlichen Gesellschaft,* Vol. 85, pp. 631-634.

Witter, E., Gong, P., Bååth, E., and Marstorp, H., 2000, "A Study of the Structure and Metal Tolerance of the Soil Microbial Community 6 years After Cessation of Sewage Sludge Applications," *Environmental Toxicology and Chemistry,* Vol. 19, pp. 1983-1991.

T. Sudhakar Babu,[1] Sridevi Tripuranthakam,[1] and Bruce M. Greenberg[1]

Synergistic Toxicity of a Mixture of 1,2-dihydroxyanthraquinone and Copper on the Aquatic Plant *Lemna gibba*

Reference: Babu, T. S., Tripuranthakam, S., and Greenberg, B. M., "**Synergistic Toxicity of a Mixture of 1,2-dihydroxyanthraquinone and Copper on the Aquatic Plant** *Lemna gibba,*" *Environmental Toxicology and Risk Assessment: Science, Policy, and Standardization - Implications for Environmental Decisions: Tenth Volume, ASTM STP 1403,* B. M. Greenberg, R. N. Hull, M. H. Roberts, Jr., and R. W. Gensemer, Eds., American Society for Testing and Materials, West Conshohocken, PA, 2001.

Abstract: Polycyclic aromatic hydrocarbons (PAHs) and metals are toxic to animals, plants and microorganisms. Both these groups of contaminants coexist in the industrialized environments. Therefore, it is important to study the mixture toxicity of such pollutants on biological systems. In the present study, we have used the aquatic higher plant *Lemna gibba* as a test organism to study the mixture toxicity of an oxy-PAH 1,2-dihydroxyanthraquinone (1,2-dhATQ), and the metal copper. 3 μM1,2-dhATQ inhibited photosynthetic electron transport downstream of photosystem II at the cytochrome b_6/f complex. Such an inhibition results in the alteration of the redox status of the chloroplast to a reduced state because the plastoquinone pool goes to a net reduced state. Under such circumstances, when 4 μM $CuSO_4$ was administered to *L. gibba*, there was a synergistic inhibition of growth and protein expression. We infer from these results that the synergistic toxicity caused by the mixture of 1,2-dhATQ plus $CuSO_4$ is due to the catalytic transfer of electrons by Cu^{2+} from the reduced plastoquinone pool to O_2. Such a mediation of electrons leads to the generation of reactive oxygen species, which could cause greater toxicity of 1,2-dhATQ.

Polycyclic aromatic hydrocarbons (PAHs) and metals are common contaminants in industrialized environments. Both these groups of chemicals are highly toxic to a variety of biological organisms (Martineau et al. 1994, McConkey et al. 1997, Wetzel and Werner 1995). In addition to their direct effects on biological systems, most PAHs have been shown to undergo photomodification under sunlight and they have an increased toxicity following photomodification (Arfsten et al. 1996, Huang et al. 1997b).

Keywords: copper, 1,2-dihydroxyanthraquinone, photosynthetic electron transport, polycyclic aromatic hydrocarbon, reactive oxygen species

[1]Postdoctoral fellow, postdoctoral fellow, and Professor, respectively, Department of Biology, University of Waterloo, Waterloo, Ontario N2L 3G1, Canada.

In this direction, we have earlier shown that several photomodified PAHs are increasingly toxic to plants, animals and bacteria (Huang et al. 1993, 1997b, McConkey et al. 1997, Tripuranthakam et al. 1999). One such photomodified PAHs is 1,2-dihydroxyanthraquinone (1,2-dhATQ) that is formed when anthracene is exposed to simulated solar radiation (Mallakin et al. 1999). This compound has been shown to cause inhibition of plant growth (Mallakin et al. 1999) and impede mitochondrial electron transport (Tripuranthakam et al. 1999).

In an attempt to further understand the toxic nature of PAHs and their possible interaction with other pollutants in natural environments, we have started studies to characterize the combined toxicity of PAHs and metals. These two groups of compounds are known to occur as co-contaminants in industrial environments (Amodio-Cocchieri et al. 1993, Wey et al. 1996). Therefore, in the present study, we have chosen to examine the co-toxicity of the oxy-PAH, 1,2-dhATQ, and the metal, copper on the aquatic plant *Lemna gibba*. 1,2-dhATQ inhibits respiratory electron transport in the cytochrome bc1 complex (Tripuranthakam et al. 1999). Because the cytochrome bc1 complex of mitochondria is homologous to the cytochrome b_6/f (Cyt b_6/f) complex in photosynthetic thylakoid membranes, it is likely that 1,2-dhATQ will be a potent inhibitor of the photosynthetic electron transport downstream of photosystem II (PS II).

When photosynthetic electron transport at Cyt b_6/f is inhibited, the redox-status of the chloroplast will be modified to a more reduced state. Under such reducing conditions, there will be formation of reduced plastoquinone pool (PQH_2) inside the chloroplast. When such a supply of electrons becomes available in biological systems, interaction with redox-active metals like copper might change the path of electrons by catalytically transferring them to a readily available acceptor such as O_2. Thus, interaction of redox-active metals with PAHs that alter the redox status of a biological system could pose an extreme danger to living cells due to the formation of reactive oxygen species (ROS). In this communication, we describe the enhanced toxicity of the combined presence of PAHs and metals and extrapolate this toxicity as being caused by the formation of ROS.

Experimental Methods

Plant Growth and Chemical Treatment

Lemna gibba (L.) G-3 (a gift from Dr. Marvin Edelman, Weizmann Institute of Science, Israel) was cultured axenically on half-strength Hutner's medium under 100 μmol m^{-2} s^{-1} of continuous cool-white fluorescent light at 25°C (Huang et al. 1993). For the chemical treatments, unless stated otherwise, plants were grown in nutrient medium supplemented with 4 μM $CuSO_4$, or 3 μM 1,2-dhATQ, or a mixture of 4 μM $CuSO_4$ plus 3 μM 1,2-dhATQ. 1,2-dhATQ was added by a 1000 fold dilution of a stock solution in dimethylsulfoxide (DMSO). DMSO up to 0.5% (v/v) does not affect growth or photosynthesis of *L. gibba*, nor does it alter PAH toxicity (Huang et al. 1993, Huang et al. 1997b). Copper was added to the media by dilution from a stock solution of 1 mM $CuSO_4$ in reverse osmosis purified H_2O. For 1,2-dhATQ, a concentration of 3 μM is close to its EC50 for plant growth inhibition (Mallakin et al. 1999). 4 μM $CuSO_4$ inhibits only 7% of the growth of *L. gibba*. All chemical treatments of *L. gibba* were performed under 100 μmol m^{-2} s^{-1} of continuous cool-white fluorescent light. Medium for control and copper-treated plants contained 0.1% DMSO, equivalent to the amount in the 1,2-dhATQ-treated plants.

Photosynthetic Electron Transport

Lemna gibba fronds were homogenized in a pre-chilled mortar at 4°C to isolate thylakoid membranes. The homogenization buffer consisted of 50 mM HEPES-NaOH (pH 7.5), 0.3 M sucrose, 20 mM NaCl and 5 mM $MgCl_2$. The homogenate was filtered through two layers of Miracloth (Calbiochem, La Jolla) and the filtrate was centrifuged at 3000 g for 1 min. The resulting pellet was resuspended in a buffer containing 20 mM HEPES-NaOH (pH 7.5), 5 mM $MgCl_2$ and 150 mM NaCl and centrifuged at 35,000 g for 5 min. Thylakoid membranes were collected as a pellet and resuspended in a small volume of reaction buffer containing 20 mM HEPES-NaOH (pH 7.5), 10 mM NaCl and 5 mM $MgCl_2$. All the isolation procedures were performed under subdued light at 4°C.

PS II, PS I and intersystem electron transport were measured in the reaction buffer at 25°C according to Babu et al. (1992) and Sabat et al. (1991) using a Clark-type O_2 electrode (Hansatech, King's Lynn, U.K.). The thylakoid suspension in all the electron transport measurements contained a chlorophyll concentration of 10 μg/ml of the reaction buffer. PS II electron transport was quantified as O_2 evolution using 0.5 mM p-benzoquinone (pBQ) as an electron acceptor and H_2O as an electron donor. PS I activity was measured using 0.1 mM reduced 2,6-dichlorophenol indophenol (DCPIP) as an electron donor and methyl viologen (MV) as an electron acceptor. Intersystem electron transport from the plastoquinone (PQ) pool to PS I was measured using reduced duroquinone (DQH_2) as an electron donor to PQ and MV as an electron acceptor (Izawa and Pan 1978, Sane et al. 1979). Light-induced electron transport measurements were taken from thylakoid membranes treated with 4 μM $CuSO_4$, or 3 μM 1,2-dhATQ, or a mixture of 3 μM 1,2-dhATQ plus 4 μM $CuSO_4$ for 1 min in the dark.

Phosphorylation of Membrane Proteins and Protein Expression in vivo

Lemna gibba were treated with 3 μM 1,2-dhATQ for 3 h under 100 μmol m^{-2} s^{-1} cool white fluorescent light. Control plants without chemical treatment were kept under similar conditions. Both phosphorylation and synthesis of proteins in *L. gibba* were studied after the 3 h pre-treatment with the toxicant at 25°C. Phosphorylation of proteins was performed by labeling two plants with 100 μCi/ml of $^{32}P[H_3PO_4]$ under 640 nm (red) light for 2 h (Elich et al. 1992). To study protein expression, two plants were labeled with 50 μCi/ml of ^{35}S-[methionine + cysteine] under 100 μmol m^{-2} s^{-1} cool white fluorescent light for 2 h (Greenberg et al. 1989). After labeling, plants were frozen in liquid N_2 until further analysis.

Isolation and Analysis of Soluble and Membrane Proteins

Frozen radiolabeled plants were thawed, homogenized, and soluble and membrane proteins were isolated as previously described (McCormac et al. 1994). Both soluble and membrane proteins were separated by SDS-PAGE, and visualized by autoradiography. The synthesis and phosphorylation of proteins was quantified by densitometry (Greenberg et al. 1989).

Whole Organism Toxicity

Axenic *L. gibba* fronds (2 plants) were placed in nutrient medium supplemented with 4 μM $CuSO_4$, or 3 μM 1,2-dhATQ, or a mixture of 4 μM $CuSO_4$ plus 3 μM 1,2-dhATQ. The plants were grown for eight days under 100 μmol m^{-2} s^{-1} of continuous cool white fluorescent light at 25°C. The medium with the test chemicals was replenished by static renewal every two days (Greenberg et al. 1992). At the end of eight days, fronds were counted to assess the growth (Greenberg et al. 1992).

Results and Discussion

We evaluated the effect of 1,2-dhATQ and copper on the photosynthetic electron transport. One can dissect photosynthetic electron transport into three parts. Photosystem II (PS II), intersystem and PS I (see Fig. 1).

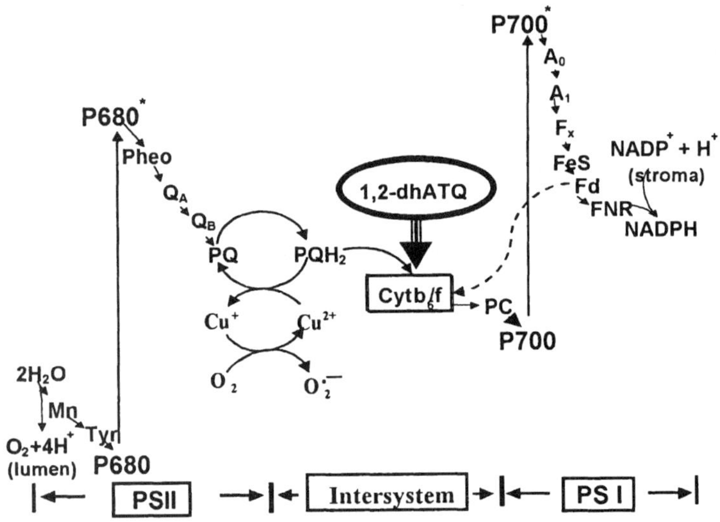

Figure 1-*Schematic of the redox-dependent Cu^{2+} mediated formation of ROS.*

The results indicate that 1,2-dhATQ did not inhibit PS II electron transport, but it strongly inhibited intersystem electron transport (Table 1). 1,2-dhATQ also inhibited PS I electron transport to some extent. Conversely, 4 μM $CuSO_4$ at the concentrations used did not inhibit any part of photosynthetic electron transport (Table 1). Thus, of these two classes of chemicals, 1,2-dhATQ is toxic to *L. gibba* by inhibiting photosynthetic electron transport.

Because 1,2-dhATQ inhibited intersystem electron transport and PS I electron transport, it is clear that this oxyPAH inhibited electron transport downstream of PS II. The inhibition in intersystem electron transport may indicate that 1,2-dhATQ blocks the

Table 1-*Effect of 1,2-dhATQ and copper on photosynthetic electron transport.*

Treatment	% Electron transport*		
	PS II	Intersystem	PS I
Control	100 ± 4	100 ± 7	100 ± 5
$CuSO_4$	97 ± 4	95 ± 5	102 ± 6
1,2-dhATQ	105 ± 6	60 ± 4**	86 ± 5

*1,2-dhATQ = 3 μM; $CuSO_4$ = 4 μM. Each value ± S.E. represents the average of 3 separate experiments. ** indicates that values were significantly different ($p < 0.05$, ANOVA, pre-planned contrast using Tukey's test of significance).

Cyt b_6/f complex and the inhibition of the PS I electron transport may indicate that P700 or components downstream of P700 are targeted by 1,2-dhATQ. However, 1,2-dhATQ inhibited the intersystem electron transport (40% inhibition) more than the PS I electron transport (14% inhibition) (Table 1). Moreover, $DCPIPH_2$ is thought to be a partial donor of electrons to the Cyt b_6/f complex (Gould, 1975). Therefore, the partial inhibition of PSI electron transport by 1,2-dhATQ could have been contributed by the electron transport to PS I through the Cyt b_6/f complex. Thus, it appears that the primary target of 1,2-dhATQ inhibition is the Cyt b_6/f complex.

This notion was tested by phosphorylation of the light harvesting chlorophyll protein complex II (LHCP II). LHCP II is known to be phosphorylated when the Cyt b_6/f complex

Table 2-*Effect of 1,2-dhATQ on the phosphorylation of LHCP II.*

Treatment	%LHCP phosphorylation*
Control	100 ± 6
0.4 μM 1,2-dhATQ	60 ± 2
1.0 μM 1,2-dhATQ	37 ± 1
2.0 μM 1,2-dhATQ	33 ± 2
3.0 μM 1,2-dhATQ	29 ± 2
4.0 μM 1,2-dhATQ	27 ± 3

*Each value ± S.E. represents the average of 3 separate experiments. All values were significantly different ($p < 0.05$, ANOVA, pre-planned contrast using Tukey's test of significance).

is active and has an occupancy site available for PQ (Bennett et al. 1988, Zito et al. 1999). Phosphorylation of LHCP II is strongly inhibited by 1,2-dhATQ, and the inhibition of phosphorylation of LHCP II was dependent on 1,2-dhATQ concentration (Table 2). Thus, the inhibition of phosphorylation of LHCP II also indicates that the site of inhibition of 1,2-dhATQ is probably at the Cyt b_6/f complex. In this context, it should be mentioned that we have earlier reported that 1,2-dhATQ inhibited mitochondrial electron transport at the Cyt bc1 complex (Tripuranthakam et al. 1999) and that the counterpart of this mitochondrial component in chloroplasts is the Cyt b_6/f complex. Thus, it becomes all the more evident that 1,2-dhATQ inhibits Cyt b_6/f in chloroplasts.

We next studied the mixed toxicity of 1,2-dhATQ (which inhibited photosynthetic electron transport) and $CuSO_4$ (which had no inhibitory effect on electron transport) (Table 1). A mixture of 1,2-dhATQ plus $CuSO_4$ inhibited the growth of *L. gibba* in a synergistic manner (Table 3). Thus, the mixture toxicity was greater than the added toxicity of individual chemicals. Similarly, the mixture of 1,2-dhATQ plus $CuSO_4$ caused an enhanced inhibition of protein synthesis as quantified by the expression of the large subunit of ribulosebiphosphate carboxylase (LSU) enzyme in the soluble fraction (Table 3). We chose to study this enzyme expression because it is the most abundant protein in plants and is involved in CO_2 fixation. Copper alone did not affect growth or synthesis of LSU

Table 3-*Effect of a mixture of 1,2-dhATQ and copper on growth and LSU synthesis.*

Treatment	%Growth	%LSU synthesis
Control	100 ± 4	100 ± 7
$CuSO_4$	93 ± 6	120 ± 5
1,2-dhATQ	60 ± 4*	60 ± 4*
1,2-dhATQ + $CuSO_4$	30 ± 2*	40 ± 3*

1,2-dhATQ = 3 μM; $CuSO_4$ = 4 μM. Each value ± S.E. represents the average of 3 separate experiments. * indicates that values were significantly different ($p < 0.05$, ANOVA, pre-planned contrast using Tukey's test of significance).

(Table 3). This observed decreased synthesis of LSU could be due to the down regulation of gene expression. Alternatively, under the mixture treatment, LSU could be subject to rapid degradation so that little accumulates in the chloroplast. Some studies have shown that under oxidative stress, ribulosebiphosphate carboxylase enzyme is subject to degradation (Penarrubia and Moreno 1990, Mehta et al. 1992, Moreno and Spreitzer 1999).

It is important to examine the probable mechanism associated with the synergistic inhibition caused by the mixture of 1,2-dhATQ plus $CuSO_4$. In this direction, it may be pointed out that metals like Cu^{2+} and Fe^{3+} are very powerful redox active metals (Halliwell and Aruoma 1991, Held et al. 1996, Stohs and Bagchi 1995). That is, these metals go from the Cu^{2+} or Fe^{3+} state to Cu^{+} or Fe^{2+} state by accepting electrons from electron donors. Thus, these metals would have the capabilities to accept and donate electrons, participating in the generation of ROS. Although the presence of such metals alone can cause oxidative damage, the synergistic inhibition of the growth of *L. gibba* by the toxicant mixture may indicate that, under these conditions there is an ample opportunity for Cu^{2+} to participate in the redox cycling of electrons. Because 1,2-dhATQ inhibited electron transport, it appears that the synergistic mechanism of toxicity is originating from this site. In fact, when 1,2-dhATQ inhibits the Cyt b_6/f complex, there would be an accumulation of PQH_2 as this molecule now can not pass electrons on to Cyt b_6/f. Thus, the inhibition of Cyt b_6/f results in the availability of a reservoir of electrons in the form of PQH_2 and creates a highly reduced state inside the chloroplasts (Fig. 1).

Under highly reduced conditions, redox active metals like copper would readily accept electrons from PQH_2 and pass them to a nearby acceptor, most probably O_2 (Fig. 1). Cu^{2+} is known to generate superoxide ($O_2^{\bullet-}$) when it passes electrons to O_2 (Aust et al. 1985, Hayakawa et al. 1997, Pecci et al. 1997). One may predict that the synergistic toxicity of the mixture of 1,2-dhATQ plus $CuSO_4$ is due to the generation of $O_2^{\bullet-}$. However, in living cells $O_2^{\bullet-}$ can be detoxified by either superoxide dismutase (SOD) or spontaneous dismutation into H_2O_2, which is very stable and is also highly toxic to biological systems. Alternatively, Cu^{2+} itself can interact with H_2O_2 to produce hydroxyl radical ($OH^{\bullet}$). Further studies are required to establish which species of ROS is likely involved in the synergistic toxicity caused by the mixture of 1,2-dhATQ plus $CuSO_4$. Thus, in the present communication, we propose that the cause for enhanced toxicity by the mixture of 1,2-dhATQ and $CuSO_4$ is due to the formation of ROS, either $O_2^{\bullet-}$ from O_2 or $OH^{\bullet}$ from H_2O_2.

Acknowledgment

This research was supported by grants from the Natural Sciences and Engineering Research Council of Canada (NSERC) and the Canadian Network of Toxicology Centres to B.M. Greenberg.

References

Amodio-Cocchieri, R., Del Prete, U., Arnese, A., Giuliano, M., and Roncioni, A., 1993, "Heavy Metals and Polycyclic Aromatic Hydrocarbons (PAHs) in Marine Organisms from Ionian Sea (Italy)," *Bulletin of Environmental Contamination and Toxicology*, Vol. 50, pp. 618-625.

Aust, S. D., Morehouse, L. A., and Thomas, C. E., 1985, "Role of Metals in Oxygen Radical Reactions," *Free Radical Biology and Medicine*, Vol. 1, pp. 3-25.

Arfsten, D. P., Schaeffer, D. J., and Mulveny, D. C., 1996, "The Effects of Near Ultraviolet Radiation on the Toxic Effects of Polycyclic Aromatic Hydrocarbons in Animals and Plants: A Review," *Ecotoxicology and Environmental Safety*, Vol. 33, pp. 1-24.

Babu, T. S., Sabat, S. C., and Mohanty, P., 1992, "Heat Induced Alterations in the Photosynthetic Electron Transport and Emission Properties of the Cyanobacterium *Spirulina platensis,*" *Journal of Photochemistry and Photobiology*, Vol. 12, pp. 161-171.

Bennett, J., Shaw, E. K., and Michel, H., 1988, "Cytochrome b_6f Complex is Required for Phosphorylation of Light-Harvesting Chlorophyll a/b Complex II in Chloroplast Photosynthetic Membranes," *European Journal of Biochemistry*, Vol. 171, pp. 95-100.

Elich, T. D., Edelman, M., and Mattoo, A. K., 1992, "Identification, Characterization, and Resolution of the in vivo Phosphorylated Form of the D1 Photosystem II Reaction Center Protein," *Journal of Biological Chemistry*, Vol. 267, pp. 3523-3529.

Gould, J. M., 1975, "The Phosphorylation Site Associated with the Oxidation of Exogenous Donors of Electrons to Photosystem I," *Biochimica et Biophysica Acta*, Vol. 387, pp. 135-148.

Greenberg, B. M., Gaba, V., Canaani, O., Malkin, S., Mattoo, A. K., and Edelman, M., 1989, "Separate Photosensitizers Mediate Degradation of the 32-kDa Photosystem II Reaction Center Protein in the Visible and UV Spectral Regions," *Proceedings of the National Academy Sciences, U.S.A.*, Vol. 86, pp. 6617-6620.

Greenberg, B. M., Huang, X- D., and Dixon, D. G. 1992, "Applications of the Aquatic Higher Plant *Lemna gibba* for Ecotoxicological Assessment," *Journal of Aquatic Ecosystems and Health*, Vol. 1, pp. 147-155.

Halliwell, B., and Aruoma, O. I., 1991, "DNA Damage by Oxygen-Derived Species. Its Mechanism and Measurement in Mammalian Systems," *FEBS Letters*, Vol. 281, pp. 9-19.

Hayakawa, F., Kimura, T., Maeda, T., Fujita, M., Sohmiya, H., Fujii, M., and Ando, T., 1997, "DNA Cleavage Reaction and Linoleic Acid Peroxidation Induced by Tea Catechins in the Presence of Cupric Ion," *Biochimica et Biophysica Acta*, Vol. 1336, pp. 123-131.

Held, K. D., Sylvester, F. C., Hopcia, K. L., and Biaglow, J. E., 1996, "Role of Fenton Chemistry in Thiol-Induced Toxicity and Apoptosis," *Radiation Research*, Vol. 145, pp. 542-553.

Huang, X- D., Dixon, D. G., and Greenberg, B. M., 1993, "Impacts of UV radiation and Photomodification on the Toxicity of PAHs to the Higher Plant *Lemna gibba* (Duckweed)," *Environmental Toxicology and Chemistry*, Vol. 12, pp. 1067-1077.

Huang, X- D., Krylov, S. N., Ren, L., McConkey, B. J., Dixon, D. G., and Greenberg, B. M. 1997a, "Mechanistic Quantitative Structure-Activity Relationship Model for the Photoinduced Toxicity of Polycyclic Aromatic Hydrocarbons: II. An Empirical Model for the Toxicity of 16 Polycyclic Aromatic Hydrocarbons to the Duckweed *Lemna gibba* L. G-3," *Environmental Toxicology and Chemistry*, Vol. 16, pp. 2296-2303.

Huang, X- D., McConkey, B. J., Babu, T. S., and Greenberg, B. M. 1997b, "Mechanisms of Photoinduced Toxicity of Photomodified Anthracene to Plants: Inhibition of Photosynthesis in the Aquatic Higher Plant *Lemna gibba* (duckweed)," *Environmental Toxicology and Chemistry*, Vol. 16, pp. 1707-1715.

Izawa, S., and Pan, R. N., 1978, "Photosystem I Electron Transport and Phosphorylation Supported by Electron Donation to the Plastoquinone Region," *Biochemical and Biophysical Research Communications*, Vol. 83, pp. 1171-1177.

Mallakin, A., McConkey, B. J., Miao, G., McKibben, B., Snieckus, V., Dixon, D. G., and Greenberg, B. M., 1999, "Impacts of Structural Photomodification on the Toxicity of Environmental Contaminants: Anthracene Photooxidation Products," *Ecotoxicology and Environmental Safety*, Vol. 43, pp. 204-212.

Martineau, D., De Guise, S., Fournier, M., Shugart, L., Girard, C., Lagace, A., and Beland, P., 1994, "Pathology and Toxicology of Beluga Whales from the St. Lawrence Estuary, Quebec, Canada: Past, Present future," *Science of the Total Environment*, Vol. 154, pp. 201-215.

McConkey, B. J., Duxbury, C. L., Dixon, D. G., and Greenberg, B. M., 1997, "Toxicity of a PAH Photooxidation Product to the Bacterium *Photobacterium phosphoreum* and the Duckweed *Lemna gibba*: Effects of Phenanthrene and its Primary Photoproduct, Phenanthrenequinone," *Environmental Toxicology and Chemistry*, Vol. 16, pp. 892-899.

McCormac, D., Bruce, D., and Greenberg, B. M., 1994, "Connection Between State Transitions, LHC II Phosphorylation and LHC II Migration in vivo in the Higher Plant *Spirodela oligorrhiza*," *Biochimica et Biophysica Acta*, Vol. 1187, pp. 301-312.

Mehta, R. A., Fawcett, T. W., Porath, D., and Mattoo, A. K., 1992, "Oxidative Stress Causes Rapid Membrane Translocation and in vivo Degradation of Ribulose-1,5-Biphosphate Carboxylase/Oxygenase," *Journal of Biological Chemistry*, Vol. 267, pp. 2810-2816.

Moreno, J., and Spreitzer, R. J., 1999, "C172S Substitution in the Shloroplast-Encoded Large Subunit Affects Stability and Stress-Induced Turnover of Ribulose-1,5-

Biphosphate Carboxylase/Oxygenase," *Journal of Biological Chemistry*, Vol. 274, pp. 26789-26793.

Pecci, L., Montefoschi, G., and Cavallini, D., 1997, "Some New Details of the Copper-Hydrogen Peroxide Interaction," *Biochemical and Biophysical Research Communications*, Vol. 235, pp. 264-267.

Penarrubia, L., and Moreno, J., 1990, "Increased Susceptibility of Ribulose-1,5-Biphosphate Carboxylase/Oxygenase to Proteolytic Degradation Caused by Oxidative Treatments," *Archives of Biochemistry and Biophysics*, Vol. 281, pp. 319-323.

Sabat, S. C., Babu, T. S., and Mohanty, P., 1991, "N,N-Diethylhydroxylamine: A New Electron Donor to Photosystem II," *Biochemical and Biophysical Research Communications*, Vol. 179, pp. 1127-1133.

Sane, P. V., Johanningmeier, U., and Trebst, A., 1979, "The Inhibition of Photosynthetic Electron Flow by DCCD: An Indication for Proton Channels," *FEBS Letters*, Vol. 108, pp. 136-140.

Stohs, S. J., and Bagchi, D., 1995, "Oxidative Mechanisms in the Toxicity of Metal Ions." *Free Radical Biology and Medicine*, Vol. 18, pp. 321-336.

Tripuranthakam, S., Duxbury, C. L., Babu, T. S., and Greenberg, B. M., 1999, "Development of a Mitochondrial Respiratory Electron Transport Bioindicator for Assessment of Hydrocarbon Toxicity," In *Environmental Toxicology and Risk Assessment*, Eds. Henshel, D., Black, M.C. and Harris, M.C., ASTM STP 1364, Vol. 8, pp. 350-361.

Wetzel, A., and Werner, D., 1995, "Ecotoxicological Evaluation of Contaminated Soil Using Legume Root Nodule Symbiosis as an Effect Parameter," *Environmental Toxicology and Water Quality*, Vol. 10, pp. 127-134.

Wey, M- Y., Chao, C- Y., and Yu, L- J., 1996, "The Influences of Heavy Metals on PAH Formation During Incineration," *Toxicology and Environmental Chemistry*, Vol. 56, pp. 35-45.

Zito F., Finazzi, G., Delosme, R, Nitschke, W., Picot, D., and Wollman, F. A., 1999, "The Q0 Site of Cytochrome b_6f Complexes Controls the Activation of the LHC II Kinase," *EMBO Journal*, Vol. 18, pp. 2961-2969.

L. E. J. Lee,[1] A. McDonald,[1] J. Stassen,[1] and K. Lee[2]

Effects of Oil-Spill Bioremediation Strategies on the Survival, Growth and Reproductive Success of the Mystery Snail, *Viviparus georgianus*

Reference: Lee, L. E. J., McDonald, A., Stassen, J., and Lee, K., "**Effects of Oil-Spill Bioremediation Strategies on the Survival, Growth and Reproductive Success of the Mystery Snail, *Viviparus georgianus*,**" *Environmental Toxicology and Risk Assessment: Science, Policy, and Standardization – Implications for Environmental Decisions: Tenth Volume, ASTM STP 1403*, B. M. Greenberg, R. N. Hull, M. H. Roberts, Jr., and R. W. Gensemer, Eds., American Society for Testing and Materials, West Conshohocken, PA, 2001.

Abstract: In situ bioremediation is now being considered as an operational oil-spill countermeasure technology. While the effects of treatment strategies on microbial populations have been studied extensively, information on bioconcentration and effects on survival, growth and reproduction of higher level macrobiota are limited. Mystery snails, *Viviparus georgianus*, are attractive wetland biomonitors because they are abundant, short-lived, dioecious, ovoviviparous, easy to collect and grow rapidly during summer months feeding on sediment debris. *V. georgianus* was used as biomonitors in a controlled oil spill experiment at a wetland site along the St. Lawrence River (Ste. Croix, QC) to assess the impact of crude oil and efficacy of bioremediation treatments. Snails were placed at various time intervals in special enclosures deployed within five treatments and control background plots (n=50/treatment/collection time). Treatments consisted of A: oiled control (natural attenuation), B: as A + ammonium nitrate + triple superphosphate + culling of plants, C: as B but plants left intact, D: as C but sodium nitrate instead of ammonium nitrate, and E: as C with no oil treatment. Although snails could survive in the presence of oil for up to two months, fertilizer treatments brought about increased mortality. Generalized tissue damage with edema and hemocytic infiltration was seen consistently in snails from treatment D and reproduction was impaired in all treatments with or without oil. These findings disclose the need to further evaluate bioremediants in oil-spill response operations for appropriate recovery.

Keywords: In situ toxicology, oil-spill bioremediation, snails, wetland biomonitors

---

[1]Associate Professor and Honours Thesis Students, respectively, Department of Biology, Wilfrid Laurier University, Waterloo, Ontario, Canada N2L 3C5.

[2]Research Scientist, Department of Fisheries and Oceans, Environmental Science Division, Maurice Lamontagne Institute, Mont-Joli, Quebec, Canada G5H 3Z4.

Introduction

Approximately 15 million tons of petroleum products are transported annually through the St. Lawrence River/Seaway (St. Lawrence Centre 1996a). These are transported in carrier ships with an average capacity of 160000 tons thus traffic of oil is heavy. The St. Lawrence is also one of the hardest freshwater passages to navigate with areas of strong currents, narrow channels, shallow waters and changing tides (St. Lawrence Centre 1996a,b). Consequently the risk of oil spills is high and although a catastrophic incident has not occurred through this waterway, minor spills are common place. In 1993, 75 accidental spills were recorded from vessels and the average quantity of oil spilled by vessel was 475 gallons (St. Lawrence Centre 1996b).

Some wetlands along the St. Lawrence's shore have been declared "World Heritage Sites" with over 140 rare species among its biota. Hence there is a major need to protect these wetlands. Information on oil spills in north- temperate freshwater wetland ecosystems is limited in comparison to marine oil-spill studies (Prince 1993, Swannell et al. 1996, Jones 1998, Head and Swannell 1999). A major oil spill along these shores could cause irreparable and catastrophic damage unless remediation technologies are in place.

Bioremediation is a cleanup technology that relies on chemical degradation brought about by living organisms. This technology is a publicly favourable countermeasure for cleaning up oil spills as opposed to the traditional chemical or physical removal of contaminants (Hoff 1993, Swannell and Head 1994, Lee and De Mora 1999). It is also less disruptive and economically viable (Korda et al. 1997, Lee 1999). However, there are some concerns associated with its application, mainly due to a lack of studies in areas such as: 1) potential production of toxic metabolic byproducts from the bioremediating organisms, 2) possible toxic components in the formulation of biostimulants used to trigger growth of bioremediating organisms, and 3) incomplete degradation of highly toxic components within residual oil which can be pervasive in the environment (Lee and De Mora 1999). Indicators are thus needed to determine the well-being of natural wildlife populations among these wetlands, especially from a field perspective.

In situ experiments can provide information of high ecological relevance not attainable from laboratory work (Korda et al. 1997). The present study investigates the suitability of a resident snail, the mystery or banded snail, *Viviparus georgianus*, as a possible biomonitor of ecosystem recovery following a controlled oil-spill and bioremediation using nutrient amendments along a stretch of beach 50 km south of Quebec City, near St Croix, Quebec, Canada. Nutrient addition (e.g. nitrogen and phosphorus) has been shown to stimulate biodegradation of crude oil on contaminated shorelines (Lee et al. 1993, Venosa et al. 1996). Yet, field-monitoring programs still need to be implemented to validate treatment effectiveness and assess ecological recovery without detriment to the environment (Lee 1999).

Molluscs, especially bivalves, have been used extensively as indicators of contaminants in marine and freshwater environments (Lagadic and Caquet 1998), and programs such as the Mussel Watch advocates its usefulness. However, freshwater mussels are scarce in the intertidal marshland habitats and their usefulness is thus limited.

Viviparus georgianus, commonly known as the mystery snail, because they migrate to deep waters in wintertime and thus appear to have disappeared mysteriously, are the dominant second trophic level macrofauna (Vincent 1979) found at the experimental site and show characteristics that could make them ideal wetland biomonitors. These freshwater snails are relatively abundant and easy to collect, grow rapidly during summer months feeding on sediment detritus, algae, diatoms and decaying organic material (Duch 1976). They are slow moving prosobranch gastropods but can cover a good range and can grow at high densities. Up to 864 snails per square meter have been reported to occur some streams (Pace and Szuch 1985). They can tolerate prolonged periods of dryness by closing their operculum during low tides. They are ovoviviparus (Vail 1978), thus their young stay in the area and they have distinct sexes that can be readily recognized in the field. Males have a distinct truncated right tentacle that functions as a penis whereas females have two slender tentacles. Females live for up to 3 years and are usually larger than males whose life span is only 2 years (Jokinen et al. 1982). These species have been shown to be good laboratory biomonitors for metal toxicity (Tessier et al. 1994, 1996).

Materials and Methods

Experimental Design

A controlled oil-spill along the south shore of the St. Lawrence River at St. Croix, QC, Canada, was performed on June 10, 1999. Four replicates of 5 treatments were set up at the intertidal zone (Fig. 1). Each replicate was set in blocks of 5 square plots each measuring 4 x 5 m. A distance of 10 m separated each plot. Along with the monitoring of snails in this study which was done in one of the replicate blocks, the efficacy of bioremediation was also monitored by plant growth (the dominant species was *Scirpus pungens*) and sediment analysis which included chemical analysis, bacterial communities and a battery of toxicity tests which are reported elsewhere (Lee at al. 2001).

Weathered medium sulphuruous oil (MESA) obtained from the Petro Canada refinery in Montreal was sprayed uniformly with atomizer sprayers attached to hose and pump at approximately 12 L/plot (0.6 L/m^2) and raked into the sediment (top 2 to 3 cm of soil to prevent loss by tidal flow) during low tide. The nutrients added were granular ammonium nitrate, NH_4NO_3 fertilizer, granular triple super phosphate, $Ca(H_2PO_4)_2.H_2O$ fertilizer, both Nutrite brand (Hydro Agri Canada), and industrial grade sodium nitrate ($NaNO_3$) from Chilean Nitrate Corporation (Norfolk, VA). The ratio of nitrogen to phosphate was set at 10:3 per plot and the amounts applied per plot using a shoulder bag broadcast spreader was 2854 g NH_4NO_3 or 6061 g $NaNO_3$ with 1220 g of triple super phosphate. Nutrients were applied just before oiling on June 10 and at regular intervals thereafter to ensure that nutrient limitation was not a factor suppressing treatment effects within the plots designated nutrient amended. Interstitial nitrogen content was not allowed to fall below 5-10 mg/L.

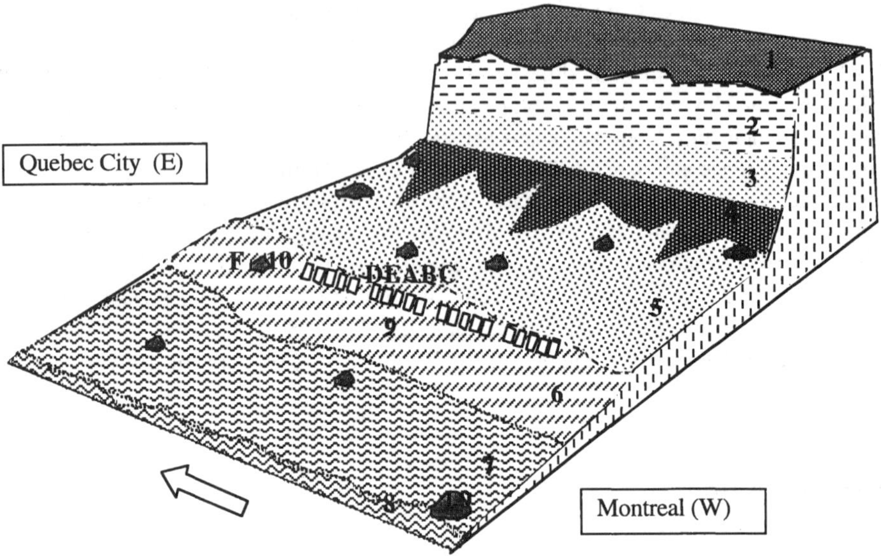

Figure 1- *Schematic diagram showing site of experimental set-up with typical zonation of the St. Lawrence River Fluvial Estuary indicated by numbers 1 to 8. Not to scale. 1. Upper terrace. 2. Shale cliff. 3. Talus slope. 4. Rocky beach. 5. Intertidal platform. 6. Marsh wetland in lower tidal zone. 7. Rocky shore at mean low tide zone. 8. Lowest low water level of river shore. 9.Treatment set-up area within marshland. 10. Boulders. Letters indicate location of plots in the block treatment where snails were located. Arrow indicates direction of water flow.*

Plot Treatments

The 5 treatments and controls were alphabetically labelled as follows:
A - Oil Only (natural attenuation, no nutrients)
B - Oil + Ammonium nitrate with plants cut (to investigate for effect of phytoremediation)
C - Oil + Ammonium nitrate
D - Oil + Sodium nitrate
E - Unoiled + Ammonium nitrate (nutrient control)
F - Control * outside of treatment area
** B,C,D,E have also super triple phosphate

Sampling and Exposure Times

Banded and non-banded specimens of *Viviparus georgianus* were collected from the surrounding area and caged in polypropylene baskets with lids that were originally designed as autoclaving baskets (Scienceware, VWR Canlab) with square mesh (1 x 1 cm) and placed (3 per treatment with 50 snails in each per sampling time) in one of the treatment blocks. A background control site was chosen near a large boulder approximately 200 m downstream. All cages were secured to the ground by attachment to wooden stakes (5 x 5 x 50 cm) driven into the sediment (~30 cm) to prevent drifting with movement of tides and current. Short- and long- term exposures were monitored , which included 1 week exposure (5 days), consecutive 1, 2 and 3 month exposures, and two staggered exposures of one month following 1 month of the spill, and one month exposure after 2 months of the spill.

Measured Parameters

Biotic parameters were measured prior to being placed in cages and following exposures. Wet weight of snails was recorded using a portable scale and shell height, width and thickness were measured using a vernier caliper (Kanon). Survival was recorded by observing snail movement following placement in buckets with fresh river water after recovery from cages (mortality overestimated) and by presence of intact operculum (mortality underestimated). Live snails were preserved for histological analysis by placing relaxed snails which had been in water with clove oil, in either 4% formalin or 70% EtOH. Some snails were starved for 3 days in distilled water at 4°C prior to freezing at -80°C for ulterior chemical analysis. Routine histological processing was followed after removing shells from the soft tissue portions by cracking open with a table vice. Hematoxylin and Eosin stained tissues were examined microscopically for signs of pathological changes and tissue degeneration. These included hemocyte infiltration, proliferation, fibrotic changes, edema, tissue hypertrophy, hypotrophy or necrosis. Brood sizes were recorded from gravid females by observation of visible young within the pallial oviduct.

Statistical Analysis

InStat, v. 2.01 (GraphPad, San Diego, CA) was used for statistical analysis. Average snail wet weight, shell height, width and thickness for each time point and treatment were compared. Analysis of variance (ANOVA) tests at the 95% confidence level were used and P values equal or less than 0.05 were considered significant. If significant results were obtained with ANOVA, then Student-Newman-Keuls multiple comparisons test were performed.

Results

Growth

Total sample size was 1800 snails. Average sizes were 1.96 g wet weight for mass, range 0.98 to 3.48 g; 19 mm shell height, range 13 to 28 mm; 13 mm shell width, range 10 to 18 mm; 0.47 mm shell thickness, range 0.15 to 0.50 mm. Significant growth ($P < 0.001$) occurred during the study period in wild snails. Changes in terms of wet weight is represented in Fig. 2. However, there were no significant differences ($P > 0.05$) between control and treated snails at any of the sampled time points in any of the measured parameters.

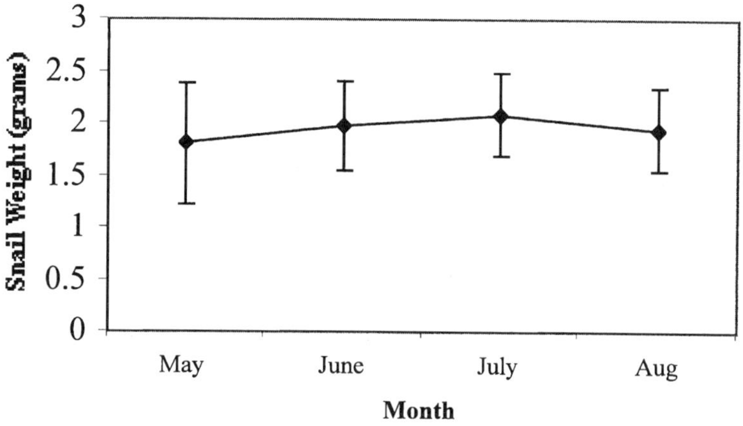

Figure 2-*Changes in wet weight of V.georgianus collected from wild at monthly intervals during the summer of 1999. May data is the mean of 10 snails, all others are means of 300. Each time point was significantly different ($P < 0.001$).*

In situ experimentation with caged snails was successful despite the constant flow of tides and extreme summer weather conditions. No cages were lost during the 3 month duration of the experiment, although some snails managed to escape from the cages.

Survival After Continuous Exposure

Snails under adverse conditions have been shown to retract into their shells and show no motility for prolonged periods of time. Taking this response mechanism into account, gastropod survival and vitality was quantified by two methods. Observation of motility provides an assessment of a relatively healthy population, but mortality may be overestimated as live, but perhaps moribund or stressed animals may be counted as dead. Whereas, vitality assessed by presence of operculum may underestimate mortality, as freshly dead snails may still show an intact operculum. Percent survival was thus calculated using both methods and although slight differences can be seen, the trend is maintained with the various treatments (Fig. 3). No surviving snails were found in the continuously caged snails after 3 months in either control or treatments.

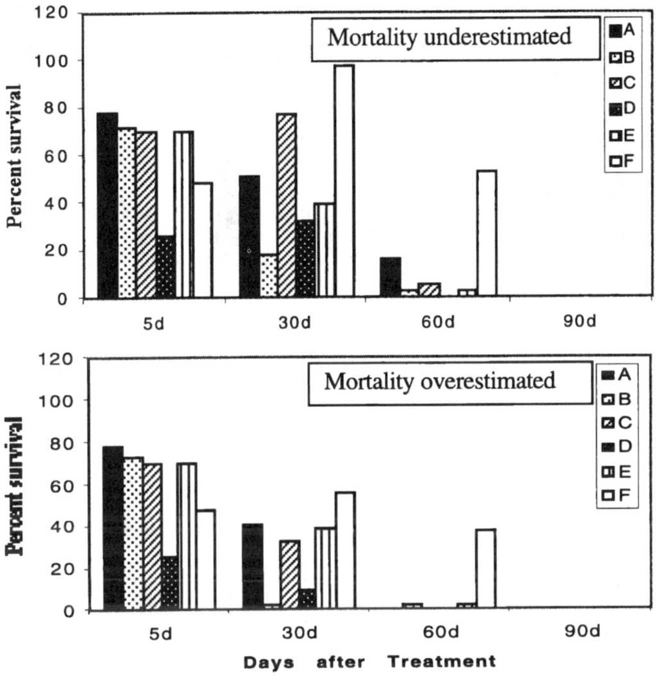

Figure 3-*Percent survival of V. georgianus following continuous exposure to bioremediation treatments with mortalities underestimated (presence of operculum) or overestimated (evidence of motility). A: oiled control (no bioremediation treatment), B: as A + ammonium nitrate + triple superphosphate + culling of plants, C: as B but plants left intact, D: as C but sodium nitrate instead of ammonium nitrate, and E: as C with no oil treatment. F: control no treatments.*

Survival with Staggered Exposures

Snails caged for a month immediately following spill or after 1 or 2 months of the spill showed survival of approximately 50% or more in those plots that did not receive fertilizers even with oil (Fig. 4). Although, treatment C showed higher survival when evaluated by the presence of operculum, only 32% showed mobility and these were still very sluggish. On average, mortality was higher with less than 25% survival in snails exposed to fertilizers even without oil. Overall, highest mortality was seen in treatment D, followed by treatments B, C, E, A and control.

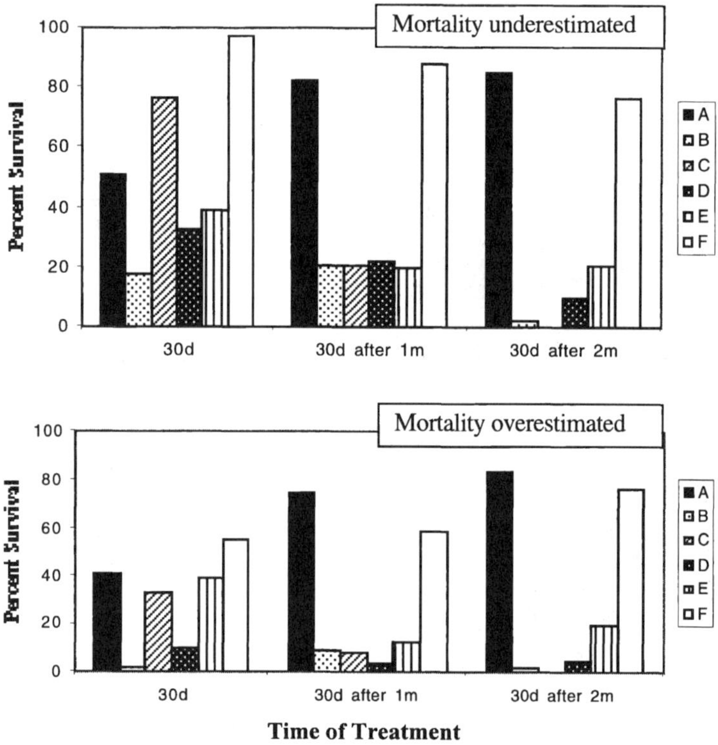

Figure 4-*Percent survival of V. georgianus following staggered exposures to bioremediation treatments with mortalities underestimated (presence of operculum) or overestimated (evidence of motility). A: oiled control (no bioremediation treatment), B: as A + ammonium nitrate + triple superphosphate + culling of plants, C: as B but plants left intact, D: as C but sodium nitrate instead of ammonium nitrate, and E: as C with no oil treatment. F: control no treatments.*

Reproduction

The sampled snails consisted of a biased population of mostly females (approximately 80%) due to size selection at capture to fit cage mesh size or perhaps to lower life span of males (Browne 1978). Gravid females (n=32) contained on average 10 young (range 3 to 15) visible with the naked eye. At 1 week post oil exposure, gravid females showed some degenerating embryos ("mushy" appearance) in all but the controls. This was also true for some of the 1 month post exposure gravid females, but the number of gravid females with macroscopic embryos decreased.

Histologic Analysis

All tissues show degenerative changes with time in snails exposed to fertilizers. Pathological changes were most obvious within lining epithelial cells of such tissues as gills, intestine and digestive gland but some degenerative changes were also observed in non-lining organs such as gonads. Most dramatic changes were observed with snails from treatment D (Na-nitrate) (Fig. 5). Although not presented here, increased lipid droplets, vacuolation of digestive cells and increase in lysosomal activity, which had been commonly observed in bivalves (Berthou et al. 1987), was also noted in these snails.

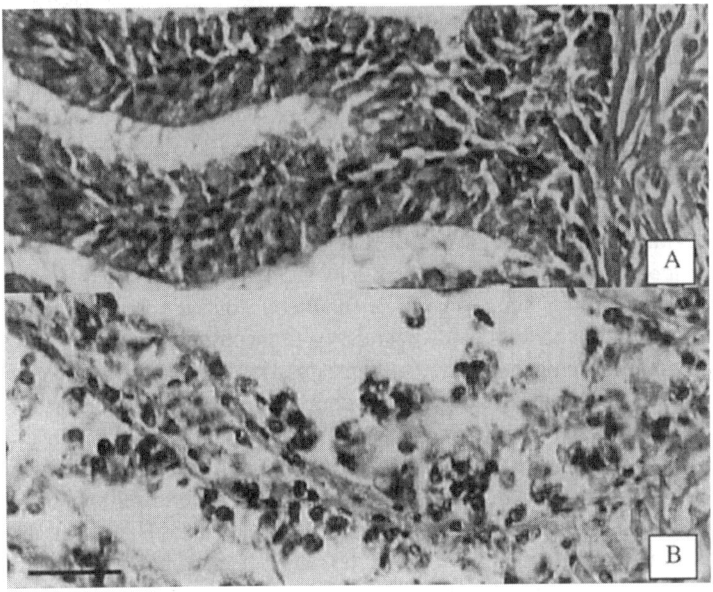

Figure 5- *Representative sections through the intestine of V. georgianus showing normal villi seen in control snails (A) and degenerated villus with hemocytic infiltration as seen in snails with treatment D after 1 month exposure (B). Bar = 75 μm.*

Discussion

Although many organisms have been used as sentinels or biomonitors of environmental contaminants (LeBlanc and Bain 1997), there is still a need to identify and exploit alternative species that are sensitive and amenable to ecotoxicological testing. Molluscs are abundant and widely distributed and their use as in situ biomonitors has been on the rise (Lagadic and Caquet 1998), especially with reports of specific syndromes in response to specific chemicals such as the imposex phenomenom (imposition of male characteristics) observed in response to tributyltin exposure in some susceptible marine snails (LeBlanc and Bain 1997). Recent reports show snails being used as indicators of metal toxicity (Gomot 1998, Svedsen and Weeks 1994), pesticides (Legierse et al. 1998) and various other chemicals including oil and oil dispersants (Gulec et al. 1997). *Viviparus georgianus* have been used as bioindicators of mercury and cadmium pollution (Tessier et al. 1996) under laboratory conditions, but their use as in situ biomonitors has not been reported.

Viviparus georgianus are suitable organisms for the evaluation of the efficacy of in situ bioremediation in northern-temperate wetland sites in terms of survival as they are numerous, easy to collect, relatively sedentary, can live in large densities and feed from organic debris in sediments. They are also useful for growth and reproduction studies as they grow rapidly during summer months, are short lived, and are ovoviviparous, thus their young remain in the area and have distinct and recognizable sexes. However, appropriate standards for their application as in situ bioindicators still need to be assessed. For instance, if they are to be used in cages, appropriate precautions should be taken to prevent their escape, especially for long-term exposures. Although there were no snails escaping after 5 days exposure, there were fewer snails left in the containers after longer exposures and after 90 days in captivity, up to 28 snails had escaped from their containers. The low sample sizes precluded statistical validation of trends seen in response to treatments and times of exposure. Either more replicates will need to be placed or individual snails should be tagged. The density of snails per cage was a bit higher than that observed under natural conditions 1250/m^2 compared to 864/m^2 (Pace and Szuch 1985), thus density of animals per cage should be reduced or size of cages should be larger. This may have contributed to poor survival in control cages, where snail activity was high influencing mortality. This appears to be the case for 5 day exposures at the control site F where mortality was higher than in the oil-treated plots, but the surviving 24 were very active crawlers compared to the survivors of oil and/or treatments, which were a bit more sluggish. Mortality after 5 days was highest with treatment D, with only 13 survivors, however this may be due to amount of fertilizer applied (more than double the ammonium nitrate levels to ensure equivalent total N levels in the interstitial water between nutrient amended plots) rather than sodium nitrate toxicity. This is supported by the longer term exposures where mortality was 100% with D at 2 months compared to the other treatments.

Toxicity of nitrogenous compounds at high levels has been noted with various organisms. Among invertebrates, ammonia toxicity was assessed with a freshwater snail

(Hickey and Vickers 1994). Acute values were derived for the snail and found to be 0.15g/m ammonia compared to the U. S. EPA value of 0.52 for salmonids, and they found that the snail was more sensitive than the normally accepted sensitive species such as mayflies and stoneflies. Inasmuch as ammonia was found to be usually more toxic than nitrates for amphibians (Schuytema and Nebeker 1999), perhaps the enhanced mortality and overall histological irregularity observed with treatment D (sodium nitrate) in the amphibious viviparus may be due to anoxic conditions brought about by the efficient enhancement of bacterial growth (Lee and DeMora 1999). The results from the staggered exposures appear to support this. All treatments containing nutrients with or without oil caused higher mortalities than with control or oil alone. Remediation strategies following oil spills need to be monitored as in many instances toxic side effects could be observed. For example, the addition of dispersants in semi-static bioassays using marine snails showed that the dispersants were significantly more toxic than the water-accommodated fraction of crude oil (Gulec et al. 1997). In the present study the side effect of eutrophication (Lee et al. 2001) may have brought about the observed snail mortality perhaps due to oxygen depletion although the compounding effect of petrochemicals can not be ruled out as survival in the staggered exposures was slightly better without oil in those plots that received nutrients. Bioremediation using nutrients in situ will need to take the above into consideration.

When organisms are exposed to xenobiotics, cellular changes have been observed to occur. Evaluation of histological changes can provide important information as to the stress of the organism and mode of action of pollutants. Although few toxicological studies in snails have dealt with histological observations, changes in the digestive gland have been reported. Klobucar et al. (1997) reported vacuolization and degeneration of digestive gland tubules in response to pentachlorophenol exposure in a pulmonate snail. The observed long term histological changes which included vacuolization of digestive glands, edema, hemocytic infiltration and overall tissue lysis are more consistent to anoxic changes than to chemical toxicity although the short-term exposures may have shown chemical irritability in lining tissues. In addition, the compounding effects of weather should also be taken into consideration. Bioconcentration of Cd and Hg has been shown to increase with temperature in viviparus (Tessier et al. 1994); perhaps the uptake of organopollutants may also increase with temperature. This will need to be further elucidated.

Another aspect that will need to be investigated is to examine the tissue content of the snails for petrochemicals. In the Australian gastropod *Austrocochlea constricta*, organopollutants were found in distinct compartments (Walsh et al. 1994). Abietic acid, a common resin acid found in pulp and paper mill effluents as well as in some crude oils, was detected only in the shell and not in soft tissue. The authors suggest that the shell may act as a "toxic waste sink" to facilitate the removal of potentially harmful compounds from the more metabolically active soft tissue and they conclude that *Austrocochlea* may be a useful biomonitor of pollutants from marine environments. The mystery snail, although not so mysterious, may be the freshwater counterpart in northern-temperate wetlands.

Conclusions

Mystery snails are useful in situ biomonitors of sediment quality in northern temperate wetlands. Various biotic characteristics, including abundance, ease of collection, short life span, dioecious, ovoviviparous, make these species suitable for survival, growth and reproductive evaluation of contaminants in situ, however standardized protocols for their evaluation remain to be defined.

Acknowledgments

Logistical and financial support from US EPA (Dr. Al Venosa) and Fisheries and Oceans Canada is gratefully acknowledged. We would also like to thank Jenny Wojtukiewicz and Katharine Haberstroh for technical help with this project.

References

Berthou, F., Balquet, G., Bodennec, G., and Marchand, M. (1987) "The Occurrence of Hydrocarbons and Histopathological Abnormalities in Oysters for Seven Years Following the Wreck of the Amoco Cadiz in Brittany (France)," *Marine Environmental Research,* Vol. 23, pp. 103-133.

Browne, R. A., 1978, "Growth, Mortality, Fecundity, Biomass and Productivity of Four Lake Populations of the Prosobranch Snail, *Viviparus georgianus*," *Ecology*, Vol. 59, pp. 742-750.

Duch, T. M., 1976, "Aspects of the Feeding Habits of *Viviparus georgianus*," *Nautilus*, Vol. 90, No. 1, pp. 7-10.

Gomot, A., 1998, "Toxic Effects of Cadmium on Reproduction, Development and Hatching in the Freshwater Snail *Lymnaea stagnalis* for Water Quality Monitoring," *Ecotoxicology and Environmental Safety*, Vol. 41, pp. 288-297.

Gulec, I., Leonard, B., and Holdway, D. A., 1997, "Oil and Dispersed Oil Toxicity to Amphipods and Snails," *Spill Science and Technology Bulletin*, Vol. 4, pp. 1-6.

Head, I. M. and Swannell, R. P., 1999, "Bioremediation of Petroleum Hydrocarbon Contaminants in Marine Habitats," *Current Opinions in Biotechnology*, Vol. 10, pp. 234-239.

Hickey, C. W. and Vickers, M. L., 1994, "Toxicity of Ammonia to Nine Native New Zealand Freshwater Invertebrate Species," *Archives of Environmental Contamination and Toxicology*, Vol. 26, pp. 292-298.

Hoff, R., 1993, "Bioremediation: An Overview of its Development and Use for Oil Spill Cleanup," *Marine Pollution Bulletin*, Vol. 26, pp. 476-481.

Jokinen, E. H., Guerette, J., and Kortmann, R. W., 1982, "The Natural History of an Ovoviviparous Snail, *Viviparus georgianus* (Lea), in a Soft-Water Eutrophic Lake," *Freshwater Invertebrate Biology*, Vol. 1, No. 4, pp. 2-17.

Jones, W. R., 1998, "Practical Applications of Marine Bioremediation," *Current Opinions in Biotechnology*, Vol. 9, pp. 300-304.

Klobucar, G. I. V., Lajtner, J., and Erben, R., 1997, "Lipid Peroxidation and Histological Changes in the Digestive Gland of a Fresh Water Snail *Planorbarius corneus* L. (Gastropoda, Pulmonata) Exposed to Chronic and Sub-Chronic Concentrations of PCP," *Bulletin of Environmental Contamination & Toxicology*, Vol. 58, pp. 128-134.

Korda, A., Santas, P., Tenente, A., and Santas, R., 1997, "Petroleum Hydrocarbon Bioremediation: Sampling and Analytical Techniques, in situ Treatments and Commercial Microorganisms Currently Used," *Applied Microbial Biotechnology*, Vol. 48, pp. 677-686.

Lagadic, L and Caquet, T., 1998, "Invertebrates in Testing of Environmental Chemicals: Are They Alternatives?" *Environmental Health Perspectives*, Vol. 106, pp. 593-561.

LeBlanc, G. A. and Bain, L. J., 1997, "Chronic Toxicity of Environmental Contaminants: Sentinels and Biomarkers," *Environmental Health Perspectives*, Vol. 105, pp. 65-79.

Lee, K., 1999, "Bioremediation of Oil Impacted Shorelines," T. Murphy and M. Munawar, Eds. *Aquatic Restoration in Canada*, Ecovision World Monograph Series, Backhuys Publishers, Leiden, Netherlands, pp. 69-85.

Lee, K. and De Mora, S., 1999, "In Situ Bioremediation Strategies for Oiled Shoreline Environments," *Environmental Technology*, Vol. 20, 783-794.

Lee, K., Tremblay, G. H., and Levy, E. M., 1993, "Bioremediation: Application of Slow Release Fertilizers on Low Energy Shorelines," *Proceedings of the 1993International Oil Spill Conference,* American Petroleum Institute, Washington, DC, pp. 449-454.

Lee, K., Doe, K. G., Lee, L. E. J., Suidan, M. T., and Venosa, A. D., 2001, "Habitat Recovery and Toxicity Reduction in an Oiled Freshwater Wetland: Efficacy of Remediation Strategies," *Proceedings of the 2001International Oil Spill Conference,* American Petroleum Institute, Washington, DC. (in press).

Legierse, K. C., Sijm, D. T., Van Leeuwen, C. J., Seinen, W., and Hermens, J. L., 1998, "Bioconcentration Kinetics of Chlorobenzenes and the Organosphosphorous Pesticide Chlorthion in the Pond Snail *Lymnaea stagnalis* - A Comparison with the Guppy *Poecilia reticulata*," *Aquatic Toxicology*, Vol. 41, pp. 301-323.

Pace, G. L. and Szuch, E. J., 1985, "An Exceptional Stream Population of the Banded Applesnail, *Viviparus georgianus,* in Michigan," *Nautilus*, Vol. 99, pp. 48-53.

Prince, R. C., 1993, "Petroleum Spill Bioremediation in Marine Environments," *Critical Reviews in Microbiology,* Vol. 19, pp. 217-242.

Schuytema, G. S. and Nebeker, A. V., 1999, " Effects of Ammonium Nitrate, Sodium Nitrate, and Urea on Red-Legged Frogs, Pacific Treefrogs and African Clawed Frogs," *Bulletin of Environmental Contamination and Toxicology,* Vol. 63: 357-364.

St. Lawrence Centre, 1996a, *State of the Environment Report on the St. Lawrence River. Volume 1: The St. Lawrence Ecosystem*. Environment Canada- Quebec Region, Montreal, QC.

St. Lawrence Centre, 1996b, *State of the Environment Report on the St. Lawrence River. Volume 2: The State of the St. Lawrence*. Environment Canada- Quebec Region, Montreal, QC.

Svedsen, C. and Weeks, J. M., 1994, " The Use of a Lysosome Assay for the Rapid Assessment of Cellular Stress From Copper to the Freshwater Snail *Viviparus contectus*," *Marine Pollution Bulletin*, Vol. 31, pp. 139-142.

Swannell, R. P. and Head, I. M., 1994, "Bioremediation comes of age," *Nature,* Vol. 368, pp. 396-397.

Swannell, R. P., Lee, K. and McDonagh M., 1996, "Field Evaluations of Marine Oil Spill Bioremediation," *Microbiology Reviews,* Vol. 60, pp. 342-365.

Tessier, L., Vaillancourt, G., and Pazdernik, L.,1994, "Temperature Effects on Cd and Hg Kinetics in Freshwater Molluscs Under Laboratory Conditions," *Archives of Environmental Contamination and Toxicology*, Vol. 26, pp. 179-184.

Tessier, L., Vaillancourt, G., and Pazdernik, L.,1996, "Laboratory Study of Cd and Hg Uptake by Two Freshwater Molluscs in Relation to Concentration, Age and Exposure Time," *Water, Air & Soil Pollution*, Vol. 86, pp. 347-357.

Vail, V. A., 1978, "Seasonal Reproductive Cycles in 3 Viviparid Gastropods," *Malacologia*, Vol. 17, pp. 73-97.

Venosa, A., Suidan, M., Wrenn, B., Strohmeier, K., Haines, J., Eberhart, B., King, D., and Holder, E.,1996, "Bioremediation of an Experimental Oil Spill on the Shoreline of Delaware Bay," *Environmental Science & Technology*, Vol. 30, pp. 1764-1775.

Vincent, B., 1979, "Etude du benthos d'eau douce dans le haut-estuaire du Saint-Laurent (Quebec)," *Canadian Journal of Zoology*, Vol. 57, pp. 2171-2182.

Walsh, K., Dunstan, R. H., Murdoch, R. N., Conroy, B. A., Roberts,T. K. and Lake, P., 1994, "Bioaccumulation of Pollutants and Changes in Population Parameters in the Gastropod Mollusc *Austrocochlea constricta*," *Archives of Environmental Contamination and Toxicology*, Vol. 26, pp. 367-376.

Yves Dudal[1] and Louise Deschênes[2]

Development of a Method to Estimate the Mass and Toxic Bioavailabilities of Pentachlorophenol during its Transport through Saturated Porous Media

---

Reference: Dudal, Y., and Deschênes, L., "**Development of a Method to Estimate the Mass and Toxic Bioavailabilities of Pentachlorophenol during its Transport through Saturated Porous Media,**" *Environmental Toxicology and Risk Assessment: Science, Policy, and Standardization - Implications for Environmental Decisions: Tenth Volume, ASTM STP 1403*, B. M. Greenberg, R. N. Hull, M. H. Roberts, Jr., and R. W. Gensemer, Eds., American Society for Testing and Materials, West Conshohocken, PA, 2001.

Abstract: Bioavailability of organic contaminants in soil has recently been a focus of interest but a lack of knowledge of its behavior during contaminant transport through saturated porous media, such as aquifers, is observed. This research presents a method, based on a generally accepted definition of bioavailability, that quantifies mass and toxic bioavailabilities of organic contaminants during their transport in terms of bioavailability rates. Elutions of pentachlorophenol (PCP) were performed using inoculated laboratory columns at two different pore-water velocities and on two different media. Both PCP and the toxic response (Microtox) were monitored at the exit of the columns for quantification of the rates. Results show that the non-dimensional mass bioavailability rate decreased with increasing pore-water velocity (from 0.52 to 0.15) and with increasing retention (from 0.15 to 0.02). The non-dimensional toxic bioavailability rate decreased with increasing retention (from 0.59 to 0.22). Results indicate that this method shows a potential for quantifying contaminant bioavailability according to both outcomes: biodegradation and toxicity.

Keywords: mass and toxic bioavailability rates, quantification method, organic contaminants, saturated porous media, aquifers, pentachlorophenol, transport

Introduction

Bioavailability of contaminants in the environment has become a topic of interest in the last few years (Baveye et al. 1999), in two different fields of research. Environmental engineers who are using biotechnology to remediate contaminated sites are often faced with limitations to contaminant biodegradation. Recent developments have shown that these limitations were mainly due to the sorption phenomena between the contaminant

[1] Ph.D. Candidate and [2] Professor, NSERC Industrial Chair for Site Remediation and Management, École Polytechnique de Montréal, Chemical Engineering Department, C.P. 6079, succ. centre-ville, Montréal (Québec) H3C 3A7 Canada.

and the subsurface matrix (Weber Jr et al. 1991). More precisely, slow sorption of the contaminant within the micropores of the natural particles are supposed to be the main mechanism limiting microbial degradation of the pollutant (Nam and Alexander 1998). Secondly, environmental toxicologists have been focusing on contaminant bioavailability to superior organisms. They found that similar mechanisms are limiting contaminant bioavailability, mostly its sorption on sediments or soil organic matter (Hamelink et al. 1994, Standley 1997). An important aspect to be underlined in both approaches is that bioavailability is organism-dependent. Two different microorganisms, both degrading a specific contaminant, will lead to two different evaluations of the bioavailable fraction (Guerin and Boyd 1992). The same result was observed with superior organisms (Davies et al. 1999).

These two approaches to determine contaminant bioavailability in the environment have been brought together with the emergence of the risk-based approach to site remediation. In this approach, the knowledge and understanding of contaminant fate and transport, hence bioavailability, is required as well as the assessment of the result of the exposure between the contaminant and a targeted organism. The notion of risk is now directly associated with the contaminant bioavailability (Alexander 1995, Kelsey and Alexander 1997). However, differences in the definition of bioavailability tend to bring difficulties in the application of the concept and mostly in quantifying bioavailability.

Definitions of Bioavailability

The fact that bioavailability is organism-dependent makes it difficult to define. From the chemistry point of view, the knowledge of contaminant partitioning is sufficient to assess bioavailability, which is in fact a chemical availability. From the biology point of view, bioavailability should include the contaminant uptake as well as the activity of all the metabolic enzymes (Baveye and Bladon 1999), which is pharmacological bioavailability. A general definition of the contaminant bioavailable fraction is usually given as the fraction found in the aqueous phase (Cuypers et al. 1999). This definition appears to be limiting when assessing bioavailability to superior organisms like earthworms and when assessing the bioavailability of very hydrophobic and almost non-soluble molecules like hexadecane, which is easily biodegradable in a soil. A refined definition would be the uptake flux of contaminant by the target organism (Baveye and Bladon 1999). Despite the fact that the uptake flux is not easily measured and quantified, this definition is very interesting because it introduces the concept of time in bioavailability which seems to be a key factor in the overall process. A more general definition of bioavailability was proposed by Hrudey et al. (1996) as the extent of organism exposure to the contaminant. The notion of exposure links the two approaches that were presented earlier in their common interest in the contaminant fate and transport. But, this definition is faced with a quantification problem.

Quantification of Bioavailability

The main method used to quantify bioavailability is based on the concentration of the contaminant in the aqueous phase. Such a concentration may be predicted from the knowledge of the contaminant partition coefficient (Kp) between water and a certain type of subsurface material. This partition coefficient is usually estimated between water and subsurface organic matter (K_{om}). This thermodynamic datum gives an approximation of the equilibrium state that can be reached by the contaminant between the two phases. Another set of methods has been developed that are based on a relationship between the contaminant extractability and its uptake by organsims. Supercritical fluid extraction was carried out by Loibner et al. (1999) at two different levels, and the ratio of the amount obtained in the two cases was correlated with biodegradation and ecotoxicity measured on the samples. The same development of chemical assays to assess bioavailability was done by Kelsey et al. (1997), but, this time, using organic solvents. These tests have shown good results for correlating biological responses and chemical extractability but it is not clear how such correlations may be used in different situations (contaminants and media) and with different biological receptors. Based on this instantaneous quantification approach, probes are being developed, either chemically based or even biologically based. Reversed-phase chromatography (C-18 probes) was used to model biopartitioning processes, mostly bioaccumulation (Hsieh and Dorsey 1995, van Loon et al. 1996). Whole-cell living biosensors are being developed to directly assess bioavailability of pollutants to degrading-microorganisms (Jaspers et al. 1999, Ripp et al. 2000). Bioconcentration or bioaccumulation are also usually used to assess bioavailability in terms of environmental toxicity (Morrison et al. 2000).

However, it is now clear that slow sorption mechanisms, driven by kinetic data, are responsible for the non-equilibrium partition observed between the contaminant in the aqueous phase and the solid phase (Pignatello and Xing 1996). Thus, bioavailability to any organism is regulated partly by these sorption-related mass transfer (Zhang et al. 1998). Bioavailability tends to be quantified by a ratio between the kinetics that appear to be the limiting factors to bioavailability: mass transfer of the contaminant to the cell and microbially-catalysed transformation of the contaminant. In non-dynamic systems or in systems where hydrodynamics are negligible, the bioavailability factor or number has been developed as the ratio of the biodegradation kinetic to the slow sorption kinetic (Chung et al. 1993, Bosma et al. 1997, Zhang et al. 1998). This effort in modeling bioavailability is based on a chemical engineering approach characterized by the use of the Thiele modulus, expressed as the ratio of two kinetics limiting a system (Ramaswami and Luthy 1997). This kinetic aspect of bioavailability has also been applied to the environmental toxicology side of the problem (Landrum et al. 1994). The authors proposed to quantify environmental bioavailability as the ratio of the contaminant uptake clearance to the encounter rate.

These kinetic approaches to bioavailability have not yet been applied to dynamic systems, such as groundwater, where hydrodynamic is not negligible. The research presented in this paper proposes a quantification method applicable to bioavailability of organic contaminants during their transport through saturated porous media, based on a generally accpeted definition of environmental bioavailability.

Method Development

From what was described above, a general definition of bioavailability must be applicable to the two aspects of environmental bioavailability (biodegradation and ecotoxicity) and should also address the kinetical aspect of it. Such a definition, based on the one proposed by Hrudey et al. (1996) states bioavailability, not as the extent of exposure, but as the rate of exposure of an organism to the contaminant (Dudal et al. 1999). When the organism is a contaminant-degrading microorganism, the response is an actual decrease in the contaminant mass over time: this is mass bioavailability. When the organism exposure to the contaminant leads to a toxic response, it is toxic bioavailability. Bioavailability is thus expressed in terms of a rate of exposure, but depending on the receptor, will be quantified as a rate of mass or toxic bioavailability. The definition given here takes into account the kinetic aspect of bioavailability and links the concept of rate to bioavailability. Hence, mass and toxic bioavailability rates are introduced.

When assessing contaminant fate and transport, dynamic studies are often carried out either on site or at the lab-scale, using flow-through columns. Contaminant is eluted through the columns at a certain concentration and monitored at the exit of the column. The results from such studies are contaminant breakthrough curves (BTC), which are helpful to understand the different mechanisms responsible for the shape of the curve. Hydrodynamic phenomena such as contaminant dispersion and advection, physico-chemical phenomena such as contaminant retardation and diffusion in pores and biological phenomena such as biodegradation or bioaccumulation all have a direct impact on the breakthrough curves. In an attempt for an integrative analysis, two observations can be made on a BTC. First, there is its horizontal extent, integrating dispersion, advection and retardation as well as slow sorption mechanisms. The more outspread the curve is, the more retained the contaminant is and the slower it passes through the column. The horizontal extent can thus be seen as the residence time distribution of the contaminant in the column. Secondly, biological mechanisms such as biodegradation or bioaccumulation will act on the vertical extent of a BTC. The more biodegradation occurs within the section, more flat the curve will be. In order to translate mathematically these observations, two parameters are set up. The first parameter, extensively used in pharmacokinetic studies is the area under the curve (AUC), qualified as a robust parameter, for its good independance from experimental variations (Ritschel 1988). The AUC is directly linked to the vertical extent of a breakthrough curve. In the case of a contaminant eluting through a section of an aquifer or a column, the area under the curve obtained represents the fraction of contaminant that was able to migrate through the column without being biodegraded, thus without showing any mass bioavailability, whatever residence-time distribution was observed. The uneluted fraction of what was injected at the entrance of the section represents the mass bioavailable fraction of contaminant. The second mathematical parameter, describing the residence time distribution has to take into account the overall curve, not only the average distribution, in order to cope with asymetric curves generated by slow sorption mechanisms. Thus, this parameter is set as the product of the average residence time with the variance of the residence time distribution.

The rate of biological exposure to the contaminant, defined as bioavailability, can then be quantified using these two parameters. As the uneluted fraction (1-AUC) is biodegraded during the overall time taken by the contaminant to pass through the section, the mass bioavailability rate is quantified as the ratio of the amount that was biodegraded to the time it took to biodegrade it, according to Equation 1.

$$\tau_{massBioA} = \frac{1 - AUC_{mass}}{\bar{t}_{mass}\sigma^2_{mass}} \qquad (1)$$

where

AUC_{mas} = area under the contaminant breakthrough curve
t_{mas} = average of the contaminant residence-time distribution
σ^2_{mass} = variance of contaminant residence-time distribution.

The amount of contaminant that was able to migrate through the column could also be considered to be bioavailable. Indeed, if a superior organism is exposed to this effluent, it may lead to the expression of toxicity. Hence, on top of monitoring the mass of contaminant, a second breakthrough curve is built up by monitoring the toxic response of an organism placed at the exit of the column, imitating a groundwater resurgence at a well, lake or river. A toxic breakthrough curve is generated and the area under such curve is calculated leading to *AUCtox*. The same quantification can be done to obtain the toxic bioavailability rate according to Equation 2.

$$\tau_{toxBioA} = \frac{AUCtox}{\bar{t}_{tox}\sigma^2_{tox}} \qquad (2)$$

where

AUC_{tox} = area under the toxicity breakthrough curve
t_{tox} = average of the toxicity residence-time distribution
σ^2_{tox} = variance of toxicity residence-time distribution.

The use of the product of the average time to the variance allows all the measured values of the distribution to be taken into account, differentiating two curves, similar in their average distribution time but exhibiting a very different range of values. This product is a better representative of the time of exposure between the contaminant and the biological receptor than the average residence time alone.

The actual values of the mass and toxic bioavailability rates may not be very easy to analyse. Hence, a non-dimensional version of these rates can be obtained by reporting them to extreme scenarios. For the mass rate, the best-case scenario is given when all of the contaminant is biodegraded within the section leading to an *AUCmass* equal to 0 and when no retardation is observed (contaminant behaves like a non-reactive tracer through standard sand). This leads to the maximum mass bioavailability rate. The ratio between the mass bioavailability rate and its maximum value gives a non-dimensional mass bioavailability number, ranging from 0 to 1. The same process is carried out on the toxic bioavailability rate, this time to the worst-case scenario, where all of the contaminant is eluted through the section with no retention in the section (equivalent to an elution through standard sand). A non-dimensional toxic bioavailability number is thus obtained. The same reference medium is used (standard sand) allowing comparison between different data sets. Therefore, an experimental study at lab-scale was carried out to show

how this method can be applied to different scenarios of contaminant fate and transport and to show the sensitivity of the method to changes in either retention capacity of the medium or in hydrodynamics.

Materials and Methods

Three columns were used in this study. Column 1 was a standard sand column on which the PCP elution was performed at 1 mL/min, Column 2 was a 0.2% resin-amended standard sand column used at the same flow rate and Column 3 was like Column 1 but the PCP elution was performed at half the flow rate, 0.5 mL/min. On each column, three elutions were performed: a non-reactive tracer test, an abiotic elution (NaPCP in the absence of microorganisms) and a biotic elution, after inoculation with PCP-degrading microorganisms. Step elutions of contaminant were performed, but the analysis, according to Equations 1 and 2, was carried out on the derivatives of the BTC, thus on the equivalent of a pulse elution. However, it is difficult, and often technically impossible to perform a true pulse elution on a column. Performing a step elution, leading to a stable response, solves this difficulty. The derivative of this BTC is then computed and the mathematical analysis presented in equations 1 and 2 can be performed on this response, corresponding to an artificial pulse elution (Levenspiel, 1972). The integral of this derivative, the area under the curve, gives the fraction of contaminant that migrated through the column, while the primitive of this derivative would lead back to the step elution response. This extra mathematical step greatly enhances the accuracy of the method by allowing the analysis of a robust experimental response.

Production of PCP-Degrading Microorganisms

PCP-degrading microorganisms (coming from a sample of a PCP-contaminated soil) were grown by sequential addition of 90 % pure NaPCP (Omega Inc., Lévis, QC) in a fed-batch slurry bioreactor, using a mineral salt medium (MSM) at pH 7.15 (Greer et al. 1990). The aqueous phase from this slurry was then filtered through an 8µm Whatman (Millipore, Bedford, MA) filter paper. The remaining bacterial suspension was then bioactivated to obtain a richer suspension. This process was carried out in an aerated (5 L/min) amber glass jar (4 L) by sequential spikes of NaPCP at concentrations increasing from 5 to 25 mg/L. A higher concentration spike of NaPCP was added when the remaining concentration was less than 1 mg/L. In order to monitor NaPCP concentration in the suspension, 4mL-samples were taken daily, filtered through a 0.25 µm filter, and analyzed in the UV-spectrophotometer at 319 nm.

Study Columns

The columns used for all the experiments were pre-chromatography Chromaflex™ columns (Kontes, Vineland, NJ), made of Kimax™ borosilicate glass and polytetrafluoroethylene (PTFE). The columns were 15cm long with a 4.8cm inside diameter. Both ends included a 20µm PTFE filter as well as a PTFE grid for bed support and accurate flow distribution. Model solids used for column packing consisted of standard Ottawa sand (Anachemia, Montreal, QC) and Amberlite XAD-4 resin (Sigma,

St Louis, MO). This resin was used to accurately control the retention capacity and kinetics of the medium for the theoretical development of bioavailability quantification. PCP is very soluble at the pH of the experiments (7.15) and its hydrophobicity is thus reduced. The resin will specifically retain hydrophobic molecules from aqueous media. Its pore size is between 20 to 60 mesh with a specific area of 715 m^2/g and an average inside pore diameters of 50Å. 400 g of dry sand were solely used in Column 1 and 3, while 399 g were mixed with 1 g of resin prior to packing in Column 2, making it a 0.25 % of retentive matter column.

Column Hydrodynamics

The columns were packed with their composition of model solids and then saturated with MSM. Different masses were measured on each column: empty column, column with dry material, column filled with MSM and saturated column. Simple calculations performed on these masses allowed the estimation of the column saturation, the pore volume and the porosity. Pore water velocity, *v*, was fixed at 2.3×10^{-3} cm/s. The hydrodynamic elution was a step tracer test using $^3H\text{-}H_2O$ (25 mCi/g, Sigma, St Louis, MO) based MSM at a continuous inflow of 10 000 dpm . Fractions were collected at the exit of the column and counts per minute were monitored using a liquid scintillation counter (Wallac 1409). The test was carried out until the counts at the exit of the column were equal to the ones for the inflow.

Abiotic Breakthroughs

Abiotic breakthroughs were carried out and consisted of step elutions of PCP (continuous inflow of PCP at 25 mg/L in MSM) in the absence of PCP-degrading microorganisms. Fractions were collected at the exit of the columns and, after filtration at 0.45μm (Millipore, Bedford, MA), the contaminant concentration was monitored by UV spectrophotometry at 319 nm. Abiotic breakthroughs were performed on Columns 1 and 2. As Columns 1 and 3 consisted of the same medium, their abiotic profiles were identical.

Biotic Breakthroughs

The same protocol as for the abiotic experiments (step elution of 25 mg/L PCP solution and monitoring of PCP) was used for the biotic elutions, but this time, the columns were inoculated with the PCP-degrading microorganisms prior to the elution. This was carried out by recirculating the suspension during 20 pore volumes (PV) followed by a flush during 2 PV to wash non-fixed cells (Herman et al. 1997). The biomass was monitored at the exit of the column during the flush by protein analysis using the micro-BCA (bicinchoninic acid) method (Pierce Chemicals, Rockford, IL). For this purpose, samples were centrifuged (13000 rpm for 10 minutes) and the deposit was washed with MSM in order to avoid interference between the reagent and PCP. After a second centrifugation, bacteria were lysed by using a 1%-triton (Union Carbide, Danbury, CT) solution, which is compatible with the reagent.

Toxicity Measurement

Toxicity of elution samples was assessed by using the Microtox® test (Azur Environmental, Carlsbad, CA). This test uses a bioluminescent marine bacterium (*Vibrio fisheri*) and measures the inhibition to luminescence caused by the presence of contaminant in the sample. Results are collected in terms of the logarithm of the EC10, expressed in percent of the sample that causes a 10% decrease of the bioluminescence. The minimum value is 100% leading to a non-dimensional toxicity (log EC10) of 2.

Results

Results are presented for the three columns in terms of contaminant fate and transport as well as toxicity elutions. Bioavailability is finally quantified according to the method presented above.

Pentachlorophenol Fate and Transport in the Columns

Hydrodynamics – The three columns were hydrodynamically similar, showing a porosity of 0.4, typical of sand columns. All experiments were performed with a saturation of 98±1%. The hydraulic conductivity was fixed with the flow rate and was calculated according to the porosity at a value of 2.3×10^{-3} cm/s for Columns 1 and 2 and 1.15×10^{-3} cm/s for Column 3. Pore volumes were 110 ± 2 mL. The symmetry of the tracer test response (results not shown) showed that neither flow-bypass nor dead volumes were observable. This implies that dissolved oxygen and nutrients were uniformly fed to the columns.

Abiotic Controls – Elutions of PCP in the absence of any degrading microorganisms were carried out to investigate PCP sorptive behavior towards the matrices. Figure 1 shows that no retardation was found when PCP was eluted through standard sand (Columns 1 and 3). The abiotic responses of these two columns are identical in the non-dimensional forms, as represented in Figure 1. Partitions as well as rate-limited sorption were observed when resin was added to the sand (Column 2). This resulted in a broken elution curve, with a first part similar in shape to the non-retarded curve and a second part that was linear and controlled by the rate-limited sorption (diffusion). Such a sorptive behavior is understandable when looking at the structure of the resin. Indeed, its surface area is quite large (715 m^2/g) and the size of its pores (50Å) allows slow diffusion of the contaminant.

BioticBreakthroughs – Results from PCP elutions after column inoculation with specific microorganisms are presented in Figure 1. No biomass was detected at the exit of the columns during the flush performed before the PCP elution. Both Columns 1 and 3 showed significant biodegradation: approximately 18% of PCP was degraded in column 1 while almost 55% of initial PCP was degraded in Column 3. This is a direct result of the competition between the two kinetics involved in these columns: biodegradation and hydraulic conductivity. In Column 2, little biodegradation was measured (the difference between the abiotic control and the biotic elution, 5 %) showing that microorganisms' access to the contaminant was limited by the presence of the resin. Here again, this result may be seen as a kinetic competition between biodegradation and rate-limited sorption.

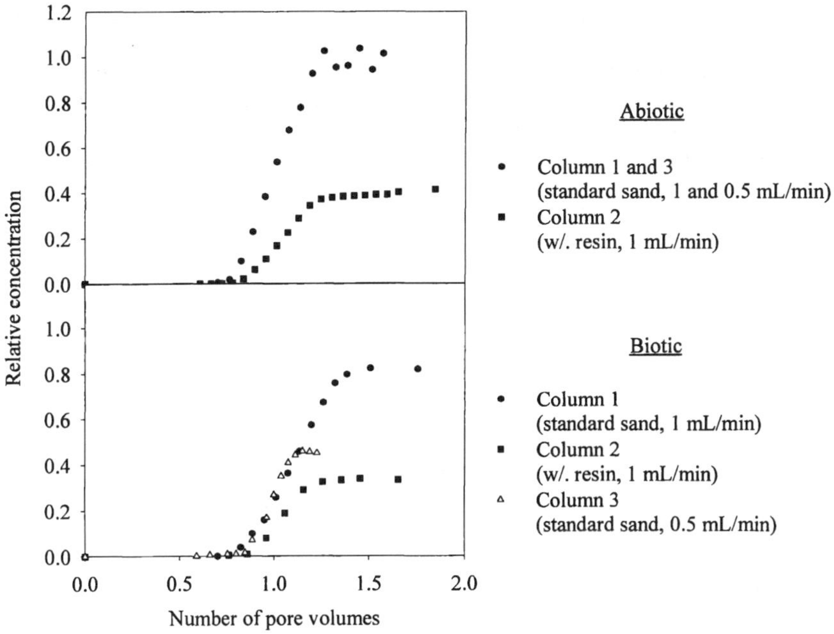

Figure 1 – *Abiotic and biotic breakthroughs for the three columns.*

Toxicity Elutions

Figure 2 presents the toxicity elution curves obtained for Columns 1 and 2.

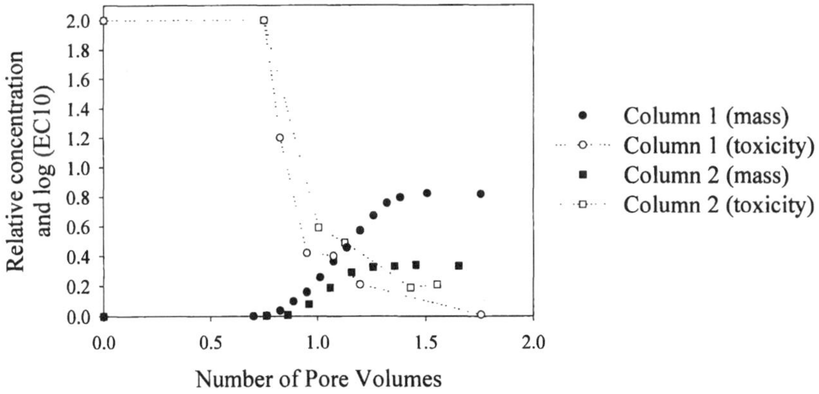

Figure 2 – *Toxicity response to PCP elutions for Columns 1 and 2.*

Toxicity responses to PCP elutions reveal that toxic pattern is closely related to the mass pattern for both columns. The lower the toxic breakthrough curve is, the higher the toxicity, because a smaller fraction of the sample is needed to reach 10% of decrease in the bioluminescence. For Column 1, despite the observed biodegradation, the toxicity reaches the maximum value (the one measured for the influent solution), while the retention action of the resin, limits the outcome in concentration as well as in toxicity, which stabilizes after 1.4 pore volumes.

Quantification of Bioavailability Rates

From these biotic mass and toxic breakthroughs, derivatives are calculated and plotted, as non-dimensional breakthrough rates (per Pore Volume, Vp^{-1}) to allow calculation of the areas under the curves, according to Figure 3.

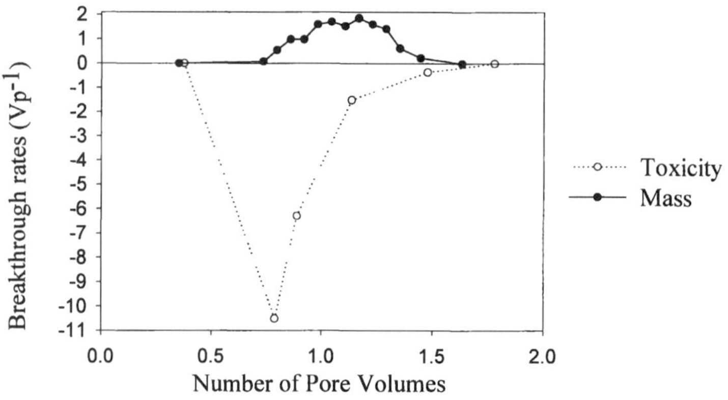

Figure 3 – *Mass and toxic elutions and derivatives for Column 1.*

The described steps are performed for the three columns and mass and toxic bioavailabilitiy rates are drawn from these calculations. These rates are then compared to the best or worst-case scenarios, in order to obtain non-dimensional bioavailability numbers, as explained in the method development section. The numbers are found in Table 1.

Table 1 – *Summary of bioavailability numbers.*

	Column 1 (sand, 1mL/min)	**Column 2** (w/. resin, 1mL/min)	**Column 3** (sand, 0.5 mL/min)
massBioA	0.15	0.02	0.52
toxBioA	0.59	0.22	N.A.

In order to calculate the toxic bioavailability in column 2, results from the PCP and toxicity elutions for this column were linearly extrapolated to obtain the area under the curve. This extrapolation was motivated by the fact that PCP elution in the second phase of the curve is controlled by rate-limited sorption, exhibiting linear outflow of contaminant.

Overall results show a great influence of a decrease in the pore-water velocity on mass bioavailability (from 0.15 to 0.52 for Columns 1 and 3, respectively). Contaminant retention by the medium led to a sharp decrease in mass bioavailability (from 0.15 to 0.02 for Columns 1 and 2, respectively) as well as for the toxic bioavailability (from 0.57 to 0.22 for Columns 1 and 2, respectively).

Discussion

Results obtained in terms of mass bioavailability (Table 1) show the two different kinetic competitions previously mentioned. If Column 1 is set as the standard, it is clear that a decrease in the flow rate favors biodegradation and thus mass bioavailability (from 0.15 to 0.52). Such a phenomenon was already observed (Angley et al. 1992) but has never been quantified in terms of bioavailability. Inversely, when resin is added to standard sand, mass bioavailability of the contaminant sharply decreases (from 0.15 to 0.02). Such a result is in total agreement to general studies of bioavailability showing that sorption of the contaminant leads to a decrease in biodegradation. These two kinetic competitions have been described previously by a set of non-dimensional numbers: the Damkohler numbers (Ramaswami and Luthy 1997). The knowledge of kinetic parameters can lead to the calculation of these numbers allowing to know what kinetic was limiting the overall process, hence bioavailability. In a similar manner, Chung et al. (1993) used a Thiele modulus as a non-dimensional number. Unfortunately, for those methods, no link was created between the numbers and the actual bioavailability. Bosma et al. (1997) created a bioavailability number (*Bn*), defined as the ratio between intraparticle diffusion and biodegradation rate and then quantified bioavailability from the knowledge of the kinetic parameters. Their *Bn* is in fact the equivalent of the mass bioavailability of this research, but estimated for static systems. The method described here quantifies mass bioavailability as a whole result of the three kinetics controlling the system (hydrodynamic, slow sorption and biodegradation) and quantifies a toxic bioavailability as well.

In terms of toxic bioavailability, the results from (Table 1) show an interesting aspect of the method based on the definition of bioavailability rates. Even though PCP concentration is rather low at the exit of Column 2, the overall rate of toxic bioavailability ends up being higher than for the standard Column 1 (0.72 compared to 0.57, respectively). This is due to the fact that a constant flow of PCP is coming out and over time leads to the equivalent of a chronic toxicity. A static look at the system would have shown a decrease in the toxic bioavailability in the presence of a retention matrix (Kelsey and Alexander 1997), but when the hydrodynamics are also taken into account, the opposite result is obtained. The estimation of the resulting hazard would be quite different. Most of the research done on toxic bioavailability uses a contaminant distribution coefficient to assess the bioavailable fraction of pollutant. Research works correlate K_{OM} values to measured toxicity (Gobas et Zhang, 1994). Again, this method is based on a thermodynamic view of the phenomenon and is usually applicable to static or pseudo-static systems such as lakes or sediments (Standley 1997). The effect of hydrodynamics on toxic bioavailability is also seen in the difference between the results obtained for Columns 1 and 3. A decrease in the flow rate leads to a strong decrease in the toxic bioavailability rate (from 0.57 to 0.31).

On a more fundamental note, it is important to realize that bioavailability is organism dependent. Whatever the quantification method is, the organism exposed to the contaminant in its actual distribution (chemical availability) will express its version of what is bioavailable. In the research presented here, a focus was made to use contaminant-sensitive organisms in order to obtain a response in terms of environmental bioavailability (mass or toxic) that would be the most accurate. Indeed, if the organisms do not respond as soon as they are exposed to the contaminant, the gathered response will not be representative of environmental bioavailability. So, in order to get as close as possible to environmental bioavailability, sensitive organisms are needed to make the organism limitation, which is pharmacological bioavailability (Dickson et al. 1994), as negligible as possible. Therefore, to measure mass bioavailability, a microbial consortium that was stimulated with PCP prior to its inoculation within the columns, was used. In the same purpose, to measure toxic bioavailability, the Microtox test was used and proved to be very sensitive to the presence of PCP in the water. However, it is clear that other receptors would have led to different results in terms of bioavailability. Nevertheless, it seems important to probe bioavailability using biological receptors. A better approach would be to use a battery of receptors and gather a general response for environmental bioavailability from this group of receptors.

Another consequence of the fact that bioavailability is organism dependent is that the results obtained with this method and organisms exposure methods in general are not really comparable to results obtained with extraction methods simply because they do not measure the same thing: a biological availability on one side and a chemical availability on the other side. .

One limitation of the method presented here resides in the way the organism is exposed in order to gather the toxic bioavailability. The degrading microorganisms are inside the column and their response to contaminant exposure is a result of multiple micro-exposures dependent on time, leading to a clear evaluation of a bioavailability rate. However, the toxicity test used to measure toxic bioavailability requires a certain exposure time, identical for all samples. Hence, the notion of time created in the evaluation of the toxic bioavailability is less representative of the reality than for the mass bioavailability.

Research is presently being carried out to further investigate the link between the different kinetics controlling the contaminant fate and transport (hydrodynamic, physico-chemical and biological) and the mass and toxic bioavailabilities obtained with this method. Results in this direction may lead to the possible prediction of bioavailabilities.

Acknowledgments

The authors acknowledge the guidance of Professor Réjean Samson and his knowledgeable input in the progress of the research. The help of Jacques Bureau in regard to toxicity analysis was greatly appreciated. The authors acknowledge the financial support from the industrial Chair partners: Alcan, Bell Canada, Cambior, Centre québécois de valorisation de la biomasse et des biotechnologies (CQVB), Hydro-Québec, Petro-Canada, Elf Aquitaine, Solvay, Ville de Montréal, Canadian Pacific Railway and the Natural Science and Engineering Research Council (NSERC).

References

Alexander, M., 1995, "How Toxic are Toxic Chemicals in Soil ? ," *Environmental Science and Technology,* Vol. *29*, No. 11, pp. 2713-2717.

Angley, J. T., Brusseau, M. L., Lamar Miller, W. and Delfino, J. J., 1992, "Nonequilibrium Sorption and Aerobic Biodegradation of Dissolved Alkylbenzenes during Transport in Aquifer Material: Column Experiments and Evaluation of a Coupled-Process Model," *Environmental Science and Technology,* Vol. *26*, No. 7, pp. 1404-1410.

Baveye, P. and Bladon, R., 1999, "Bioavailability of Organic Xenobiotics in the Environment: a Critical Perspective," *Bioavailability of Organic Xenobiotics in the Environment - Practical Consequences for the Environment*, P. Baveye, J.-C. Block and V. V. Goncharuk, Eds., Dordrecht, The Netherlands, Kluwer Academic Publishers, pp. 227-248.

Baveye, P., Block, J.-C. and Goncharuk, V. V., 1999, *Bioavailability of Organic Xenobiotics in the Environment - Practical Consequences for the Environemnent*, P. Baveye, J.-C. Block and V. V. Goncharuk., Eds., Kluwer Academic Publishers, Dordrecht, The Netherlands.

Bosma, T. N. P., Middeldorp, P. J. M., Schraa, G. and Zehnder, A. J. B., 1997, "Mass Transfer Limitation of Biotransformation: Quantifying Bioavailability," *Environmental Science and Technology,* Vol. *31*, No. 1, pp. 248-252.

Chung, G.-Y., McCoy, B. J. and Scow, K. M., 1993, "Criteria to Assess when Biodegradation is Kinetically Limited by Intraparticle Diffusion and Sorption," *Biotechnology and Bioengineering,* Vol. *41,* pp. 625-632.

Cuypers, M. P., Grotenhuis, J. T. C. and Rulkens, W. H., 1999, "Prediction of PAH Bioavailability in Soils and Sediments by Ppersulfate Oxidation, " *Bioremediation Technology for PAH Compounds*, Leeson A and Alleman BC, Eds., Batelle Press, Colombus Ohio, pp. 241-246.

Davies, N. A., Edwards, P. A., Lawrence, M. A. M., Taylor, M. G. and Simkiss, K., 1999, "Influence of Particle Surfaces on the Bioavailability to Different Species of 2,4-Dichlorophenol and Pentachlorophenol," *Environmental Science and Technology,* Vol. *33*, No. 14, pp. 2465-2468.

Dickson, K. L., Giesy, J. P., Parrish, R. and Wolfe, L., 1994, "Summary and conclusions," *Bioavailability - Physical, Chemical and Biological Interactions*, J. L. Hamelink, P. F. Landrum, H. L. Bergamn and W. H. Benson, Eds., CRC Press, Boca Raton, FL, pp.221-230

Dudal, Y., Deschênes, L. and Samson, R., 1999, "Quantifying the Intrinsic Biormediation Potential and the Hazard Index of Organic Xenobiotics in Aquifers Based on their Bioavailability Rates," *Bioavailability of Organic Xenobiotics in the Environement - Practical Consequences for the Environment*, P. Baveye, J.-C. Block and V. V. Goncharuk, Eds., Kluwer Publishers, Dordrecht, The Netherlands, pp.147-151.

Gobas, F. A. P. C. and Zhang, X., 1994, "Interactions of Organic Chemicals with Particulate and Dissolved Organic Matter in the Aquatic Environment," *Bioavailability. Physical, Chemical and Biological Interactions*, , J. L. Hamelink, P. F. Landrum, H. L. Bergamn and W. H. Benson, Eds., CRC Press, Boca Raton, FL, pp.83-91.

Greer, C. W., Hawari, J. and Samson, R., 1990, "Influence of Environmental Factors on 2,4-Dichloropenoxyacetic Acid Degradation by *Pseudomonas cepacia* Isolated from Peat, " *Archives Microbiology*, Vol. *154*, pp. 317-322.

Guerin, W. F. and Boyd, S. A., 1992, "Differential Bioavailability of Soil-Sorbed Naphtalene to Two Bacterial Species," *Applied and Environmental Microbiology,* Vol. *58*, No. 4, pp. 1142-1152.

Hamelink, J. L., Landrum, P. F., Bergman, H. L. and Benson, W. H., 1994, *Bioavailability. Physical, Chemical and Biological Interactions*, CRC Press, Boca Raton, FL.

Herman, D. C., Lenhard, R. J. and Miller, R. M., 1997, "Formation and Removal of Hydrocarbon Residual in Porous Media: Effects of Attached Bacteria and Biosurfactants," *Environmental Science and Technology,* Vol. *31*, No. 5, pp. 1290-1294.

Hrudey, S. E., Chen, W. and Rousseaux, C. G., 1996, *Bioavailability in Environmental Risk Assessment*, CRC Press, Boca Raton, FL.

Hsieh, M.-M. and Dorsey, J. G., 1995, "Bioavailability Estimation by Reverse-Phase Liquid Chromatography: High Bonding Density C-18 Phases for Modeling Biopartitioning Processes," *Analytical Chemistry,* Vol. *67*, No. 1, pp. 48-57.

Jaspers, M. C. M., Totevova, S., Demnerova, K., Harms, H. and Van Der Mer, J. R., 1999, "The Use of Whole-Cell Living Biosensors to Determine the Bioavailability of Pollutants to Microorganisms," *Bioavailability of Organic Xenobiotics in the Environment - Practical Consequences for the Environment*, P. Baveye, J.-C. Block and V. V. Goncharuk, Eds., Kluwer Academic Publishers, Dordrecht, The Netherlands.

Kelsey, J. W. and Alexander, M., 1997, "Declining Bioavailability and Inappropriate Estimation of Risk of Persistent Compounds," *Environmental Toxicology and Chemistry,* Vol. *16*, No. 3, pp. 582-585.

Kelsey, J. W., Kottler, B. D. and Alexander, M., 1997, "Selective Chemicals Extractants to Predict Bioavailability of Soil-Aged Organic Chemicals," *Environmental Science and Technology,* Vol. *31*, No. 1, pp. 214-217.

Landrum, P. F., Hayton, W. L., Lee II, H., McCarty, L. S., Mackay, D. and McKim, J. M., 1994, "Synopsis of Discussion Session on the Kinetics Behind Environemntal Bioavailability," *Bioavailability - Physical, Chemical and Biological Interactions*, J. L. Hamelink, P. F. Landrum, H. L. Bergman and W. H. Benson, Eds., CRC Press, Boca Raton, FL, pp. 203-219.

Levenspiel, O., 1972, *Chemical Reaction Engineering*, John Wiley and Sons, New York.

Loibner, A. P., Gartner M, Schlegl M, Hautzenberger I and Braun R., 1999, "PAHs: Rapid Estimation of their Bioavailability in Soil," in *In situ and On site Bioremediation Volume 5*, Leeson A and Alleman BC, Eds., Batelle Press, Colombus Ohio, pp. 617-622.

Morrison, D. E., Robertson, B. K. and Alexander, M., 2000, "Bioavailability to Earthworms of Aged DDT, DDE, DDD, and Dieldrin in Soil," *Environmental Science and Technology,* Vol. *34*, No. 4, pp. 709-713.

Nam, K. and Alexander, M., 1998, "Role of Nanoporosity and Hydrophobicity in Sequestration and Bioavailability: Tests with Model Solids," *Environmental Science and Technology,* Vol. *32*, No. 1, pp. 71-74.

Pignatello, J. J. and Xing, B., 1996, "Mechanisms of Slow Sorption of Organic Chemicals to Natural Particles," *Environmental Science and Technology*, Vol. *30*, No. 1, pp. 1-11.

Ramaswami, A. and Luthy, R. G., 1997, "Measuring and Modeling Physicochemical Limitations to Bioavailability and Biodegradation," *Manual of Environmental Microbiology*, C. J. Hurst, Ed., ASM Press, Washington, D.C.

Ripp, S., Nivens, D. E., Ahn, Y., Werner, C., Jarrell IV, J., Easter, J. P., Cox, C. D., Burlage, R. S. and Sayler, G. S., 2000, "Controlled Field Release of a Bioluminescent Genetically Engineered Microorganism for Bioremediation Process Monitoring and Control," *Environmental Science and Technology,* Vol. *34*, No. 5, pp. 846-853.

Ritschel, W. A., 1988, "Pharmacokinetic and Biopharmaceutical Aspects in Drug Delivery," *Drug Delivery Devices. Fundamentals and Applications*, P. Tyle. New York, Marcel Dekker Inc. Vol. *32*, pp. 17-79.

Standley, L. J., 1997, "Effect of Sedimentary Organic Matter Composition on the Partitioning and Bioavailability of Dieldrin to the Oligochaete Lumbriculus variegatus," *Environmental Science and Technology,* Vol. *31*, No. 9, pp. 2577-2583.

Van Loon, W. M. G. M., Wijnker, F. G., Verwoerd, M. E. and Hermens, J. L. M., 1996, "Quantitative Determination of Total Molar Concentrations of Bioaccumulatable Organic Micropollutants in Water Using C18 Empore Disk and Molar Detection Techniques," *Analytical Chemistry,* Vol. *68*, pp. 2916-2926.

Weber Jr, W. J., McGinley, P. M. and Katz, L. E., 1991, "Sorption Phenomena in Subsurface Systems: Concepts, Models and Effects on Contaminant Fate and Transport," *Water Research,* Vol. *25*, No. 5, pp. 499-528.

Zhang, W-X, Bouwer, E. J. and Ball, W. P., 1998, "Bioavailability of Hydrophobic Organic Contaminants: Effects and Implications of Sorption-Related Mass Transfer on Bioremediation," *GWMR,* Vol. *Winter*, pp. 126-138.

Author Index

Subject Index